MENTAL HEALTH

Psycho-Social Pespectives

VOLUME TWO: Multi Group Analysis

The details of the forthcoming volumes are:

Volume 1: Issues and Interventions
Volume 2: Multigroup Analysis
Volume 3: Strength of Human Resources
Volume 4: Therapeutic Applications

About the Editors

Aradhana Shukla is Prof. and former Head Department of Psychology, Kumaun University Campus, Almora Uttarakhand. Currently she is Campus Dean (Arts) at Kumaun University Campus, Almora. She has served in Department of Pediatrics of Banaras Hindu University, Post Doctoral fellow (U.G.C.) at University of Gorakhpur and has been serving here for last 27 years. She has published 100 research papers of national and international repute, ten books in which nine are published by national agencies and one from Germany (LAP). She has carried out 4 major projects from ICSSR and UGC and co-worked in UNICEF and GFATM-round 7 projects. She has guides 45 Ph.D. students and prepared 26 psychological tests. Moreover, she has attended 40 Seminars of national and international repute and organized 4 seminars in her department. Her major thrust areas are: developmental psychology, personality psychology, cultural psychology, environmental psychology and mental health care system.

Anubhuti Dubey is Associate Professor of Psychology at Department of Psychology, DDU Gorakhpur University, Gorakhpur. Her research interest includes Health Psychology, Applied Social Psychology, Gender and health and Counselling. She had published a book entitled "Psychological Perspectives on Chronic Illness". She had also completed a research project sponsored by ICSSR on "Psychological Dynamics of Health and Illness in Women of Eastern Uttar Pradesh." She had published 25 research papers in journals of national and international repute and also contributed 11 chapters in different edited volumes. Four students had been awarded their Ph.D. thesis under her supervision. She had received university gold medals at under-graduate and post-graduate levels. She is also a Master Trainer and Supportive Supervisor for Training HIV/AIDS counsellors under GFATM-Round 7 programmes.

MENTAL HEALTH
Psycho-Social Perspective

Volume Two
Multigroup Analysis

Edited by

Anubhuti Dubey
Aradhana Shukla

CONCEPT PUBLISHING COMPANY PVT. LTD.
NEW DELHI-110059

ISBN-13: 978-93-5125-173-6 (Series)
ISBN-13: 978-93-5125-170-5 (Vol. II)

First Published 2015

Published and Printed by

Concept
Since 1974

Concept Publishing Company Pvt. Ltd.
A/15-16, Commercial Block, Mohan Garden
New Delhi-110059 (India)
T: 25351460, 25351794, *F*: 091-11-25357109
E: publishing@conceptpub.com, W: www.conceptpub.com
Editorial Office: H-13, Bali Nagar, New Delhi-110 015, India.

Cataloging in Publication Data--Courtesy: D.K. Agencies (P) Ltd. <docinfo@dkagencies.com>

Mental health : psycho-social perspectives / edited by Aradhana Shukla, Anubhuti Dubey.
volumes 1-2 cm
Contributed articles.
Includes bibliographical references and indexes.
Contents: volume one. Issues and interventions -- volume two. Multigroup analysis
ISBN 9789351251736 (Series)
ISBN 9789351251699 (Vol. I)
ISBN 9789351251705 (Vol. II)

1. Mental health--Social aspects--India. 2. Mental health--Social aspects. I. Shukla, Aradhana, editor. II. Dubey, Anubhuti, editor.

DDC 300.72 23

Preface

We desire to live a healthy and happy life. It is a common and well accepted fact that everyone desires to live a healthy life. The mind and bodily functions are closely embedded hence, the relative significance of mental health along with physical wellness cannot be denied. As mind and bodily functions are closely embedded we cannot deny the relative significances of mental health a long with physical wellness. Mental health is an integral part of health, mental health is more than the absence of mental illness, and mental health is intimately connected with physical health and behaviour. Mental health is the foundation for well-being and effective functioning for an individual and for a community. Good mental health is a sense of well-being, confidence and self-esteem. It enables us to fully enjoy and appreciate other people, day-to-day life and our environment.

Mental health is the sheer responsibility of a person himself. The mental health field aims to deal with (1) mentally ill people, (2) people at risk, and (3) promoting mental health of normal people so that their normality can be sustained.

If we go back into the history of mental health we can see that it was treated either as "boon of God" (good or positive mental health) or "curse of Gcd" bad or negative mental health). Both the eastern and western evidences support the notion. Not only in abroad but our ancient evidences also support this notion. The Western literatures on mental health were seen hallucinations as communication of humans with bad souls, ghosts and witches. Moreover, in the ancient Indian literature of Ayurveda, Mental disorders are represented as various forms. The aetio-genesis of these disorders was thought to be endogenous because of provoked humours like *Vat*, *Pitta* and *Kaph*. Exogenously the causes were attributed to sudden fear or association with ill influence of certain mythological gods or demon. *Charak Samhita* listed Psychiatry as *'Bhuta Vidya'*. Psychotherapy was known as *Ilaj-I-Nafsani* in Unani Medicine. But time never remains stable. Years and years were passed and the outlook of people towards mentally ill people become more and more aversive and they were treated like an undesirable social being for whom only such behaviour was required that was only meant for animals or criminals. Even with the advent of modern scientific methods and practical thoughts, the stigma and discrimination against mentally illnesses prevail the society. However, the advocates of Psychology started to cola soft touch and healing approach for the mentally ill people. Again it took decades to develop behaviour and psycho-therapies against tying mentally ill people with iron chain, and treat them like prisoners. A complete soft and medico-human environment under single roof was constructed for them and it was termed as asylum or mental hospital. Psychologists attempted such patients to get out from the boundaries and from the trap of *ojhas, neem-haquims* and other such traditional healers and placed them at asylum. The patients were properly medicated along with different psychotherapies and many of them got complete recovery. At first the asylums were established in abroad but in India the first asylum was established in 1787 by Surgeon Kenderline in Calcutta and thereafter many asylums were made. This period was relatively longer but it opened the doors of a new era for the support and care of mental ill-health. They not only paid attention to treat the mentally ill people but also concentrated on maintaining and nurturing public health, and trying to eradicate the stigma and discrimination faced by people with mental disorders. Psychologists and mental health care professionals are still trying to launch innovative programmes for the same. The focal theme of these developmental programmes are the utilization of community resources for mental health care. These programmes have given new vision to the mental health care professionals to prevent mental disorders and promote mental health. This also needs a greater role for the non-medical mental health care professionals and better utilization of cultural resources in terms of belief, practice and important social institutions like family and community groups. The contemporary world's realization about mental health and mental illness has come to a point where we find passionate discussions and caring mental health professionals to deal with mental disorder and promote well-being.

Keeping these views into consideration the innovative thought of this series appeared in our mind and we decided to pool the thoughts of psychologists and health care professionals regarding various concerns of mental health. The basic aim of this series was: (i) to bring concepts, issues, strengths and treatment in a single jacket, (ii) bring a sense of mental health awareness in people so that they can make their health safe with additional attention on social health, (iii) to carve the research competence in young researchers, and (iv) to put forth the mental health policies before the readers, so that a better understanding of mental health can be developed.

About the series Mental Health: Psycho-Social Perspectives

It is a series on the psychology of mental health and we have tried to cover as many areas as possible and we could justify its name, i.e. rethinking. Many traditional notions of mental health have been reconceptualised and many concepts in a new framework have been introduced. This series has four volumes:

1. ***Mental health: Psychological Issues and Interventions:*** In this volume we have covered various issues that foster or hamper mental health. Also, strategies to minimize negative mental health and improve positive mental health are discussed.
2. ***Mental health: Multigroup Analysis:*** This volume covers the conceptual background and psycho-social perspective of mental health in various social settings.
3. ***Mental health: Strength of Human Resources:*** In this volume we have tried to throw light on the promotional strategies of mental health following which a person can be relieved from negative mental health.
4. ***Mental Health: Therapeutic Applications:*** This volume covers a range of behavioural therapies which were found effective to minimize or overcome mental ill health.

We have exercised our best attempt to seek out as many experiences as possible and we also anticipate that this will open new foresight for the researchers. However, we will be highly blessed to obtain the healthy and critical comments from our colleagues, seniors and friends and we will appreciate them from the bottom of our hearts.

Anubhuti Dubey
Aradhana Shukla

Acknowledgements

We, the editors, feel immense pleasure to present our series on mental health before the august readers. We hope that it will be admired by you all and the comments will be highly appreciated.

We feel our deep sense of gratitude and thankfulness to our respected contributors. It was only their support that the volumes came in the shape. We are thankful to Mr. Abhishek and Mr. Pankaj Tewari for computer task.

Last but not least, we are thankful to Mr. Ashok Mittal, M/s. Concept Publishing Company Pvt. Ltd., New Delhi to shape our dreams in concrete form.

15 January 2015
Makar Sankranti

Anubhuti Dubey
Aradhana Shukla

Contents

Introduction

Mental health is a state which is free from all sorts of disease or infirmity and it is full of complete physical, mental and social well-being. A person when thinks about the well-being of others more than his own he is considered more mentally healthy. In addition, proper adjustment with the surrounding in particular, and society in general, is also an important feature of good mental health.

Our balanced mental state, socially desirable behaviour, positivity in behaviour, alertness and making positive bond even with negative conditions are the indicators of good mental health, but a person will always be happy and cheerful is not possible for anyone. A person having consistent balanced, physical and mental state can reveal the symptoms of impulsivity, sleeplessness, irritably and emotional inconsistency as per demand of the circumstances.

Some psychologists have considered adaptability and adjustment as the criteria of good mental health because it has observed that mental disorders produce illness in mental health, otherwise, desirable behaviour and adaptability are the consequences of good mental health. Level of satisfaction is an important feature of mental health. There are many resources that arise competitiveness in us and it causes dissatisfaction. If a person accepts his own capacity and limitation, he will behave accordingly and surely be successful. In this way he will make a consistent progress and his satisfaction will be retained.

There is one more truth that needs to be thought. Mental illness or mental circumstances are not common for all. Every segment of society has its own problem, own worry and own way of solution. Whether rich or poor, child or adolescent, old or young, male or female, persons living in joint or nuclear family, are surrounded by their own problem(s) and they have their own way to get rid of.

One strange situation which we have seen is the oscillation of a person between illness and health. "We are not ill but we are not healthy". It is impossible sometimes because we have no time to take care about us. We just take us to meet with the demands of daily life and people think that we are absolutely fine but the situation is entirely reversed. We suppress our disease and deal with other priorities of life because we think them more important than us. This is a major cause that affects our mental health. As the time and situation appears they show their signs in us.

Although similar attempts have been made in India and in abroad to study concept, etiology and prevention of mental health yet in India it is being studied till the ancient time. Indian psychology stress more on the positive aspect of mental health state that being happy and balanced in every circumstance and converting negative into positive is the best sign of mental health. *Atharvaveda* states the causes and remedy of mental disorder. The aim of this Veda is to guide the humanity to worldly welfare.

Atharvaveda states three attributes of mental health. They are *Satogun*, *Rajogun* and *Tamogun*. They provide mental balance and purity (*Satogun*), dominant and work orientedness (*Rajogun*) and anger and mental retardation (*Tamogun*). All sorts of treatment are based on meditative *Artharvanic* therapy, *Kaushik tantra*, transference, consolation, desensitization, *tap* and *divya havan*. *Yoga* has also become successful to maintain and cultivate positive mental health. *Hathyoga*, *Mantrayoga*, *Bhaktiyoga*, *Ayanyoga*, *Karmyoga, Layayoga* are the main schools of yogic science. In addition, Abhidhamma theory of Buddhism also focuses on mental health and describes it through two factors, namely skilled factor and unskilled factor. Both are necessary for proper development and a person establishes good mental health by making a balance between these two factors.

There are many more factors which influence mental health, for example age, sex, emotional stability, adjustment, autonomy, le[illegible] satisfaction, feeling of security/insecurity, but the most import[illegible] not discussed yet is economic status. Here we cannot ignore the notion of "disease of poverty and disease of affluence". We often see that some "*sukhrog*" go in the part of affluent while incurable diseases are most often shared by the poor. When the poor finds that any disease, by which he or his family members are surrounded, is more expensive than his pocket, he becomes anxious and this anxiety influences his mental health. This notion has similarly been investigated in India and abroad.

A close perusal of above mentioned discussion reveals that in Indian system preventive aspect of mental health is discussed thoroughly but curative and promotive aspects are still to be explored.

Keeping these views in consideration the editors thought to pen and decide to cover as many aspects of mental health as they can. Their endeavour came an end and "Mental health: Psychosocial Perspectives" came in existence.

The aim of this volume is to bring out the young talents in the light and take the senior ones to get more experience, knowledge and thought through their wise contributions in this volume. Our next aim is to ravel the unravelled aspects of mental health and how much we have got success will be decided by our esteemed readers.

There are seventeen research papers in this volume. They are empirical and review based both. In the introductory article Anubhuti Dubey and Aradhana Shukla have tried to introduce the concept of mental health and its social significance. The second paper is written by Rajbir Singh and Sandeep Kumar. They explored health and healthiness in psychosocial perspective. Aradhana Shukla in her empirical research paper has shed light on the hazards of mental health and cross-cultural perspective of mental health is presented by Anubhuti Dubey and Dhananjay Kumar.

Rajneesh Chaubisa and Tanu Shukla have elaborated reckoning linkages, needs and agenda of positive psychological and economic development. Mukta Rani Rastogi has adopted Indian approach and discussed the pattern and functioning of well-being among elderly Indians. Swaran Lata, Varsha Rani and Shikha Verma have shed light on the orphans and they have very successfully described the mental health of child and adolescent groups, which have also been considered by Neelam Verma and she has discussed their mental problem along with the etiology. Mental health in adolescent has also been discussed by Rupali Srivastava.

Aradhana Shukla has elaborated the concept of happiness and studied in family and cultural perspective. Women's mental health and their social position is described by Anubhuti Dubey. Shraddha Joshi Kapoor and Aradhana Shukla have studied quality of life and related its poverty and scholastics. Tanu Shukla and Kalyan Kumar have thrown light on dynamic construct and static gender through the construction of higher education by deconstructing well-being. Positive mental health is discussed by V.N. Pathak, Priyanka Singh and S.K. Singh and a fine correlation among rituals, religiosity, spirituality and health is revealed by Teenu Nandal and Nav Rattan Sharma. In this sequence Shilpa Kumari and Shobhana Joshi have explored the relationship between spirituality and mental health.

The concluding remark has been made by Anubhuti Dubey in which she has viewed psychosocial perspectives of mental health.

Although, we have done our sincere endeavour to put forth the views of ours and other contributors before the readers yet we feel that some limitations may be visited by them. Their healthy suggestions will be highly admired. We, the editors, hope that this volume will open a new door before the readers and a fresh breeze to enjoy the concept of mental health.

Anubhuti Dubey
Aradhana Shukla

List of Contributors

Anubhuti Dubey is Associate Professor of Psychology, DDU Gorakhpur University, Gorakhpur.
E-mail: anubhutiddu@rediffmail.com

Aradhana Shukla is Professor of Psychology and Dean (Arts), Kumaun University Campus, Almora.
E-mail: aradhana.shukla5@gmail.com

Dhananjay Kumar, Associate Professor of Psychology, DDU Gorakhpur University, Gorakhpur. E-mail: dk_ddugu@yahoo.co.in

Kalyan Kumar is Assistant Professor, Department of Sociology, South Asian University, New Delhi. E-mail: 3k.kalyan@gmail.com

Mukta Rani Rastogi is Former Head & Professor of Psychology, Deparment of Psychology, Lucknow University, Lucknow.
E-mail: mrrlkouniv@gmail.com

Nav Rattan Sharma is Professor of Psychology, Maharishi Dayanand University, Rohatak, Haryana. E-mail: sharmanr5@gmail.com

Neelam Verma is Clinical Psychologist, Child and Adolescent Guidance Clinic, Noormanzil. Psychiatric Centre, Lucknow.
E-mail: neelampsycho.86@gmail.com

Priyanka Singh is Research Scholar, Department of Psychology, Mahatma Gandhi Kashi Vidyapeeth, Varanasi.
E-mail: priya786_singh@rediffmail.com

Rajbir Singh is Professor of Psychology, Maharishi Dayanand University, Rohatak, Haryana. E-mail: rajbirsinghmdu@gmail.com

Rajnish Chaubisa is Assistant Professor of Psychology, Department of Humanities & Social Sciences, Birla, Institute of Technology and Sciences (BITS), Pilani, Rajasthan. E-mail: rajnish.chaubisa@gmail.com

Rupali Srivastava is Professor in Psychology, Department of Psychology, Faculty of Social Sciences, Banaras. Hindu University, Varanasi. E-mail: kashi.bhu@gmail.com

Sandeep Kumar is Research Scholar, Department of Psychology, Maharishi Dayanand University, Rohatak, Haryana.
E-mail: sandeepkumarmdu@gmail.com

Santosh Kumar Singh is Post Doctoral Fellow (ICSSR), Department of Psychology, Mahatma Gandhi Kashi Vidyapeeth, Varanasi.
E-mail: santosh.singh.psych@gmail.com

Shikha Verma is Post Doctoral Fellow, Department of Psychology, Banaras Hindu University, Varanasi. E-mail: shikha22bhu@gmail.com

Shilpa Kumari is Post Doctoral Fellow, Department of Psychology, Banaras, Hindu University, Varanasi. E-mail: chaudhary_shipla@yahoo.com

Shobhana J. Kapoor is Associate Professor, Department of Psychology, Banaras, Hindu University, Varanasi. E-mail: getshobhna@yahoo.com

Shraddha J. Kapoor is Project Fellow (U.G.C.), Department of Psychology, Kumaun University Campus, Almora, Uttarakhand.
E-mail: shraddhajoshi1808@gmail.com

Swaran Lata is Assistant Professor at Department of Psychology, Banaras Hindu University, Varanasi. E-mail: swaran80@gmail.com

Tanu Shukla is Assistant Professor of Psychology, Department of Humanities and Social Sciences, BITS, Pilani, Rajasthan.
E-mail: tanushukla8@gmail.com

Teenu Nandal is Lecturar, Department of Psychology, Government College, Meham, Haryana.

Varsha Rani is Part-time Lecturer, Department of Psychology, Navyug Kanya Mahavidyalay, Lucknow. E-mail: varsharaj@gmail.com

Vijendra Nath Pathak is Research Assistant in Department of Psychology Mahatma Gandhi, Kashi Vidyapeeth, Varanasi.
e-mail 14pathak@gmail.com

1

Psycho-Social Perspectives on Mental Health

Anubhuti Dubey and *Aradhana Shukla*

Mental and physical health is indivisible and both social and psychological aspects play an important role in human functioning. About 14 per cent of the global burden of disease has been attributed to neuropsychiatric disorders, mostly due to the chronically disabling nature of depression and other common mental disorders, alcohol-use and substance-use disorders, and psychoses (Prince *et al.*, 2007). The World Health Organization (WHO)'s Mental Health Atlas (2005) surveyed the resources available and found fewer than one psychiatrist per 100,000 population across India, China and much of the rest of South and South East Asia, and fewer than one psychiatrist per million population in most of sub-Saharan Africa.When Nunnally (1960) explored public conceptions of mental illness in the United States and asserted on the two possible results, that (1) the public was "misinformed" in the sense that the "average" person held numerous misconceptions about mental illness or (2) the public was uninformed in the sense that the average person had little information, correct or incorrect, about many of the problems related to mental illness. Furthermore, The World Health Organization's Ottawa Charter for Health Promotion establishes health as multidimensional and advocates a social model of health. It defines health as '*a positive concept emphasizing social and personal resources, as well as physical capacities.*' Mental health is the capacity of the individual, the group and the environment to interact with one another in ways that promote subjective well-being, the optimal development and use of mental abilities (cognitive, affective, and relational), the achievement of individual and collective goals consistent with justice and the attainment and preservation of conditions of fundamental equality (WHO, 1986).

A Report of the Surgeon General (U.S. Department of Health and Human Services [*DHHS*], 1999) defined mental health, mental illness and mental health problems. *Mental health* refers to the successful performance of mental health function resulting in productive activities fulfilling relationships with other people and the ability to adopt to change and to cope with adversity (DHHS, 1999). *Mental Illness* refers collectively to all diagnosable mental disorders characterized by alterations in thinking or behaviour (or some combination thereof) associates with distress and/or impaired functioning (U.S. Department of Health and Human Services, 2010). *Mental Health Problems* refers to signs and symptoms of insufficient intensity or duration to meet the criteria for any mutual disorder (U.S. Department of Health and Human Services, 2010).

The biopsychosocial model is based on is the notion of multiple simultaneous causes of mental disorder. The biopsychosocial model is usually interpreted as implying that biological, social and psychological factors are co-equal partners in the aetiology of mental disorder. The psychological model of mental disorder presented here suggests that disruption or dysfunction in psychological processes is a final common pathway in the development of mental disorder. It is important that this research is properly integrated with psychological and social accounts of mental disorder. The psycho-social determinants of health occur at the individual, subjective level. The prevalence rates of various types of psychiatric disorders varied consistently by gender, socio-economic status, and locale (urban *vs*. rural).

Psychological View of Mental Illness

A variety of psychological theories have attempted to explain abnormal behaviour. The psychological view of mental illness does not exclude a biological etiology, however, the psychological approaches to mental disorders offer alternative perspectives and can also be integrated with biological perspectives. Academic reviews of the role of psychosocial influences on mental illnesses and psychotic experiences (British Psychological Society, 2000) and randomised controlled trials have repeatedly demonstrated the effectiveness of psychological therapeutic approaches in a range of mental health problems (Department of Health, 2001). When people refer to psychological issues, they sometimes refer to the effects of potentially life-shaping experiences that impact on mental health such as childhood sexual abuse (Palmer, 1992), bullying (Kaltiala-Heino *et al.*, 2000), attachment relations with parents (Riggs & Jacobvitz, 2002), assault (Jacobson, 1989) and all other major and minor interpersonal experiences. Although these are disparate kinds of event, it remains true that life events in general contribute to mental disorder (Kendler *et al.*, 1995).

Social (Cultural) View of Mental Illness

In a social and cultural view of mental illness suggest that an individual is seen as "ill" when he or she is unable to find a sense of purpose, harmony, and health for themselves in their surroundings (Axelson, 1993). Maladjustment conversely is seen as the inability of an individual to develop the behavioural patterns necessary for personal and social success. A cultural view of mental illness allows to recognize the role of personality and culture in the production of patterns of adjustment or maladjustment. Hall (1985) explored the relationships between ethnicity, the conception of mental illness, and attitudes associated with seeking psychological help among black and white school teachers. The analysis of the study indicated significant differences between African Americans and Whites teachers in their conception of mental illness. The responses of Blacks reflected a more stereotypic view of mental illness, and those of Whites were closer to those of mental health professionals. African American teachers were more likely than White teachers to believe that the mentally ill look and act differently than *normal* individuals. They also strongly endorsed the notion that will power can cure mental disorders and that women are more likely than men to suffer from mental illness. Blacks more than Whites believed that mental illness can be controlled by the avoidance of morbid thoughts and that guidance and support of strong persons in the community are needed to maintain mental health. Whites were more likely than Blacks to seek counselling for problems related to sexual issues, parenting, and truancy in a school child. Hence, Blacks have a much narrower view of what problems warrant psychological interventions. The major difference between the two cultural groups was what constituted a type of mental illness that necessitated psychological intervention. Puerto Rican and other Hispanics underutilize mental health services (Padilla & Ruiz, 1973). Greek-Americans (Samouilidis, 1978) tend to perceive mental illness as a stigma. Caribbean islanders tend to have a very narrow view of mental illness (Hall, 2002).

Gender and Mental Health: Psychosocial Perspective

The gender perspective into the health sector necessitates a broad-based definition of health for women as well as for men that refers well-being across the life cycle and in domains of both physical and mental health. Gender is a measure of both biological/genetic and social differences. Health inequalities between men and women indicate both sex-related biological and social factors, and the interplay between them (Bird & Rieker, 1999; Verbrugge, 1989). Women have lower rates of mortality but, paradoxically, report higher levels of depression, psychiatric disorders, distress, and a variety of chronic illnesses than men (Baum & Grunberg, 1991; McDonough & Walters, 2001; Verbrugge, 1985). Gender considerations in health promotion and healthcare have to highlight the mental health risks and the socio-economic and cultural determinants of mental health. Apparently, economic independence, physical, sexual, and emotional safety and security are primarily needed for good mental health.

Women and Mental Health: Psychosocial Perspective

Women's health is inextricably linked to their status in society. It benefits from equality, and suffers from discrimination. Today, the status and well-being of countless millions of women worldwide remain tragically low. As a result, human well-being suffers, and the prospects for future generations are dimmer [World Health Report (WHO), 1998]. Women who were poor and those who were less educated were also found to be at increased risk of poor mental health. Heise and Garcia-Moreno (2002) postulated that poverty probably acts as a marker for a variety of social conditions that combine to increase the risk of violence faced by women. Women in better jobs than their husbands were also found to be at risk of poor mental health, a feature that is not unique to India. Socio-economic circumstances, social support and health-related behaviours all have independent effects on health, but cluster together and are mutually reinforcing (Srivastava, 2012). Violence against women is like an endemic in society. It is estimated that 14-20 per cent of women will experience rape at some point in their lives (Tjaden & Thoennes, 2000). Mental health sequels to spousal violence are significant and have long-term health implications. Battered women were found to have more depressive symptoms than other women (Campbell & Lewandowski, 1997). Studies have found the relationship between severity of abuse and physical and mental health. Women's mental health concerns extend beyond specific conditions or problems. They incorporate the structures that rule the requirement of health related education, information and health care delivery, the processes that influence women's interactions with the health care system and the factors that determine whether the treatment they receive is gender sensitive.

Children and Mental Health: Psychosocial Perspective

Bronfenbrenner (1979) emphasized the importance of the environment in which children grow up, and conceptualizes environmental influences at different nested levels—for example the individual (ontogenic system), the meso-system, exo-system, and macro-system—depending, for instance, on the amount of direct interaction that a child has with these social systems. When resources at any level are compromised, the risk of poor developmental outcomes and poor mental health adjustment increases. Among children and youth exposed to conflict, adverse mental health outcomes triggered by exposure to horrific events are compounded by war-related damage to the extended support systems (family, social, economic, political) that usually foster healthy child development (Ellis *et al.*, 2012; Tol *et al.*, 2009; 2013). When resources across the social ecology are vigorous (e.g. family and community acceptance, access to school), children can achieve more positive outcomes, even in the face of extreme hardship (Rutter, 1985; Masten, 2001). Theoretical framework with children in adversity have focused on transactions taking place between risk and protective factors at different socio-ecological levels—that is, the family, peer, school, and wider-community levels (Betancourt & Khan, 2008; Tol *et al.*, 2009; 2013). McCloskey, Figueredo and Koss (1995) found that different forms of abuse in the home were highly interrelated and that children of battered women were at risk for child abuse. Domestic violence predicted children's general psychopathology. Mothers experiencing conjugal violence were more likely to have mental health problems; their mental health did not mediate the children's response to family conflict. Finally, there was less sibling and parental warmth in families marked by aggression, although when it was present, family social support failed to buffer children. A few studies have examined barriers to children's mental health care (Kazdin, 2003; Kazdin & Wassell, 2000), children's mental health services researchers have focused on characteristics of children, parents, and families (socio-demographics, health and mental health problems, other family members' use of mental health services, perceived parental burden) associated with mental health service utilization.

Elderly and Mental Health: Psychosocial Perspective

Elderly mental health is potentially useful area of study that has remained relatively less explored in India and empirical works are needed to support a developmental approach to psychiatric or mental health nursing and care for elderly. For older people, mental health conditions are significant reason of morbidity and premature mortality. Growing numbers of elderly in countries of the developing world signify a rise in those influenced by organic, age-related mental diseases such as dementia. A simultaneous rise in the burden of non-organic mental disorders in elderly populations is likely because stressors in many countries are affecting the mental health of the elderly directly and/or indirectly by altering the ability of families to provide care for them (Levkoff, Macarthur & Bucknall, 1995). Depression is a major contributor to chronic disability and is one of the most prevalent psychiatric problems among older adults.

Mental Health Professionals: Psychosocial Perspective

With escalating globalization, mental health professionals are being challenged with decisions related to culture-specific aspects of diagnosis, validity of diagnostic entities, and variability of symptoms (Minas, 2001). It is important to be able to evaluate the role of culture in explaining differences in symptom manifestation and to be aware of the interaction between culture and depressive symptomatology when assessing a depressed patient (Kastrup, Machleidt, Behrens & Calliess, 2009). Key challenges to addressing mental health needs include the shortage of mental-health professionals, the fairly low capacity and motivation of non-specialist health workers to provide quality mental-health services to young people, and the stigma associated with mental disorder. Psychiatrists' training should incorporate the use of biological, social and psychological treatments. Mental illness is a pattern of behaviours that is troubling to the person or the community where the individual lives hence, a psychosocial assessment is needed and such assessment is an evaluation of an individual's mental health and social well-being. Mental health problems are only just ever limited to one sphere of human experience. Instead, the majority of mental health problems are predisposed to multiple spheres of human experience, and have biological (medical), psychological (mental) and social/ spiritual impacts.

Conclusion

Epidemiological increases in mental disorders and associated emotional and financial costs to individuals, families, and communities. Prevention within the mental health field needs to include not only minimizing mental disorders, but also enhancing positive qualities of daily functioning. The socio-economic and cultural context of positive mental health is emphasized with particular attention given to the interrelatedness of individual, family and community "collective sense of well-being" (Magyary, 2002).

References

Baum, A., and Grunberg, N.E. (1991). Gender, stress and health. *Health Psychology* 10 (2), 80-85.

Betancourt, T.S., and Khan, K.T. (2008). The mental health of children affected by armed conflict: protective processes and pathways to resilience. *International Review of Psychiatry*, 20, 317-28.

Bird, C., and Rieker, P. (1999). Gender matters: An integrated model for understanding men's and women's health. *Social Science and Medicine*, 48, 745-755.

British Psychological Society Division of Clinical Psychology (2000). *Understanding mental illness and psychotic experiences: A report by the British Psychological Society Division of Clinical Psychology*. Leicester: British Psychological Society.

Bronfenbrenner, U. (1979). *The ecology of human development: experiments by nature and design.* Cambridge, MA: Harvard University Press.

Campbell, J.C. and Lewandowski, L.A. (1997). Review mental and physical health effects of intimate partner violence on women and children. *Psychiatry Clinic North America*, 20 (2), 353-74.

Department of Health (2001). *Treatment choice in psychological therapies and counselling: Evidence based clinical practice guideline*. London: Department of Health.

Ellis, B.H., Fogler, J., Hansen, S., Forbes, P., Navalta, C.P., and Saxe, G. (2012). Trauma systems therapy: 15-month outcomes and the importance of effecting environmental change. *Psychology & Trauma*, 4, 624-30.

Hall, L.E. (2005). *Issues in multicultural psychology. In* Iowa, Kendall/Hunt.

Heise, L. and Garcia-Moreno, C. (2002). Violence by intimate partners. In Krug,

E.G., Dahlberg, L.L., Mercy, J.A. (Editors) *World Report on Violence and Health*. Geneva: World Health Organization, pp. 89-121.

Jacobson, A. (1989). Physical and sexual assault histories among psychiatric outpatients. *American Journal of Psychiatry*, 146: 755-758.

Kaltiala-Heino, R., Rimpela, M., Rantanen, P., and A. Rimpela, (2000). Bullying at school: An indicator of adolescents at risk for mental disorders. *Journal of Adolescence*, 23, 661-674.

Kastrup, M., Machleidt, W., Behrens, K., and Calliess, I. (2009). Cultural aspects of depression. In Maj. M., *et al.*, (Eds) *The WPA Educational Series on Depressive Disorders. Volume 4: Depression in Population Groups* (pp. 208-237). Geneva, Switzerland: WPA.

Kazdin, A.E. (2003). Psychotherapy for children and adolescents. *Annual review of psychology*, 54(1), 253-276.

Kazdin, A.E., and Wassell, G. (2000). Therapeutic changes in children, parents, and families resulting from treatment of children with conduct problems. *Journal of the American Academy of Child & Adolescent Psychiatry*, 39(4), 414-420.

Kendler, K.S., Kessler, R.C., Walters, E.E., MacLean, C., Neale, M.C., Heath, A.C., and Eaves, L.J. (1995). Stressful life events, genetic liability, and onset of an episode of major depression in women. *American Journal of Psychiatry*, 152, 833-842.

Levkoff, S.E., Macarthur, I.W., and Bucknall, J. (1995). Elderly mental health in the developing world. *Social Science & Medicine*, 41(7), 983-1003.

Prince, M., Patel, V., Saxena, S., Maj, M., Maselko, J., Phillips, M.R., and Rahman, A. (2007). No health without mental health. *The Lancet*, 370 (9590), 859-877.

Magyary, D. (2002). Positive mental health: A turn of the century perspective. *Issues in Mental Health Nursing*, 23(4), 331-349.

Masten, A.S. (2001). Ordinary magic: resilience processes in development. *American Psychologists*, 56, 227-38.

McCloskey, L.A., Figueredo, A.J. and Koss, M.P. (1995), the Effects of Systemic Family Violence on Children's Mental Health. *Child Development*, 66: 1239-1261.

McDonough, P., and Walters, V. (2001). Gender and health: reassessing patterns and explanations. *Social Science and Medicine* 52, 547-559.

Minas, H. (2001). Service responses to cultural diversity. In: Thornicroft, G., Szmukler, G., (eds.). *Textbook of Community Psychiatry*, pp. 192-206, Oxford, UK: Oxford University Press.

Nunnally, J.C. (1960) *Popular conceptions of mental health: Their development and change*. New York: Holt, Rhinehart and Winston, Inc.

Padilla, A. and Ruiz, P. (1973). *Latino mental health: A review of the literature*. Rockville, MD.: National Institute of Mental Health.

Palmer, R.L. (1992). Effects of childhood sexual abuse on adult mental health. *British Journal of Hospital Medicine*, 48, 9-10.

Riggs, S.A., and Jacobvitz, D. (2002). Expectant parents' representations of early attachment relationships: Associations with mental health and family history. *Journal of Consulting & Clinical Psychology*, 70: 195-204. 2002.

Rutter, M. (1985). Resilience in the face of adversity: protective factors and resistance to psychiatric disorder. *British Journal of Psychiatry*, 147, 598-611.

Samouilidis, L. (1978). Psychoanalytic vicissitudes in working with Greek patients. *The American Journal of Psychoanalysis*, 38, 223-233.

Srivastava, K. (2012). Women and mental health: Psychosocial perspective. *Industrial Psychiatry Journal*, 21 (1), 1-3.

Tjaden, P., and Thoennes, N. (2000). Prevalence and consequences of male-to-female and female-to-male intimate partner violence as measured by the National Violence against Women Survey. *Violence against Women*, 6, 142-61.

Tol, W.A., Jordans, M.J., Kohrt, B.A., Betancourt, T.S., and Komproe, I.H. (2013). Promoting mental health and psychosocial well-being in children affected by political violence: Current evidence for an ecological resilience approach. In Fernando, C., Ferrari, M., (eds.) *The handbook on resilience in children of war.* New York: Springer.

Tol, W.A., Jordans, M.J., Komproe, I.H., De Jong, J.T. (2009). Interventions for children affected by war: synthesis of cluster randomized trials in four countries. Paper presented to *International Congress for Transcultural Psychiatry*, Florence, Italy.

US Department of Health and Human Services. (1999). *Health, United States.* National Center for Health Statistics.

US Department of Health and Human Services. (2010, 2nd edition).*With understanding and improving health and objectives for improving health.* Washington DC: US Government Printing Office.

Verbrugge, L.M. (1985). Gender and health: An update on hypothesis and evidence. *Journal of Health and Social Behaviour*, 26, 156-182.

Verbrugge L.M. (1989). The twain meet: empirical explanations of sex differences in health and mortality. *Journal of Health & Social Behaviour*, 30, 282-304.

World Health Organization, Health and Welfare Canada (1986). Ottawa Charter for Health promotion Canadian Public Health Association.

World Health Organization. (1998). *The World Health Report, 1998. Executive summary*. Geneva.

World Health Organization. *Mental Health Atlas 2005*. Geneva: World Health Organization.

2

Psychological Perspective of Health and Healthiness

Rajbir Singh and *Sandeep Kumar*

The proverb, 'health is wealth' or disease eats up your health, is prevalent in its true sense. The poorest people in the world are also the ones with poorest health. Over the past decade there has been a large movement world over towards health and healthy behaviour. Regional and international agencies have made well designed actions for many years yet we all have remarkably failed to achieve the goal of the WHO-formulated 'Health for All by the Year 2000'. At the beginning of the 21st century many of nations suffer from high mortality caused by unhealthy behaviour. At the present day, majority of us eat too much fat food, drink too much alcohol and use other stimulants like tobacco and others to excess. As a result of these health risk behaviours and life styles, we have to spend vast sums of money treating a number of 'self-inflicted' diseases. So, the subject of being healthy is becoming a very important one for the individual.

Meaning of Health and Healthiness

Concept of health and illness are embodied in everyday talk and thought of people with different languages, cultures and religious groups. The word 'Health' is derived from Old High German and Anglo-Saxon words meaning 'whole', 'hole', and 'holy'. Historically and culturally there are strong associations with ideas of wholeness, holiness, cleanliness, sanity, goodness, saintliness and goodliness. An emphasis on health as wholeness and naturalness was present in ancient China, classical Greece and Ayurveda where health was seen as a state of harmony, balance/equilibrium with nature. These beliefs are found in many healing systems to the present day.

In our today's fast-paced life, there are innumerable sources such as environmental pollution, unhealthy work conditions, sources of stress, industrial smoke, unsafe water, noise and so many others that are responsible for making us unhealthy. For most of us, being healthy is the norm—most people are healthy for most of the time. Therefore, beliefs about being ill exist in the context of beliefs about being healthy (e.g. illness means not being healthy, feeling different to usual, etc.). In 1948, the World Health Organization defined health as "a complete state of physical, mental, and social well-being and not merely the absence of disease or infirmity". This definition presents a broad multidimensional view of health that departs from the traditional medical emphasis on physical health only.

Over years, there had been varied beliefs/conceptions regarding the meaning of health. Helman, a social anthropologist, in 1978 explored the extent to which beliefs inherent within the humoral theory have survived alongside those of conventional medicine. Particularly he focused on the saying 'feed a cold and starve a fever', and argued that health could be conceptualized according to the dimensions 'hot/cold' and 'wet/dry'. For example, problems with the chest were considered either 'hot and wet' (e.g. fever and productive cough) or 'cold and wet' (e.g. cold and non-productive cough). Likewise, problems could be considered 'hot and dry' (e.g. fever, dry skin, flushed face, dry throat, non-productive cough) or 'cold and dry' (e.g. cold, shivering, rigor, malaise, vague muscular aches). In a similar manner, medical sociologists have also explored lay conceptions of health. For example, Herzlich (1973) categorized the models of health into three dimensions: Ist one, health in a vacuum, which implied the absence of illness; 2nd one, the reserve of health, which was related to physical strength and resistance to illness; and last one, equilibrium, which indicated a full realization of the individual's reserve of health. Likewise, Blaxter (1990) asked individuals to describe someone whom they thought was healthy and to consider, 'What are the reasons that make you call them healthy?' and, 'What is it like when you are healthy?' A qualitative analysis was then carried out on a sub-sample of these individuals. For some of us, health simply meant not being ill. However, for many, health was seen in terms of a reserve, a healthy life filled with health behaviours, physical fitness, having energy and vitality, good social relationships with others, being able to function in an effective manner and an expression of psychosocial well-being. Further, Calnan

(1987) explored the health beliefs of women in England and found that their models of health could be conceptualized in two sets of definitions:

(a) Positive definitions which includes being energetic, doing plenty of exercise, feeling fit, eating the right things, being the correct weight, having a positive outlook and having a good life/ marriage; and
(b) Negative definitions which includes don't get coughs and colds, only in bed once, rarely go to the doctor and have check-ups – nothing wrong.

Meaning of health has also been explained by a psychological perspective with a particular focus on health and illness cognitions. For example, Lau (1995) found that when young healthy adults were asked a simple question—what is the meaning of being healthy for them?, they reported their beliefs about health which could be understood by the following presented dimensions:

- *Physiological/physical*, e.g. good condition, has energy.
- *Psychological*, e.g. happy, energetic, feel good psychologically.
- *Behavioural*, e.g. eat, sleep properly.
- *Future consequences*, e.g. live longer.
- *The absence of*, e.g. not sick, no disease, no symptoms.

According to Lau (1995), most people define health as not only the absence of illness but also include more than just physical and psychological factors. He further suggested that healthiness is most people's normal state and represents the backdrop to their beliefs about being ill. Psychological studies of the beliefs of the elderly (Hall *et al.*, 1989), those suffering from a chronic illness (Hays and Stewart, 1990) and children (Normandeau *et al.*, 1998; Schmidt and Frohling, 2000) have established that these individuals also conceptualize health as being multidimensional.

From traditional Indian view point, health can't be viewed as merely a state but a dynamic process of striving which ensures stability between inner as well as outer factors. These factors are continuously changing and therefore, there is no ideal state. There is continuity between the human body (microcosm) and universe (macrocosm) and this interconnectedness complimentarily inherent in natu``e is the key to unlock the principles of health and well-being (Misra, 2005). This fact is exemplified in the *Charak Samitha,* which defines disease as disequilibrium, of various subtle elements or *dhatus*. In *Ayurvedic* system, it is conceptualized that a living organism is made of *Panch-mahabuta*, in the form of—*Pitta, Vata, Kapha* at the physical level (*prakriti*) and *Sattva-Rajas-Tamas* at mental level (personality). This covers the psychosomatic constitutions and commonly known as the *Tridosha Theory* (Tripathi, 2000). Dwivedi (2005) considers that healthiness leads to a state of happiness and disorder leads an individual to an unhappy state. The *Susruta Samitha* describes health as a state where three humors (*Vata, Pitta and Kapha* are in balanced state), the *Agni* (digestive fire) of the body is within normal limits, the *dhatus* and the excretory mechanism is also in a balanced state and the psychic functions of the mind, sense organs and the self are in a most happy position (Jain, Sharma and Yadava, 2006; Vidyalankar, 1968).

Nature and Emergence of Health Psychology

Everyday, we see headlines about health, such as from newspapers, TV reports, magazines and various other sources. We are told that smoking is bad for us, that we need to exercise more, and that we've grown obese. We learn about new treatments for diseases about which we are only dimly aware, or we hear that a particular herbal remedy may make us feel better about ourselves. We are told that meditation or optimistic beliefs can keep us healthy or help us to get well more quickly. How do we make sense of all these claims, and which ones are personally important? Health psychology addresses important questions like these.

Health psychology is an interdisciplinary field concerned with the application of psychological knowledge and techniques to health and illness. Fundamental to research and practice in health psychology is the definition of health. The WHO (1948) definition of health, which was very forward looking for its time, is at the core of health psychologists' conception of health. Rather than defining health as the absence of illness, health is recognized to be an achievement involving balance among physical, mental, and social well-being. Many use the term wellness to refer to this optimum state of health.

Matarazzo (1980) has stated that Health psychology represents the educational, scientific and professional contributions of psychology to the promotion and maintenance of health, the prevention and treatment of illness, the identification of the causes and correlates of health, illness and related dysfunction, the improvement of health care system and health policy formation.

Many of the world's early philosophers viewed that the mind and the body were intimately connected. Close to 5,000 years ago, both the ancient Chinese Taoist sages and the ancient Indian practitioners of Ayurveda wrote about various ways the mind could calm the body and *vice versa* (Dash & Junius, 1983; Kaptchuk, 2000; Svoboda, 1992). Historically, philosophers have fluctuated between the view that mind and body are part of the same system and the idea that they are two separate from each other. Hippocrates (337 B.C.) stated that an individual gets ill/disease when the four circulating fluids/humors of the body, i.e. blood, black bile, yellow bile and phlegm—are imbalanced or out of balance. The function of treatment is to restore balance among those humors/fluids. In middle ages, however, a disease was dominantly conceptualized by mysticism and demonology which was seen as God's punishment for evil doing. Beginning in the Renaissance and continuing up to the present day, great strides have been made in the technological bases of medical practice. Rene Descartes, a French philosopher, strengthened the idea about the separation of mind from body. The hundreds of years that people believed that the mind was separate from the body helped medical sciences develop as scientists dissected dead bodies and increased our knowledge of human anatomy.

In the early 20th century psychologists started to play a part in the examination of health. Freud was the first to draw attention to the possibility that illness could have psychological causes. He found that many of his patient's illness were due to psychological reasons/issues. Once these issues were resolved, the physical symptoms disappeared. Later on psychoanalysts mainly Alaxender and Dunbar continued this approach and this movement was termed psychosomatic medicine. The realization of the potential implications of psychological knowledge for medical practice leads to the employment of psychologists in medical schools. As a result of this growing interaction between psychology and medicine, the field of Behavioural Medicine evolved. Behavioural medicine is a field that integrates knowledge from many different disciplines including medicine and psychology as well as sociology, education, nutrition and all other scientific fields that may provide information relevant to health and illness.

In recent years, more recognition is given to the social context of health and as a result of it, health psychologists are increasingly working beyond the level of individual, with families, work places, organizations and communities. The field of health psychology is already very broad but it is even becoming broader now-a-days. The realization of the importance of psychology in the field of health leads to the creation of an independent division of Health Psychology (Division 38, APA). The field has grown rapidly since then with its several branches, such as, psycho-oncology, community health psychology.

Models of Health Psychology

Biomedical Model

Proposed in 19th and 20th centuries, it assumes that health problems are rooted in physical causes, such as viruses, bacteria, injuries and biochemical imbalances (Engel, 1977; Schwartz, 1982; Wade & Halligan, 2004). This model explains illness in terms of the pathology, biochemistry and physiology of a disease (e.g. diabetes is caused by an imbalance in blood sugar, polio is caused by exposure to a virus and cancer is caused by genetic mutations). In turn, biomedical model proposes that medical treatment is needed to cure or manage the physical complaint and thereby return a person to good health. The biomedical model, therefore, focuses on the physical treatments for disease, such as a vaccine to prevent measles, medication to manage high blood pressure and chemotherapy to delay the spread of cancer.

Although the biomedical model has led to a number of benefits for our society such as advancements in immunology, public health policy, pathology yet there are evidences which proves that biological factors alone cannot account for health. The psychological and behavioural factors are associated with many of the leading causes of death, such as cancer and heart disease. People who are experiencing high level of stress at home and/or workplace—are at greater risk of experiencing a heart attack (Rosengren *et al.*, 2004). Biomedical model also fails to take into account how psychological factors, such as personality, cognitive beliefs, social support and the relationship between the patient and the health care practitioner can influence development of and recovery from illness. Thus, the shortcomings of the biomedical model are several. It has difficulty accounting for why a particular set of somatic conditions need not inevitably lead to illness. Why, for example, if six people are exposed to measles, do only three develop the disease? There are psychological and social factors that influence the development of illness, and these are ignored by the biomedical model. Whether a treatment will cure a disease is also substantially affected by psychological and social factors, and this cannot be explained by the biomedical model. As a consequence, researchers and practitioners have increasingly adopted the biopsychosocial model.

Biopsychosocial Model

This model was developed in the late 1970s and states that health is affected by both biology and social factors (Engel, 1977, 1980). In this perspective, there are two aspects which influence a person and his/her health. One aspect is physical body and other aspect is related to personality, family and society. Thus, the biopsychosocial model maintains that health and illness are caused by multiple factors and produce multiple effects. The model further maintains that the mind and body cannot be distinguished in matters of health and illness because both so clearly influence an individual's state of health. This model emphasizes health and illness rather than regarding illness as a deviation from some steady state. From this viewpoint, health becomes something that one achieves through attention to biological, psychological, and social needs rather than something that is taken for granted.

But how biological, social, and psychological variables interact with each other, particularly if biological factors are micro level processes and psychological and social factors are macro level processes? This question can be answered by a systems theory approach adopted by researchers. Systems theory maintains that all levels of organization in any entity are linked to each other hierarchically and that change in any one level will effect change in all the other levels. This means that the micro level processes (such as cellular changes) are nested within the macro level processes (such as societal values) and that changes on the micro level can have macro level effects and *vice versa*.

Consequently, health, illness, and medical care are interrelated processes involving interacting changes both within the individual and on these various levels. To address these issues impels researchers towards interdisciplinary thinking and collaboration. It also requires researchers to apply sophisticated, multivariate approaches to testing problems and to the often complex statistics needed to analyze those (Suls & Rothman, 2004).

There are several implications of the biopsychosocial model for clinical practice with patients. First, the model maintains that the process of diagnosis should always consider the interacting role of bio-psycho-social factors in assessing an individual's health or illness (Oken, 2000). Therefore, according to Suls and Rothman (2004) an interdisciplinary team approach may be the best way to make a diagnosis.

Second, this model maintains that recommendations for treatment must also involve all three sets of factors, i.e. biological, psychological and social. By doing this, it should be possible to target therapy uniquely to a particular individual, consider a person's health status in total, and make treatment recommendations that can deal with more than one problem simultaneously. Again, a team approach may be most appropriate (Schwartz, 1982).

Third, this model explores the significance of the relationship between patient and practitioner. An effective patient-practitioner relationship can improve a patient's use of services, the efficacy of treatment, and the rapidity with which illness is resolved (Belar, 1997).

In summary, for a healthy individual, the biopsychosocial model suggests that one can understand health habits only in their psychological and social contexts. These contexts may maintain a poor health habit or, with appropriate modifications, facilitate the development of healthy ones. For ill individual, biological, psychological, and social factors all contribute to recovery. This model also added that the practitioner must understand the social and psychological factors that contribute to an illness in order to treat it appropriately.

Aims of Health Psychology

There is a general agreement that the main purpose of health psychology is to reduce risks to physical and mental health. According to Matarazzo (1984 a, b), a general goal of health psychology is to identify risk factors for the most frequently occurring diseases, pathogens and immunogens, and their interactions, to explain them and to initiate appropriate behaviour changes.

Main goals of health psychology may be described as:

- ***Prevention of illness***: Health psychologists have argued strongly that it is better to prevent an illness than to cure it once it has occurred. Prevention is not only cheaper in the long-term, but it is also better for the individual. The role of health psychologists in preventing illness is to develop effective methods of behaviour change in advance. Behavioural intervention techniques such as, stopping smoking after a heart attack, during illness may prevent its further aggravation and chronicity. If we wish to stop people doing things that are bad for their health, first of all, we have to find out the reasons why they do those behaviours in the first place. Self-regulatory principles are also found to be effective for these conditions because they involve behavioural control and planning, are deliberative, reflective and consciously goal directed.

Investigation of psychological correlates of illness is an important aspect of the health psychologist's work. It involves carrying out research to gain knowledge about the specific role played by various factors which are responsible for diseases or illness. For example, the knowledge that stroke is related to smoking, high cholesterol and high blood pressure can enable practitioners to identify people at risk as early as possible.

- ***Treatment of illness***: People usually fall ill despite of preventive measures taken by them. In such circumstances, health psychologists may play an important role in developing treatments that take psychological aspects into account, e.g. a doctor may use drugs or surgery for treatment, but a health psychologist could contribute by introducing stress management programme cr could apply any other appropriate intervention technique/principle.
- ***Promotion of good health:*** As health psychologists see health as being more than just the absence of disease, they are interested in actively promoting well-being. A health psychologist may apply psychological principles and intervention techniques that will help in increasing the level of physical and mental well-being of an individual. Positive health psychology is one of them. There is a general agreement among medical practitioners and social scientists that positivity towards health can bring marvelous changes in one's life. With this positivity one can fight and deal with most terrible diseases and also maintain hope and optimism in life. Positive health is a state of complete well-being, which can be experienced when an individual becomes aware of that knowledge, that enables him to view himself as an integrated whole. A healthy individual is supposed to integrate his/her life in most meaningful and creative manner because human health is an outcome of human wholeness and organismic orientation. As we know that without unity of human being, body, mind and soul, we can't achieve positive health. Reducing stress through meditation techniques, improving vitality through balanced nutrition and developing energy through silent sittings are a few of basic approaches of mind-body healing with demonstrable health enhancing effects.

Challenges to Health Psychology and Need for Community Health Psychology

Community health psychology is an orientation that has arisen in response to growing concerns about the minimal contribution that health psychology has made to debates about the causes of health inequalities, and how to address these. While health psychologists have played a key role in exposing the individual determinants of health-related experiences and behaviour, they have too frequently ignored the way in which individual and proximal determinants of health are shaped by the broader social context.

Furthermore, while health psychologists have produced a group of graceful and rigorous explanations of health-related behaviour in the context of carefully monitored research studies, these findings often have limited significance to the challenge of designing and implementing real-world interventions and policies designed to promote health of individuals. There are more chances of happening of this challenge/problem particularly among the most marginalized social groupings where ill-health is most likely to prevail. Murray and Campbell (2003) have argued that the role of academic research should be not only to understand the world, but also to develop understandings that point towards the possibility of changing it. In other words, researchers should analyse not only the ways in which social conditions may be damaging of health, but also tries to find the possibility of alternative social relations that are less damaging to health, and map out the processes and mechanisms that would be needed to challenge and alter these. In this regard, the concept of social change is central to both the theory and the practice of community psychology. Community psychologists often align themselves with grassroots social movements working to challenge social inequalities and to promote social justice. Within this context, communities are seen as important social forces in the process of change (Nelson & Prilleltensky, 2004). Community health psychologists place strong emphasis on the importance of participation in collective action in increasing the likelihood that people will act in health-enhancing ways, and the creation of community contexts that will enable improved health.

Social/Collective Action and Community Health Psychology

In the modern era of life, psychologists have shifted their attention from individual to settings and from treatment to prevention. This established prevention orientation works as a founding principle of the field. Therefore, Health Psychology has become a science of prevention and community intervention. There is a widely agreeableness and conviction that the most humane and economical way to maintain, protect, and promote well-being of individuals is through prevention. Prevention is a globally supported concept but in Indian context in general, and in rural community in particular, everybody talks about it but a few implies preventive measures to promote health and well-being. Almost all rural communities have limited access to preventive health care. For this reason, they tend to suffer more health problems and have a higher mortality rate. Therefore, the purpose of our community health psychology is to understand and remove barriers that limit access to health care in these communities.

Community Health Psychology: Experiences from Rural Settings

One of the earliest community campaigns was initiated in 1972 for residents of a rural country in Finland with a very high incidence of coronary heart disease (Kottke, Puska, Salonen, Tuomilehto, and Nissinen, 1984). In the context of preventive programmes, wellness promoting programmes focus on factors like smoking cessation, diet and exercise regimes, as well as stress management and emotional control. The quality of life is obviously a factor, often recognized in planning for prevention. Therefore, health professionals must understand the importance of contentment, happiness, life satisfaction, optimism, and positive thoughts as preventive vaccine.

By following this approach, our research programme (SAP, Department of Psychology, M.D. University, Rohtak, Haryana) was aimed to sensitize people about their health, to provide some screening facilities, and to build positive attitude for preventive action with the basic thrust in the rural community. This health awareness programme also focused on the development of good health habits and a healthy lifestyle started in 2004 and an ongoing initiative with the grants of UGC, Delhi. We present ahead some of our findings up to 2009 to substantiate practical applications and implications of various notions of health psychology/ community health psychology.

The purpose of our community health field approach was to understand and remove barriers that limit access to health care in these communities (Singh *et al.*, 2006; Singh & Dinesh, 2007; and Singh & Dinesh, 2010). In relation to health, the first step involves the participation of a group of people in the collective development of critical understandings of how health can be promoted. Ideally, such critical understandings of the social obstacles to health and well-being form a key starting point for this group to mobilize for social change aimed at reducing such obstacles.

The two approaches were followed to achieve this goal – community health camps and community field survey. Community health camps were organized by establishing a make-shift psychological laboratory for assessing psychological parameters such as health cognitions, health beliefs, positive thoughts, happiness, optimism, and physiological parameters such as blood group, hemoglobin level, blood sugar, blood pressure etc. For this purpose, the Special Assistance Programme (SAP) team identified places (some common space, community institution, educational institution or a religious place like temple, dera etc.) and gave wide publicity about the camp through pamphlets, posters and local motivators. In this way, community health psychologists' teams go to near the villagers and make itself available to them in their vicinity and proximity, yet the initiation is from their side. We experience a massive affirmative response from their side expressing health anxieties.

In rural communities people are available in around their households, they do not exhibit xenophobic reactions to strangers and they feel secure in their village, they are receptive to messages provide these are conveyed in vernacular language even preferably in local dialect. When local motivators tell them beforehand that a team of university teachers (psychologists) and students (PG and Research Fellows) is coming rather a Governmental Organization (Health Department), their response tend to be very positive and hospitable. More so, we experienced a spontaneous collectivity among the community elements who took the roles of guide, mediators, hosts and even protectors (our esteem and regard). Village elders, chief and members of village Panchayat and other NGOs in the village come forward.

The community health psychologist can exploit such rural spirits to their advantage for delivery of programmes. Many myths are dispelled when one is among them in their settings. It was highly touching when the village folk come forward to raise a community kitchen with their own resources to take care of the food and refreshment of the entire team comprising more than 150 members (Psychologists, Physicians, Psychiatrists, Dentists, Homeopaths, Ayurvedacharyas and Yogacharyas, Technicians, logistic services and a hundred of Post-graduate and research students of Psychology). It is to be noted that it happened every time during our visit all over the years.

Then what does bind us together?

1. We prefer to go to them for their welfare, they find it good reversal.
2. The village community considers all those who visit to them as guests.
3. We offer them some screenings and initial diagnostics with referral recommendations from qualified consultants of various systems at their door step free of cost.
4. Some recommended hygiene kits and common preventive medicines are also provided free of cost.
5. We maintain continual interaction with the community.
6. The settings offer some persons to come forward, assuming leadership roles, and self-less service (*Kar-seva*).
7. We, of course, get information, training to students, experience and even esteem.

The community can be a powerful force for promoting healthy living. People are more likely to adopt health-enhancing behaviours when these behaviours are promoted by community organizations themselves. Therefore, the presence of community health psychologists' team in a remote village helps to change at the outset certain beliefs about health and disease. Indirectly, participation in collective action to improve health may result in the development of community networks capable of serving as a potent source of social support and buffering individuals from the health-damaging effects of stress. More directly, participation in such initiatives may increase the likelihood that people will engage in health-enhancing behaviours through a range of processes. Ideally, participation in collective action may also increase participants' confidence and empowerment in their ability to take control of their lives in general and their health in particular, increasing the likelihood that they will act in health-enhancing ways.

In addition, community field survey was organized by conducting a semi-structured door-to-door interview to get the Health Related Schedule filled individually after the consent of the participants. Trained investigators were employed for this purpose. These interviews were conducted in local dialect with a household setting in the presence of all the family members of the respondents by a team of investigators (one of them putting queries). In fact the purpose of house visit was to involve and sensitize the entire family. Quite often even the neighbourhood too joins. These experiences invoke varied informations about health and hygiene practices in their family and neighbourhood. Continual home made treatments since earlier generations are still prevalent and practiced.

The total sample achieved so far is 5278, which is self-selected, who participated in the health camps and in the field survey. The department organized 10 health camps in different villages (a cluster of few hundreds to thousand households). The team also visited 25 villages for field survey. These activities were organized during the five year tenure of the research programme. These villages were nearby Rohtak division (Haryana, India).

A snapshot of findings of the ongoing project is included here to give the article an empirical fervour. The results reveal that 92.8 per cent of the participants reported health to be as being free from disease, 97.1 per cent as the ability to function properly, and 89.5 per cent as balance between the nature and physique. These were the lay meanings of health. People carry multiple beliefs/meanings rather a unitary belief, however, a pragmatic functional ability with highest frequency. Even 96.5 per cent believed that they can maintain health by keep going working implying worklessness leading to ill health. It was observed that 97.7 per cent believed that having good food was a way through which one maintains and remains healthy. Followed by 94.2 per cent and 93.1 per cent of respondents reported exercise and yoga respectively. However, only 68.8 per cent of the subjects believed that meditation could help in being healthy. Results point out that 95.4 per cent of the participants value health and consider to be healthy as one's ethical responsibility (internal control). To an extent of 72.6 per cent participants reported health to be God's gift, whereas heredity was ascribed by only 58.4 per cent for one's health. About spiritual beliefs related to health, and 96.3 per cent reported that whatever health individual gets is an outcome of his/her *karma* or "so shall you sow so shall you reap", whereas 73.8 per cent participants even it to be the outcome of deeds of previous life. The perceived health in the community was almost equally distributed in three categories: good, average and so-so or bad (1/3rd). Majority of them opt for allopathic treatment while ill, whereas 13 per cent try other systems of medicine. Half of the participants (56%) attribute their present health to themselves, i.e. internal locus of control.

Community sample widely believe that 'sharing of concerns' with others keeps one healthy (83%), avoiding smoking (53%), and doing regular exercise (29%) for being healthy. During narrations participants seem to carry a myth that since they are engaged in physical work they do not require exercise. A vast majority (95%) believe that 'good work/deeds' may help them to be in good health.

There appear some contradictions in the health cognitions of people as half of them believe that they have no control of disease (52%), and even if they get sick, 60 per cent believe that 'luck' may help them in recovery.

Gender Differences

Gender differences were verified on the continuous variables selected for the present study. Results reveal that males have better usual as well as present perceived health than females. Although, females are found to be happier and have more spiritual beliefs in relation to health, like, belief in God, outcomes of previous life and *Karma*, in comparison to males. They also reported to have more somatic complaints and psychological distress than males. These findings generate a state of paradox. Further, on biological measures such as blood pressure and blood sugar, a minor difference is present between males and females. Here, females have higher blood pressure (systolic and diastolic) and higher blood sugar than males but within normal range. There is a common understanding that females usually have low level of Hemoglobin (Hb) in comparison to males, but our findings don't attest. We find that females have a high level of Hb than males. It can be attributed to iron poor diet in the sample. But a surprising fact is that the Hb level of both, males and females, represents a mild anaemic state (10-11 mg). On Body Mass Index (BMI), males have a little more BMI than females, though both fall in a normal range (21-22kg/m^2). On cognitive measures like memory forward and memory backward, females have better memory spans in comparison to males.

Age Differences

The sample was divided into three groups—21 to 40 years (group 1–early adulthood, n = 3085), 41 to 60 years (group 2–late adulthood, n = 1589) and 61 to 80 years (group 3–old age, n = 324). It is interesting and encouraging that young adults come forward in greater proportion (60%) to participate in the programme. Results reveal significant age differences in usual and present perceived health, in favour of early adults than late adult and old subjects. The usual as well as present perceived health decreased with increase in age, due to decrement in the strength of immune system, and weakening. The findings reveal that as the age of an individual increases, he/she becomes more optimistic and more satisfied with his/her life. Elders are found to be most optimistic and satisfied with life in comparison to other two younger groups. On the other hand young adults reported to be happiest than old age followed by late adults. In late adulthood, an individual has to perform multiple roles, has a lot of responsibilities, has pressure and expectations from society and has to face stress from daily hassels. It is also found that with an increase in age people have more somatic complaints and psychological distress. On BMI, all three groups differed significantly with late adults being the highest than by early adults followed by old age. On the biological dimension of blood pressure (systolic), three groups differed significantly with a continuous, but, little increment in B.P. with increase in age. Age differences are also observed in blood sugar level and it is reported that late adults and old age have nearly same, but, more blood sugar than early adults. Significant age decrements are observed on cognitive measures of both forward memory and backward memory.

Do Perceptions of Sick and Those Free from Illness Differ?

While comparing healthy (no disease) and ill (clinically diagnosed for chronic disease) subjects, it is found that the healthy participants reported significantly higher usual and present health than ill ones. Healthy subjects have better forward memory than diseased. When both groups were assessed on somatic complaints and psychological distress, the diseased group significantly reported more somatic complaints and showed more psychological distress. They also have higher diastolic BP, though in normal range. Chronic disease, thus, tend to contribute towards psychological distress in patients.

Health Locus of Control

By comparing respondents with internal and external locus, it is observed that the participants with internal locus of control reported to have better usual as well as present perceived health. They are also more optimistic, more satisfied with their life and happier than externals. They also scored higher on cognitive task of backward memory. On the other hand, participants attributing health to external factors reported greater spiritual beliefs, more somatic symptoms and were more psychologically distressed compared to internal locus respondents.

Grouping of Variables

To verify the validity of the contention that health is a multidimensional and also to justify the selection of variables in the schedule, principal component factor analysis was done on seven continuous variables obtained from 5272 respondents. The variables were: (1) Perceived present health; (2) Perceived usual health; (3) Somatic complaints; (4) Psychological distress; (5) Happiness; (6) Life satisfaction; and (7) Optimism.

Two components emerged, explaining 31.26 per cent and 15.05 per cent, respectively, the first named as perceived health and the other happiness (loading single variable significantly). Life satisfaction and optimism did not converge on either. Happiness though was contributing to general health perceptions yet had its unique variance too. Findings suggest that if we experience somatic or/and psychological complaints (symptoms), we tend to be less healthy and perceive ourselves having poor health.

In other factor analysis on 15 variables ($n = 496$) comprising biological variables (BMI, BP, Hb and blood sugar) and cognitive variables like forward and backward memory in addition to the variables described above and included in the analysis on much bigger data, three factors were obtained with 14 per cent, 13 per cent, and 11 per cent of the total variance, while other three factors were having less than 10 per cent of the variance. The main purpose was to verify the biopsychosocial model. Since the general factor loading of all variables were not obtained but the psychosocial factor, biological factor and cognitive factor had their unique variances, the model could not be empirically validated.

Conclusion

There is probably a greater emphasis on health promotion today than at any other time in history. Besides these limitations, substantial efforts are devoted to shaping the public's views on health issues through health educational campaigns and community health programmes (CHP). Thus, CHP promote health by encouraging educational campaigns in community setup. These efforts are focused at many levels, from individual to the community and to society as a whole. The goal of community based health programme is to create a social infrastructure that supports the efforts of each community member to improve the quality of his/her life (Heller, King, Arroyo & Polk, 1997). Therefore, at the heart of the wellness movement is the realization that preventing diseases is easier, cheaper and far more desirable than curing disease. In addition, we live in a country in which poverty and inequalities in wealth and access to resources are the major causes of ill-health. So, the challenge is to work with communities to overcome social deprivation and enhancement of health and well-being.

Active citizen participation can play an important role in community health programmes. Everyone must agree with the issues that the role of social context in shaping opportunities for health, and the role of participation in community level action in the challenge of creating community contexts that enable and support health enhancing behaviours, are of fore most importance.

Findings revealed that lay meanings of health, health beliefs and practices are embedded in the cultural context of the community. People come forward and participate in health programmes with enthusiasm. The scope of programmes should be beyond health awareness. Delivery of other health services at their door step help screening for some common chronic diseases and timely intervention. Employing local motivators, using vernacular language and dialects in the programme, offering opportunities to community people to decide plane, timings and other arrangements to have a sense of participation, offer some screening for common deficiency and chronic ailments, are some features to be included in the community based field programmes to be effective. Some tangibles like supplements, medicines and hygiene kits further enhances the participation for the immediate participation. Large teams of service providers seem to have initial impact. Continual contact with the same community helps building mutual trust and regard between team of service providers and the beneficiary community. Professionals in the team are also beneficiary as they enrich their knowledge with field experience and to revisit their skills and expertise.

This field study awakes the policy makers that how action at the community level can contribute to the development of community contexts that are enabling and supportive of health enhancing behaviours. Now-a-days, community health programmes are on the rise because a large body of research evidence indicated that rates of morbidity and mortality are linked to social conditions such as poverty, unstable living conditions, community disorganization, poor education, social; isolation and unemployment (Adler & Mathews, 1994; Williams & Lund, 1992). Although community campaigns are expensive to run and require massive organization efforts to reach all the residents (Susser, 1995). In addition, community campaigns must continue for several years before noticeable effects occur. Thus, today health promotion or behavioural health is perhaps the most predominantly preventive specialty area.

References

Adler, N., and Matthews, K. (1994). Health Psychology: Why do some people get sick and some stay well? *Annual Review of Psychology*, 45, 229-259.

Belar, C.D. (1997). Clinical health psychology: A speciality for the 21st century. *Health Psychology.* 16: 411-416.

Blaxter, M. (1990). *Health and Lifestyles*. London: Tavistock.

Calnan, M. (1987). *Health and illness: The lay perspective*. London: Tavistock.

Dash, B. and Junius, M. (1983). *A Handbook of Ayurveda*, New Delhi: Concept Publishing Company.

Dwivedi, C.B. (2005). The Samkhya, Yogic and Gita models of stress and coping. In R. Singh, A. Yadava and N.R. Sharma (Eds.) *Health Psychology* (pp. 295-303). New Delhi: Global Vision.

Engel, G.L. (1977). The need for a new medical model: A challenge for biomedicine. *Science*, 129-136, 196.

Engel, G.L. (1980). The clinical application of the biopsychosocial model. *American Journal of Psychiatry*, 137, 535-544.

Hall, J.A., Epstein, A.M. and McNeil, B.J. (1989) Multidimensionality of health status in an elderly population: Construct validity of a measurement battery, *Medical Care*, 27: 168-177.

Hays, R.D. and Stewart, A.L. (1990). The structure of self-reported health in chronic disease patients, *Psychological Assessment*, 2: 22-30.

Heller, K., King, C.M., Arroyo, A.M. and Polk, D.E. (1997). Community-based interventions. In A. Baum, S. Newman, J. Weinman, R. West, and C. McManus (Eds.), *Cambridge handbook of psychology, health and medicine* (pp. 203-206). Cambridge University Press.

Helman, C. (1978). "Feed a cold and starve a fever"— Folk models of infection in an English suburban community and their relation to medical treatment, *Culture, Medicine and Psychiatry,* 2, pp. 107-137.

Herzlich, C. (1973). *Health and Illness: A Social Psychological Analysis*, New York, Academic Press.

Jain, N., Sharma, N.R., and Yadava, A. (2006). Personality and Behaviour: A triguna perspective. In U. Kumar, S. Mukherjee and V. Parkash (Eds.) *Recent Developments in Psychology* (pp. 19-33). New Delhi: DIPR, DRDO.

Kaptchuk, TJ. (2000). *The Web That Has No Weaver: Understanding Chinese Medicine*. 2 ed: McGraw-Hill.

Kottke, T.E., Puska, P., Salonen, J.T., Tuomilehto, J., and Nissinen, A. (1984). Changes in perceived heart disease risk and health during a community-based heart disease prevention program: The North Karelia project. *American Journal of Public Health,* 74, 1404-1405.

Lau, R.R. (1995) Cognitive representations of health and illness, in D. Gochman (ed.), *Handbook of Health Behaviour Research,* Vol. I. New York: Plenum.

Marks, D. (1996). Health psychology in context. *Journal of Health Psychology*, 1(1), 7-21.

Marks, D. (2004). Rights to health, freedom from illness: A life and death matter. In M. Murray (Ed.), *Critical health psychology*. London: Palgrave.

Matarazzo, J.D. (1980). 'Behavioural health and behavioural medicine: frontiers for a new health psychology'. *American Psychologist*, 37, 1-14.

Matarazzo, J.D. (1984a). Behavioural immunogens and pathogens in health and illness. In B.L. Hammonds and C.J. Scheier (Eds.), *Psychology and health* (pp. 9-43). Washington D.C.: APA.

Matarazzo, J.D. (1984b). Behavioural health: A 1990 challenge for health services professions. In J.D. Matarazzo, Sh. M. Weiss, J.A. Herd, N.E. Miller and St. M. Weiss (eds.) *Behavioural health: A handbook of health enhancement and disease prevention,* pp. 3-40. New York: Wiley.

Misra, G. (2005). From disease to well-being: Perspective from an Indigenous tradition. In R. Singh, A. Yadava and N.R. Sharma (Eds.) *Health Psychology* (pp. 281-294). New Delhi: Global Vision.

Murray, M., and Campbell, C. (2003). Living in a material world: Reflecting on some assumptions of health psychology. *Journal of Health Psychology*, 8, 231-236.

Nelson, G., and Prilleltensky, I. (Eds.). (2004). *Community psychology: In pursuit of liberation and well-being*. London: Palgrave.

Normandeau, S., Kalinins, I., Jutras, S. and Hanigan, D. (1998). A description of 5 to 12 years old children's conception of health within the context of their daily life, *Psychology and Health*, 13: 883-96.

Rosengren, A., Hawken, S., Ounpuu, S., Sliwa, K., Zubaid, M., Almahmeed, W.A., INTERHEART Investigators. (2004). Association of Psychological risk factors with risk of acute myocardial infarction in 11,119 cases and 13,648 controls from 52 countries (the INTERHEART study): case control study. *Lancet*, 364, 953-962.

Schmidt, L.R. and Frohling, H. (2000) Lay concepts of health and illness from a developmental perspective. *Psychology and Health*, 15: 229-38.

Schwartz, G.E. (1982). Testing the biopsychosocial model: The ultimate challenge facing behavioural challenge? *Journal of Consulting and Clinical Psychology*. 50, 1040-1053.

Singh *et al.* (2006). Biopsychosocial Perspective of Health Psychology: An Empirical Tryout. *Journal of Indian Health Psychology*, 9: 8-28.

Singh, R., and Dinesh (2009). Health Cognitions and Subjective Well-Being in Middle-Aged and Older Adults. *Journal of Indian Health Psychology*, 4: 1-11.

Singh, R., and Dinesh (2010). Community Health Psychology: A Report of Field Study. In S. Ojha, U.R. Srivastava, and S. Joshi (Eds.). *Health and Well-Being: Emerging Trends,* pp. 23-34. New Delhi: Global Vision.

Suls, J., and Rothman, A. (2004). Evolution of the biopsychosocial model: Prospects and challenges for health psychology. *Health Psychology,* 23, 119-125.

Susser, M. (1995). The tribulations of trials-interventions in communities. *American Journal of Public Health*, 85, 156-158.

Svoboda, R. (1992). *"Ayurveda: Life, Health and Longetivity"*, New York: Penguin Books.

Tripathi, Y.B. (2000). Molecular approach to Ayurveda. *Indian Journal of Exp. Biology*, 38, 409-414.

Vidyalankar, A. (1968). *Susruta Samitha*. Varanasi: Motilal Banarsidass.

Wade, D.T., and Halligan, P.W. (2004). Do biomedical model of illness make for good healthcare systems? *British Medical Journal*, 329, 1398-1401.

Williams, A.F., and Lund, A.K. (1992). Injury control: What psychologists can contribute? *American Psychologist*, 47, 1036-1039.

World Health Organization (WHO) *Definition of Health.* Preamble to the Constitution of the World Health Organization as adopted by the International Health Conference, New York, 19-22 June 1946, and entered into force on 7 A.

3

Hazards of Mental Health

Towards Disruptive Behaviour

Aradhana Shukla

More recently health has been defined as in more positive term. Antonovsky (1979) has stated that health includes following features—

1. It is a very habitual, having to do with the persistent routine actions of people (e.g. relating to self and others).
2. It is more encompassing than the absence of specific physiological pathology.
3. It exists on a dynamic temporal continuum, fluctuating in response to the perceived demands (external as well as internal) over time.
4. It cannot be understood as independent of the particular social and physical context.
5. It involves available energy to perform certain tasks successfully.
6. It "breaks down" (i.e. disease predominates with various symptoms occurring) when there is insufficient energy or skill to satisfy demands and maintain a sense of balance and harmony.

The preamble of the constitution of WHO defines health "as a state of complete physical, mental and social well-being and not merely the absence of disease and infirmity". According to this definition health is –

(a) Something which goes beyond the mere absence of disease, and
(b) It has social and psychological characteristics. In Indian treatises health is defined in almost similar way. In accordance with *Sushrut Samhita*, "health is a state of delight or a feeling of spiritual, physical and mental well-being (Raina, 1990; Rao,

> 1983; Sharma, 1981). If we talk about the challenges of mental health, at first we describe disruptive behaviour. Defining disruptive behaviour in children is a subjective matter. Major issues that likely to be involved are: differences in conceptualization, purpose of definition, measurement of behaviour, range and variability of normal behaviour, relationship of behaviour disorders to other types of deviance, transience of behaviour problems, and problems of labelling. Thus, it is seen that identifying and defining disordered behaviour is a complex matter that depends on many factors. Since normal and abnormal behaviours are placed on the same continuum, any child may be more or less problematic only with regard to particular characteristic. Further, because the criteria for defining disorders behaviour are mainly social, these are always relative and also likely to change over a period of time.

Not only is disordered behaviour in children on the same continuum with normal behaviour, but it does not differ, by and large from normal behaviour in its development. It is, therefore, important to relate normal and disordered behaviour. It is widely believed that the developmental context can contribute a great deal to the understanding of problem behaviour in children. The process of development constitutes the crucial link between genetic determinants and environmental variables. A developmental perspective requires taking account of continuities and discontinuities between infancy, childhood and adulthood. Empirical data indicate that both occur (Rutter, 1984).

Some Queries about Disruptive Behaviour

Often we come across some people who are excessively shy or would run around incessantly with exuberant energy as would just throw a tantrum as would evince abnormal behaviour in different forms, e.g. confusion, worry, embarrassment, fear or even repulsion. In a given socio-cultural setting adults may find these behaviours as not normal, a typical strong as more often then not as annoying because they carry these forms of behaviour with themselves. Their onset of norms is treated as standards with which they evaluate the appropriateness of child behaviour. The decision of abnormality or normality is determined in family and school related environment. When the child does not get favour by these two main streams of society he thinks that he is not properly understood by them. As a result, his behaviour turns aversively. Main quarries about disruptive behaviour are given below:

(a) What are the norms on the basis of which a child is entitled disruptive in behaviour?
(b) How do children develop many sorts of behaviour and what are the underlying processes following which they are developed?
(c) How and when the behaviour of child is conceptualized as problem behaviour?

Keeping these views in consideration this study was planned. The objectives and hypotheses were as follows:

1. The first objective of this study was to find out the impact of age on disruptive behaviour. It was assumed that variation in age would cause variation in disruptive behaviour.
2. The second objective of this study was to find out the impact of sex on disruptive behaviour. It was assumed that sex difference would cause difference in disruptive behaviour.
3. The third objective of this study was to find out the impact of climateric variation on disruptive behaviour. It was contended that experience of problem behaviour would vary between home and school.

Keeping these objectives in consideration this study was planned in 2 × 2 × 2 factional design with 2 levels of age (8-9, 10-12 years), 2 levels of sex (boys, girls) and 2 types of climatic conditions (home, school).

Method

Sample: Eighty children in the age range of 8-12 years participated in this study. Half of them were studied at 'Nirvan' a voluntary organization in Haldwani Kumaun region of Uttarakhand and others were the students of public school at Haldwani. They were arranged according to the requirements of 2×2×2 factorial design with 2 levels of age (8-9, 10-12 Yrs.), 2 levels of sex (boys, girls) and 2 types of climatic condition (home, school), i.e. 10 Ss per cell. The schematic presentation of experimental design is given below in Table. 3.1.

Measures: Following measures were taken in consideration:

Table 3.1: Schematic presentation of experimental design

		A			
		A1		A2	
		B		B	
		B1	B2	B1	B2
C	C1	10	10	10	10
	C2	10	10	10	10

Legends:

A = Chronological age
A1 = 8-9 years
A2 = 11-12 years
C = Climatic Condition
C1 = Home
C2 = School

B = Sex
B1 = Boys
B2 = Girls

The Child Behaviour Checklist (CBCL)

Parental Rating Form (Achenbach, 1981) was used, which was translated in Hindi by Shukla (2002) and named as Child Behaviour Checklist (CBCL). On this standardized instrument, teachers/parents had to indicate the presence of 113 behaviour problems presented in their children (as perceived by them) using 1 to 5 on a five point scale for each item. The scale provided score on two broad dimensions of child behaviour problems – internalizing and externalizing problems. Low score presented higher level of behaviour disorders presented in the child and high score *vice versa.*

Home Environment Scale

In order to assess the patterns of family climate the HES was employed. Constructed by Dhaundiyal (1993) this measures has 74 items in Yes-No form and it deals with 10 dimensions, namely 1-Attention and care, 2-facilities, 3-impartially, 4-parental approval of adolescent actives, 5-sharing of ideas, 6-trust, 7-confidence, 8-decision making, 9-parental support and encourage and 10-harmony among family members. It is a questionnaire of True-False items. Two scores were given for the true items and one score for false items.Thus, the score ranges between 74 and 148. Low score indicated supportive family climate and high *vice versa.* Split-half reliability is 79 and retest reliability is 0.79. This scale is successfully used in other studies of child development (Dwivedi, 2000; Bhandari in progress).

Procedure

At first the investigator contacted the teachers of the target age groups at Public School and "Nirvan Institute of Haldwani". After the establishment of proper rapports she requested them to give a list of the children suffering from the disordered behaviours of everyday life. It was followed by the completion of CBCL by the teacher for each such child separately. The investigator visited the homes of such children and CBCL was filled up by the parents. Separate forms were filled up by mothers and fathers. Then the measure of home environment was given to the children. Items were convinced to the children and then the response was recorded. Normal children were also tested in the same way. Thus, the data collection was done in three subsequent phases. Data collection was done individually and best attempts were made to avoid external distractions.

Results

Obtained findings were analysed by mean, analysis of variance and correlation coefficient. Data were analysed in five subsequent phases. In phase one distribution of scores of child behaviour checklist was made followed by the distribution of scores on home environment scale in phase two. Analysis of variance was made. It was aimed to find out the impact of age, sex and climateric variation on disruptive behaviour. In phase three area-wise analysis of home environment was made. In fourth phase area-wise analysis of child behaviour was made. In fifth phase findings will be discussed accordingly:

1. **Distribution of CBCL:** Obtained data were subjected to area-wise distribution and the scores are given in Figure 3.1 and Table 3.2. Table and figure show that the scores of disruptive behaviour were effective in all areas. In schizoid, uncommunicative, social withdrawn and hyperactive the discrepancy between the scores of mothers and fathers was very less while in all other areas the discrepancy was very high. The same story was appeared by the score of teachers.
2. **Distribution of Score of Home Environment as Affected by Sex and Age:** In this phase an attempt was made to find out the

pattern of home environment as influenced by sex and age. Data of home environment scale were classified according to the dimensions and findings are given in Table 3.3. Findings show areawise similarity of home environment as affected by age and sex.

3. **Areawise analysis of home environment:** The scores of home environment scale were also analysed by correlation and findings are given in Table 3.4. Table 3.4 shows that all correlations were significant.

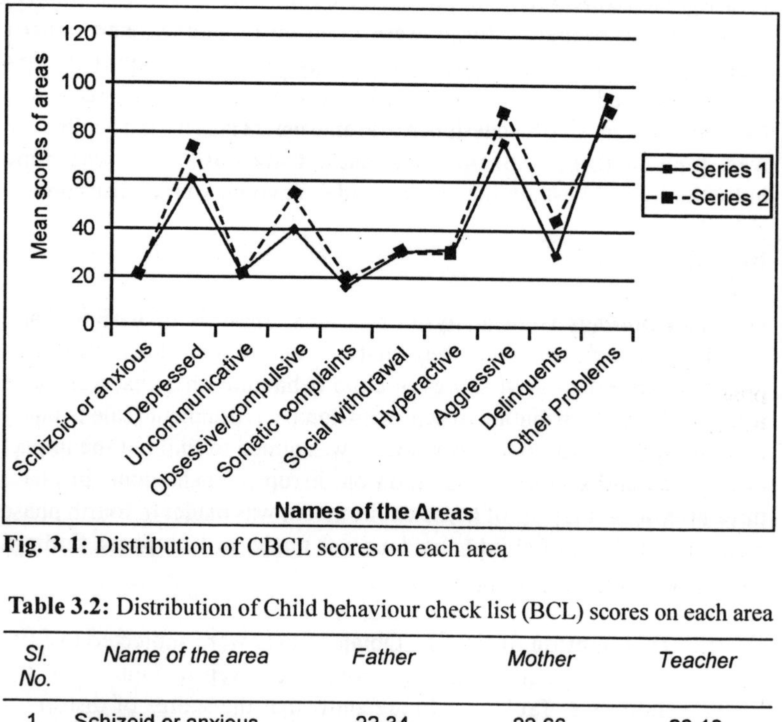

Fig. 3.1: Distribution of CBCL scores on each area

Table 3.2: Distribution of Child behaviour check list (BCL) scores on each area

Sl. No.	*Name of the area*	*Father*	*Mother*	*Teacher*
1.	Schizoid or anxious	22.34	22.66	23.19
2.	Depressed	60.19	74.76	76.44
3.	Uncommunicative	22.46	23.74	24.24
4.	Obsessive/compulsive	40.79	54.54	55.15
5.	Somatic complaints	16.15	19.16	18.17
6.	Social withdrawal	31.19	30.30	29.74
7.	Hyperactive	30.71	32.17	31 30
8.	Aggressive	76.79	90.68	89.79
9.	Delinquents	30.47	45.80	46.09
10.	Other problems	97.92	91.14	92.15

Table 3.3: Mean scores of home environment scale as affected by sex and age

Sl. No.	*Name of areas*	*Boys*		*Girls*	
		8-9 yrs	*11-12 yrs*	*8-9 yrs*	*11-12 yrs*
1.	Attention and care	17.96	16.79	18.98	19.00
2.	Facilities	12.12	10.11	13.17	14.18
3.	Impartiality	5.20	6.20	5.78	6.90
4.	Parental approval	15.85	18.18	20.01	21.17
5.	Sharing of ideas	8.55	9.01	11.90	12.08
6.	Trust	9.65	9.71	11.30	13.99
7.	Confidence	16.00	15.91	28.10	29.29
8.	Decision makers	13.40	14.49	23.22	24.08
9.	Parental support encouragement	14.90	14.00	16.14	16.00
10.	Parental harmony	16.17	15.00	20.15	21.79

Table 3.4: Areawise analysis of home environment

Sl. No.	*Name of the area*	*1*	*2*	*3*	*4*	*5*	*6*	*7*	*8*	*9*	*10*
1.	Attention and care	—	.62	.65	.70	.71	.65	.61	.70	.60	.56
2.	Facilities		—	.50	.76	.61	.64	.60	.69	.58	.68
3.	Impartiality			—	.79	.69	.56	.52	.49	.51	.60
4.	Parental approval				—	.62	.68	.56	.66	.74	.76
5.	Sharing of ideas					—	.61	.59	.62	.70	.65
6.	Trust						—	.60	.61	.59	.69
7.	Confidence							—	.59	.56	.72
8.	Decision makers								—	.64	.69
9.	Parental support encouragement									—	.71
10.	Parental harmony										—

Note: All values are significant.

4. **Areawise analysis of CBCL:** In this phase interrelation between the areas of CBCL was made. Findings are given in Table 3.5. Table shows that good relationship was maintained by all areas.
5. **Impact of age, sex and climatic condition on disruptive behaviour:** In order to find out the impact of age, sex and climatic variation analysis of variances was computed. Scores cf teachers, father and mother were pooled and average pattern of disruptive behaviour was assessed. Obtained data were analysed by three way analysis of variance and interpreted in terms of disruptive behaviour as affected by age, sex and climatic conditions. Findings are given in Table 3.2. A close perusal of the Table 3.2 indicates that the main effect of age was significant (F, 1, 72 = 6.14 P <0.01).

Table 3.5: Areawise analysis of child behaviour checklist (CBCL)

Sl. No.	*Name of the area*	*1*	*2*	*3*	*4*	*5*	*6*	*7*	*8*	*9*	*10*
1.	Schizoid or anxious	1.00	.59	.62	.69	.69	.72	.62	.69	.79	.69
2.	Depressed		1.00	.51	.49	.52	.62	.64	.64	.79	.53
3.	Uncommunicative			1.00	.56	.61	.53	.47	.62	.62	.71
4.	Obsessive compulsive				1.00	.54	.51	.62	.64	.67	.61
5.	Somatic complaints					1.00	.52	.47	.67	.62	.76
6.	Social withdrawal						1.00	.52	.52	.53	.40
7.	Hyperactive							1.00	.51	.46	.49
8.	Aggressive								1.00	.50	.48
9.	Delinquents									1.00	.70
10.	Other problems										1.00

Table 3.6: Summary table showing the impact of age, sex and climatic condition on disruptive behaviour

Sources of Variation	*Ss*	*df*	*MS*	*f*	*p*
A	6.94	1	6.94	6.74	<.10
B	6.35	1	6.35	6.17	<.50
C	4.93	1	4.93	4.79	<.10
AB	8.15	1	8.15	7.91	<.10
AC	10.03	1	10.03	9.74	<.10
ABC	6.91	1	5.31	6.17	<.10
Error (within)	74.16	72	1.03		
		79			

Mean values pooled across sex and climatic conditions were 167.24 And 230:70, respectively for young and old children. It revealed that disruptive behaviour was more evident in older children. The next main effect of sex was also significant ($F, 1, 72 = 6.17$ $P < 0.1$) and showed that boys ($x = 185.72$) and girls ($x = 213.13$) yielded significant difference in disruptive behaviour. Also, it was noticed that the magnitude of disruptive behaviour was more pronounced in girls. The third main effect of climatic conditions was also significant ($F1, 72 = 4.79$ $P < .05$) and it revealed that disruptive behaviour was more pronounced at school ($X = 206.17$) than at home ($X = 192.77$).

The age and sex interaction was significant ($F1, 72 = 7.91$, $P < .01$) and it is given in Figure 3.2.

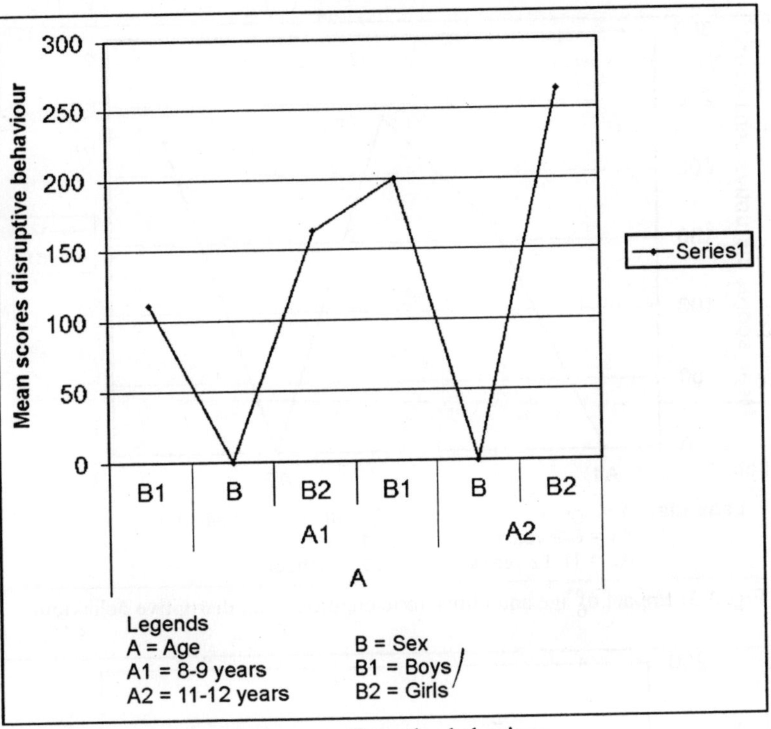

Fig. 3.2: Impact of age and sex on disruptive behaviour

Figure reveals that sex related discrepancy in disruptive behaviours was more pronounced. In addition, the trend of responses in boys and girls was entirely variant.

The age and climatic conditions interactions was also significant (F1, 72 = 9.74 P < .01) and it is mentioned in Figure 3.3.

Although the trend was similar in both groups yet the discrepancy between score was highly different. Likewise it was also, revealed that disruptive behaviour was more pronounced at school. The sex X climatic condition interaction was also significant (F, 1, 72 = 6.17) and it is revealed in Figure 3.4.

A close perusal of the data that the discrepancy revealing climatic condition was more pronounced in school.

The three-way interaction of age, sex and climatic condition was also (F, 1, 72 = 5.16 *P* < .01) significant. It was found that all variables laid their impact on disruptive behaviour. They are presented in Figure 3.5.

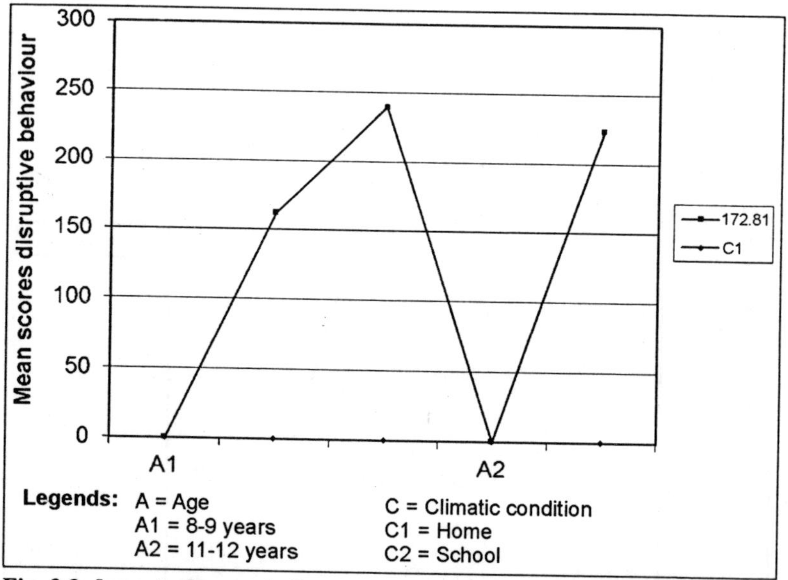

Fig. 3.3: Impact of age and climacteric conditions on disruptive behaviour

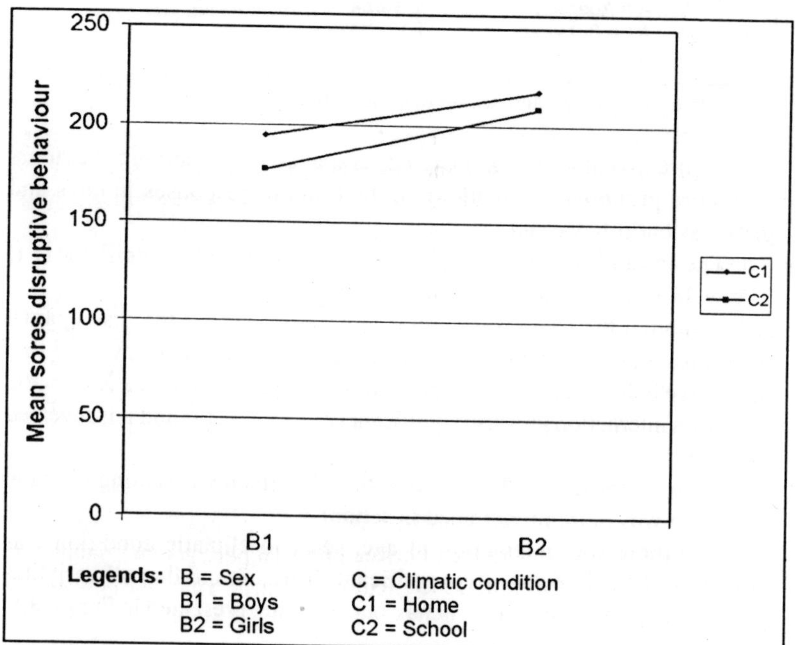

Fig. 3.4: Impact of sex and climatic conditions on disruptive behaviour

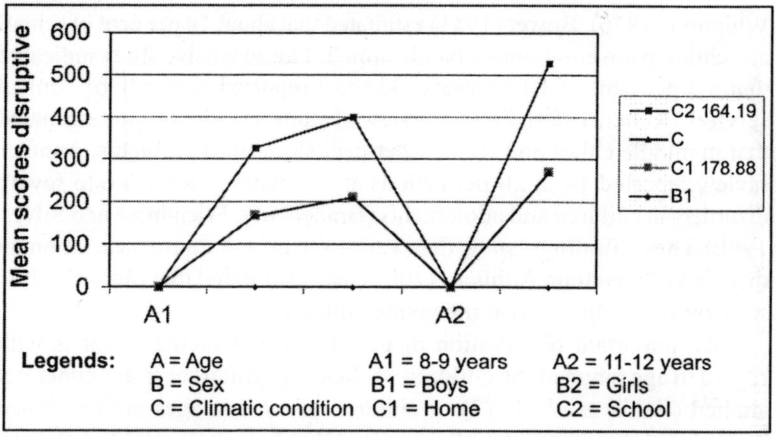

Fig. 3.5: Impact of age, sex and climatic conditions on disruptive behaviour

Findings in general state that

(1) Pattern of disruptive behaviour was highly influenced by age, sex and climatic conditions.
(2) All variables in sum, laid their influence on disruptive behaviour.
(3) Areawise analysis showed that a common trend was seen.

DISCUSSION

Obtained findings were analysed by means, ANOVA and correlation and interpreted in terms of age, sex and climateric variation as effectors of X disruptive behaviour. Prior to the test to some hypotheses were formulated and findings will be discussed in the realm of these hypotheses. Findings are discussed below:

Variation of age would cause variation in disruptive behaviour: Our first and foremost concern was related with the developmental pattern of disruptive behaviour. It was formulated that variation in age would cause variation in disruptive behaviour, therefore, children would vary in their score on disruptive behaviour, fortunately, the hypothesis was confirmed and it was found that older children showed more disruptive in behaviour.

Most of the age-related studies report a high prevalence rate of behaviour disorders. They ranged between 6 to 10 per cent (Achenbach & Edelbrock, 1981: Grahm, 1979; Rutter, Tizard, Yule, Grahm and

Whitmore, 1976). Bower (1981) estimated that about 10 per cent of school age children are emotionally handicapped. This extensive study indicated that 6.8 per cent of 10-11 years old were reported as needy of clinical services (Rutter, 1989). From a review of studies Cotler (1986) estimated that in middle childhood about 7 per cent show mild problems. Another review reported 14 to 20 per cent as an estimate of moderate to severe disorders in children and adolescents (Bradenburg, Friendman and Silver, 1990).These findings state that variation in age causes variation in disruptive behaviour, Adhikari (2002), has also stated that older children were more disruptive than the young children.

An important observation of the studies conducted so far is with regard to age range of the children studied. Age differences are either not studied (Banik *et al.,* 1972) or children of various ages are combined under a very broad group as 0-12 years (Verghese *et al.*, 1973; Adhikari, 2002; Bhandari 2005). Use of broad age is necessary to understand age trends in the problem behaviour under study. The studies where age differences have been taken into account, dealt with only one or two problems like enuresis or hyperactivity etc. is studied. As children grow and move through various stages over the years, changes that occur in them are phenomenal. Physically, intellectually, socially and emotionally, the variations are termed as lesion. Behaviour disorders of children, therefore, must be viewed in relation to their ages and developmental stages.

It is apparent that definite trends are not discernible with regard to association between age and incidence of problem behaviour among children. Many studies have reported declining trends in problem behaviour with increase in chronological age (Dagar & Singh, 1981; Werry & Quay, 1977). Muralidharan (1973) reported that problems such as sleeping and eating difficulties, habit disorders, aggression and delinquent behaviour decrease with age.

Sex difference would cause variation in disruptive behaviour: Our second hypothesis was related with the impact of sex on disruptive behaviour. It was contended that boys and girls would differ in disruptive behaviour. Fortunately, the hypothesis was confirmed and it was found that disruptive behaviour was more pronounced in girls than boys.

Almost all studies report a higher prevalence rate of problem behaviour in boys (Rubin & Balow, 1978; Werry & Quay, 1977). Evidence of conduct disorders like aggression, dislike for school, attention demanding behaviour and restlessness have been reported to be higher among boys (Banik, 1992). Incidence of such problems such as over activity, attention demanding behaviour temper tantrums and lying has been reported to be significantly higher among boys while problems such as excessive modesty, shyness and fear were fond to be more common among girls.

Variation in climatic condition would cause variation in disruptive behaviour: Last but not least was the third hypothesis where it was assumed that variation in climatic conditions would cause variation in behaviour. As a result, the magnitude of disruptive behaviour would be different in home and school. Our findings confirmed the hypothesis and we found that the level of disruptive behaviour was more pronounced at school as compared with home.

Often we see many people who are extremely shy or aggressive in behaviour on one side and cooperative and social on the other. This observation states clearly that the causes of disruptive behaviour are hidden in society and it is the society that says person to follow a particular conduct core. In addition, the decision of abnormality or normality is determined in family and school related environment. When a child does not get favour by one or both it means and he is not properly understood by them. Perhaps this notion has caused our findings. In school it is practically very difficult for a teacher to manage such a large group in which so many children are more or less disruptive in nature. Although teachers had made a continuous and appreciable effort but some constraints may have influenced them resulting to which the magnitude of disruptive behaviour was found higher in school. However, our results confirm the hypothesis.

Thus, it can be believed that the early childhood and late childhood (6-12 yrs.) are the most common period of onset reported for all childhood behaviour problems. Also, as we know, many behaviour problems can occur together in children. The research studies must be so planned that they should be built in scope for tapping various types of problems. For this purpose, use of comprehensive measures is essential. Findings in general indicate that there is a need to minimize the level of disruptive behaviour in children following the ways given below:

(1) The norm of disruptive behaviour is formed by society. It is its direction that behaviour is termed as normal on the one side of the coin and abnormal on the other side.

(2) Children develop such behaviour according to the view of the society and the underlying progress is also determined by them.

Thus, it is clear from the result of the present study that disruptive behaviour are commonly seen in children. There is a need to develop research strategies and behavioural skills to abolish it. Recent studies from various countries confirm that many behavioural problems are commonly reported.

References

Antonovski, A. (1979). Health, Stress and Coping, San Francisco: Jossey Bass.

Achenbach, T.M. and Edelbrock, C.S. (1981). Behavioural problems and competencies reported by parents of normal and disturbed children aged four through sixteen. *Monographs of the Society for Research in Child Development*, 46. (Whole No. 188).

Anderson, K.E. Lytton. H. and Romney, D.M. (1986). Mother's interactions with normal and conduct-disordered boys: Who affects whom? *Development Psychology*. 22, 604-609.

Adhikari, S. (2000). Relationship between parenting style. Problem behaviour and school performance in children, Unpublished doctoral dissertation Department of Psychology. Kumaun University, Nainital.

Banik, N.D.B.; Sushila. N.; Krishna A., and Raj, L. (1972) Behaviour problems of primary school children. *Indian Paediatrics*, 9, 757-761.

Bassa, D.M. (1962). An analysis of cases attending child guidance psychotherapy centers. *Indian Journal of Psychiatry*, 4, 139.

Bower, E.M. (1981). Early Identification of Emotionally Handicapped Children in School (3rd ed.) Springfield, Ill: Charles C. Thomas.

Brandenburg, N.A.; Friedman, R.M. and Silver, S.E., (1990). The epidemiology of childhood psychiatric disorders: Prevalent findings from recent studies. *Journal of the Academy of Child and Adolescent Psychiatry*, 29, 76-83.

Bhandari, V., Disruptive behaviour of children in Rural and Urban setting. Doctoral work in progress. Department of Psychology, Kumaun University, Nainital.

Campbell, S.B. (1982). Developmental perspective in child psychopathology, In T.H. Ollendick & M. Hersen (Eds.). *Handbook of Child Psychopathology*, New York: Plenum.

Chawala, P.; Sahasi. G.; Sunderam, K.R. and Mehta, M. (1981). A Study of prevalence and pattern of hyperactive syndrome in primary school children. *Indian Journal of Psychiatry*. 23, 313-323.

Cotler, S. (1986). Epidemiology and outcome. In J.M. Reismen (Ed.), Behaviour disorders in infant children and Adolescents. New York: Random House.

Dager, B. and Singh, M.V. (1981) Behaviour disorders in a community child guidance centre. *Archives of Child Health*, 23, 140-145.

Dhaundiyal, V.R. (1993). *Emotional disturbance in the adolescents of Himalayas.* Almora, Shyam.

Dwivedi, V. (2000). Impact of age and sex and climatic conditions on academic stress and stress management: A study of open and closed cultural. Unpublished doctoral dissertation, *Department of Psychology*, Kumaun University, Nainital.

Grahm, P.J. (1979). Epidemiological studies in H.C. Quay. and J.S. Werry (Eds) *Psychopathological Disorders of Childhood* (2nd ed.) New York: Willey.

Indian Council of Medical Reserch (1983). Multicentre study of the patterns of child and adolescent disorders; Unpublished final report of the Task Force Project. New Delhi: Author.

Malhotra, S., and Chaturvadi, S.K. (1984), Patterns of childhood psychiatric disorders in India. *Indian Journal of Paediatrics* 51, 235.

Malhotra, S. and Chadda, R. (1987). Specific development disorders in children attending child guidance clinic. *Indian Journal of Paediatrics*. 51, 235.

McMahon, R.J. and Forehand, R. (1988) conduct disorders. in E.J. Mash & L.G. Terdal (Eds.) *Behavioural Assessment of Childhood Disorders* (2nd Ed.) New York: Gulford.

Murlidharan, R. (1973), Age trends in behaviour problems of children. In T.E. Shanumagam (Ed.). *Research in Personality and Social Problems.* pp. 107-128, Madras: Madras University.

Murthy, R.S., Ghosh, A., and Verma, V.K. (1974) Behaviour disorders of childhood and adolescence. *Indian Journal of Psychiatry*. 16, 229.

Raina, B.L. (1990). Health Sciences in Ancient India. New Delhi: *Common Wealth.*

Rutter, M. (1989). ISLE of Wight revisited: Twenty five years of child psychiatric epidemiology. *Journal of American Academy of Child and Adolescent Psychiatry*. 28. 633-653.

Rao, S.K.R. (1983). The conception of stress in Indian thought: The theoretical aspects of stress in Samkhya and Yoga systems. *Nimhans Journal*. 2. 115-121.

Rubin, R.A. and Balao, B. (1978). Prevalence of teacher Identified behaviour problems: A longitudinal study. *Exceptional Children*, 45, 102-111.

Sharma, P. (1981). *Charak Samhita* (English Adition). Varanasi, Chaukhamba Sanskrit Series Office.

Shukla, A. (2002). Child behaviour checklist Unpublished Script, Department of Psychology. Kumaun University, Nainital.

Verghee, A.; B. Vig, A., Sememan, S.A.; Rao, S.S.; and Benjamin, V.A. (1973). Social and Psychiatric study of representative group of families in Vellore town. *Indian Journal of Medical Research*, 61, 608.

Werry, J. and Quary, H. (1977). The prevalence of behaviour symptoms in younger dementry school children. *American Journal of Orthopsychiatry.* 41, 13. 136-143.

4

Cross Cultural Researches on Mental Health with Special Reference to India

Anubhuti Dubey and *Dhananjay Kumar*

Health is often used to mean the absence of disease or disability, but, just as often, health may refer to a state of fitness and ability, or to a reservoir of personal resources that can be called on when needed (Naidu & Wills, 2000). Moreover, WHO (2001) had defined mental health as a state of well-being in which the individual realizes his or her own abilities, can cope with the normal stresses of life, can work productively and fruitfully, and is able to make a contribution to his or her community (WHO, 2001). Mental, physical and social functioning is interdependent. Neither mental nor physical health can exist alone. Furthermore, health and illness may co-exist. They are mutually exclusive only if health is defined in a restrictive way as the absence of disease (Sartorius, 1990). People with different backgrounds and cultures may conceptualize health differently. Some people describe it as the particular circumstances of their lives. Under some circumstances, they equate health with freedom from disease; some may equate health with autonomy or with vitality. Older people, for example, tend to define health as inner strength and the ability to cope with life's challenges, whereas younger people tend to emphasize the importance of fitness, energy, and strength. Unified theories of health such as that propounded by WHO cover wide territory, including environmental and individual factors The global burden of mental ill-health is well beyond the treatment capacities of developed and developing countries, and the social and economic costs associated with this growing burden will not be reduced by the treatment of mental disorders alone (WHO, 2001). Research evidences also pointed out that mental ill-health is more common among people with relative social disadvantage.

Social Determinants of Mental Health

The factors which can enhance or threaten an individual's or a community's health status are social determinants of health. These can be matter of individual choices, such as whether to smoke tobacco or not, or can relate to social, economic, and environmental characteristics beyond the control of individuals. Examples include the person's social class, gender, ethnicity, access to education, quality of housing, and presence of supportive relationships. A wide range of social factors are related to inequalities in health. Inequalities result to a degree from individual differences in genetics, health related behaviour, and choices regarding education, work, and play to the degree that inequalities are a consequence of social injustice. There are gross inequalities in health between and within countries. Life expectancy at birth, to take one measure, ranges from 34 years in Sierra Leone to 81.9 years in Japan (WHO, 2004). According to WHO, health promoting policies are needed not only in the health care sector, but also in the economic, environmental, and social sectors for positive impact on the determinants of health and social determinants of mental health. Many studies conducted with socio-economic variables have shown the powerful health associations of social connectedness (Putnam, 2001). The evidence on the personal, social, and environmental factors associated with mental health and mental illness has been reviewed by a number of authors (e.g. Lehtinen, Riikonen, Lahtinen, 1997; Wilkinson & Marmot, 1998; Eaton & Harrison, 2000; Patel & Kleinman, 2003; Jané-Llopis *et al.*, 2011). Advances in learning from the brain sciences and neuroscience, there have been an evolution of ideas about the social determinants of mental health and mental disorders. Low control at work and poor social support has important influences on both physical health (e.g. cardiovascular morbidity) and psychological health (e.g. depression) (Kopp, Skrabski & Szedmák, 2000). Many of the people living with HIV/AIDS and their families experience stigma and discrimination as well as depression and anxiety and other mental illnesses (WHO, 2001c).

Developing Indicators of Mental Health

A considerable body of practice informs the development and use of population indicators in mental health and mental health promotion such as epidemiological studies of mental health, cross-national studies of quality of life, findings regarding the relationship between social determinants and inequalities and health and mental health outcomes, psychometric studies, and observations from health surveillance and monitoring. In proposing mental health indicators, the different perspectives of health promotion practitioners and mental health practitioners need to be appreciated, although these are not antithetical. Thus, either through a focus on populations or a focus on individuals, both acknowledge that positive mental health is set within a larger socio-political, economic, and cultural environment which in turn influences the distribution of material and social resources through a variety of institutional and individual mechanisms. Ultimately, individual biology and genes are conditioned by and interact with these environments. As a consequence, indicators of positive mental health will of necessity reflect differing levels of influence.

Emerging frameworks or conceptual models of positive mental health, while at an early stage, already acknowledge the need to specify a range of indicators at differing levels of developmental influence on mental health (Korkeila, 2000; Lahtinen *et al.,* 1999). These influences entail multi-sectoral interests (e.g. health, welfare, education, justice). They also include four levels of measures—(i) macro-level measures of cultural, social, and political-economic structural processes, (ii) distal measures of the social organization and behaviour of communities, schools, local neighbourhoods, and workplaces, (iii) proximal measures of the demographic, material, and social circumstances and behaviours of families and peers, and (iv) direct measures of the psychological, biological, social, material, and demographic characteristics of individuals. Obviously, developing a framework to portray all or even some of this is a massive task. Some efforts in this regard have been made, however. Broad-based macro-level determinants of mental health are measured by, for example, the Human Development Index (HDI) which was reviewed in 2000 by the UN. The HDI was developed as a measure of achievement and focuses attention on human outcomes as well as the economic performance of a country. The Gender-related Development Index (GDI) and Gender Empowerment Index (GEI) are other examples of macro-level national indicators. They are relevant in characterizing some aspects of basic human development, giving measures of mental health an appropriate context.

Epidemiological Findings on Prevalence of Mental Disorders in India

From time to time the prevalence of mental disorders in the country is estimated by mental health planners in India. Such data facilitate in understanding the status of mental health in the country and in planning for prevention and treatment of disorders. The Bhore Committee (Government of India, 1946) assumed from prevalence rates in U.K. and U.S.A. and ended up that mental patients requiring hospitalization in India be taken as 2 per 1000. Yet again in 1966, the Mental Health Advisory Committee of the Government of India recommended a probable prevalence of mental illness of 20 per 1000 population in general, 18 per 1000 for semi-rural and 14 per 1000 for rural areas (Elnaggar *et al.*,1971). Ganguli (2000) analysed the fifteen epidemiological studies since 1960 to shed light on national all-India prevalence rate for all mental disorders, national prevalence rates for specific disorders, rural-urban difference, morbidity in urban industrial population as compared to rural and urban general populations and stability of schizophrenia rate. The national prevalence rates for all mental disorders was found to be 70.5 (rural), 73 (urban) and 73 (rural + urban) per 1000 population. Prevalence of schizophrenia is 2.5/1000. Schizophrenia appears to be the only disorder whose prevalence is consistent across cultures and over time. Urban morbidity in India is 3.5 per cent higher than the rural rate, but rural-urban differences are not consistent for different disease categories like depression, anxiety neurosis, hysteria and mental retardation. Mental morbidity amongst factory workers is two and half times that of the non-industrial urban inhabitants and five times the rural morbidity in Hindi speaking north India was found. In another study Madhav (2001) reported that mental retardation was observed to have national rate of 4.2 per 1000. However, the most widely prevalent disorders were depression and anxiety with the rate of 31.2 and 18.5 per 1000 respectively. In 2010, a study conducted in NIMHANS, Bangalore reported that the burden of mental and behavioural disorders ranged from 9.5 to 102 per 1000 population (Math & Srinivasaraju, 2010).

Burden of Mental Disorders in India

A study conducted in Pune (Deswal & Pawar, 2012) reported the overall life time prevalence of mental disorders to be nearly 5 per cent. Males were reported to be at higher risk. Major cause was depression followed by substance abuse and panic disorders. These findings were similar to results of the meta-analysis, which estimated the prevalence of mental disorders to be 5.8 per cent among the Indian population (Reddy & Chandrasekhar, 1998). Barua *et al.* (2007) reported that among a rural community in Karnataka reported that women had significantly higher symptoms of somatic disorders and anxiety than men, and this was strongly associated with the lack of education, poverty, low socio-economic status and also among unmarried or widowed/divorced individuals as compared with their married counterparts. The prevalence of depression was found to be 12.7 per cent among elderly in a study done in South India. On the contrary, the prevalence of mental disorders was reported to be as high as 26.7 per cent by a study in elderly with predominant depressive disorders, dementia, generalized anxiety disorder, alcohol dependence and bipolar disorder (Seby, Chaudhury & Chakraborty, 2011). Prevalence of mental depression among the elderly in West Bengal, Medinipur town, was assessed and it was found that 59.8 per cent of the subjects were suffering from depression and prevalence increased with age. Prevalence was significantly higher (83.33%) among respondents who were single and/or physically disabled (88.9%) (Dhar, 2013). In urban population of Kerala the prevalence of dementia was found to be 33.6 per 1000. Alzheimer's disease was the most common cause (54%) followed by vascular dementia (39%) (Shaji, Bose & Verghese, 2005). In their study Hackett and associates (1999) affirmed the prevalence of mental disorders in child and adolescent population was 9.4 per cent. Likewise, another study from Bangalore documented the burden of mental disorders to be 12.5 per cent. The study also showed that there were no significant differences among prevalence rates of mental disorders in urban middle class, slum and rural areas with annual incidence of 18 per 1000 population. The prevalence of mental disorders among 0-3 years old children was 13.8 per cent, most commonly due to breath holding spells, pica, behaviour disorder NOS, expressive language disorder and mental retardation. The prevalence rate in the 4-16 years old children was 12.0 per cent mainly due to enuresis, specific phobia, hyperkinetic disorders, stuttering and oppositional defiant disorder (Srinath *et al.*, 2005). In 2002, the prevalence rate of mental disorders in the Indian industrial population was estimated to be 14 to 37 per cent. On the contrary, Western world reported it to be nearly 75 per cent (Kar, Dutta & Patnaik, 2002). Another study among industrial workers mentioned the lifetime prevalence of mental disorder to be more than 50 per cent. Most common associated factor in industrial workers was substance abuse (12.3%) (Kumar, Jayaprakash, Monteiro & Bhagavath, 2011). Besides substance abuse, National Crime Record Bureau reported that suicide among young people has seen 27.7 per cent increase in recorded number of suicides between 1995 and 2005 with suicide rate of 10.5 per million. Almost 35 per cent of suicides occur amongst youth (15–29 years) with rate of 152 per lakh for girls and 69 per lakh for boys reported in a study conducted in Hyderabad (Leo, 2003). Pillai, Andrews and Patel (2009) revealed that overall 3.9 per cent youth reported suicidal behaviour. A study conducted in rural areas of south India, in 2010 reported 37 per cent of those who died by suicide had a mental disorders too. The two most common reasons were alcohol dependence (16%) and adjustment disorders (15%) (Manoranjitham *et al.*, 2010). In çomparison to studies conducted in Western world the prevalence rates of mental disorders reported in India are very low. The reason may be that the Indian epidemiological studies were not able to assess mental disorders effectively or prevalence rates of mental disorders are genuinely low in India. The explanations for the same may be attributed to the factors like genetic reasons, good family support, cultural factors, lifestyle and better coping skills and comfortable environment (Math & Srinivasaraju, 2010).

Culture in Cross-cultural Researches on Mental Illness

Cultural and ethnic groups vary pertaining to practices and activities relevant for eco-cultural adaptation and survival (Weisner, 2002). The bulk of cross-cultural psychiatric research has been carried out with an objective to demonstrate that psychiatric disorder is like other disorder (Kleinman, 1987) with the perception that mental disorders occur in all societies with somehow the same cluster of symptoms in more or less the same way in all groups and societies. Scrutinizing many clinic based comparative studies Kleinman (1987) reported that these studies applied a template of symptoms to psychotic patients in a range of societies to identify groups of patients who seemed to be similar. He finished that there is an inherent problem of these studies which leave out those patients who fail to fit the template, the patient who otherwise has greatest importance from a cultural perspective because they could be expected to reveal the greatest amount of cultural diversity. It was asserted in DSM-IV that even if disorders are rooted to internal dysfunctions, the dysfunctions may start off from contact to negative and destructive environments. Hence, the Universalist position does not cancel out the risk and/or protective factors associated to the pathogenesis of the disorder may have an effect on a number of expressions of the disorder. As a matter of fact, for each disorder DSM-IV has a section on specific culture, age and gender features which is meant to direct the clinician on variants of the disorder that may be credited to the individual's culture, sex or developmental stage. On the other hand, the relativistic standpoint upholds that culture outlines the individual's development and his/her biological and psychological recounting to a large degree, with the need to integrate culture within the diagnostic classificatory system (Lewis-Fernandez & Kleinman, 1995). According to the relativists DSM leave out important cultural symptoms and syndromes unique to particular cultural settings that result in a category fallacy or apparent homogeneity of disorders across cultures (Kleinman & Kleinman, 1991). The viability of developing a universal classificatory system for all cultures, such as the ICD-10 (WHO, 1992) was questioned by relativists (e.g. Weisz, McCarty & Valeri, 2006) as these taxonomies are developed on the assumption that syndromes or disorders are alike across cultures and what may differ is the manifestation of the symptoms. Rutter and Nikapota (2002) argued in favour of integrating both a universal and relativistic view of psychopathology depending on the specific disorder. The combined relativistic and universalistic approach in diagnostic classificatory systems for psychopathology states that some disorders (i.e., autism, schizophrenia, fragile X syndrome and other pervasive developmental disorders) are more likely to be universal in all cultures because they are mostly based on neural pathology. However, other more common disorders, even though they may share a biological or genetic substrate, are more likely to be shaped by social context, cultural norms and developmental stage (Rutter & Nikapota, 2002).

Culture and Mental Health

There are a number of approaches that endeavour to understand the psychopathology, mental illness and mental disease under the cultural framework. This area of activity has come to be known as the field of "cultural psychiatry" and "trans-cultural psychiatry". Tanaka-Matsumi and Draguns (1997) had raised the question that 'What questions arise when studying cultural universals in depression?' There is another perspective known as "cultural clinical psychology".

Three general orientations have been proposed to understand the human behaviour in a cross-cultural perspective, i.e. absolutism, universalism and relativism (Berry, Poortinga, Segall & Dasen, 1999). These orientations can also be extended to conceptualize the interplay of abnormal behaviours and cultures. Cross-cultural researchers have adopted both emic (culture-specific) and etic (pan-cultural) positions. The absolutist orientation presumes that psychological phenomena are principally the same in all cultures. The absolutists' perspective suggests that culture have little or no role in either the meaning or manipulation of human characteristics. However, relativism, which stands in sharp contact to absolutism, posits that human behaviour is shaped by culture. The third perspective Universalism stands between the previous two positions. Universalism possesses the view that "Basic psychological processes are common to all members of the species and that culture influences the development and display of psychological characteristics" (Berry, Poortinga, Segall & Dasen, 1999).

Some of the classical definitions of culture are given here. Tylor (1871) defined culture as "that complex whole which includes knowledge, beliefs, arts, morals, laws, customs" and any other capabilities and habits acquired by man as "member of society". Linton (1936) proposed that culture can be conceptualized as "the total social heredity of mankind", while Herskovits (1948) asserted that "culture is the man made part of the human environment." In his definition of culture Wissler (1923) incorporated speech, material traits, arts, knowledge, religion, society, property, government and war.

Fundamental for culture is that these shared system of knowledge, values, customs, belief and artefacts of a society, typically learned and transmitted from generation to generation. However, cultures are open dynamic systems that deal with constant change and challenges over time.

From a cross cultural perspective 'cultures' are seen as product of past human behaviour, and as shapers of future human behaviour. Thus, humans are producers of culture and, at the same time, our behaviour is influenced by it. If we found in studies a dichotomous descriptions and labelling of cultures. We list some of the examples: (1) simple-complex, (2) Western-Non-Western, (3) technologically advanced-less-advanced, (4) primitive civilized, (5) Eastern-Western cultures, and (6) Industrialized and Pre-industrialized (Tanaka-Matsumi & Chang, 2002).

Influence of Culture on Mental Health

Culture influences mental health by different ways. It influences the beliefs about how mental illness occurs, and how they are expressed, experienced, treats presented and assessed. Beliefs about practices to maintain and enhance health, the causes of illness are deeply rooted in our cultural beliefs. It varies from culture to culture and the stigmas associated with mental health problems are much stronger in some cultures than in others. Culture shapes how individuals perceive and respond to others with mental illness. Previous studies have showed that Asians and Asian Americans typically endorse greater stigma of mental illness compared to Westerners (White Europeans and Americans). However, whether these differences in stigma arise from cultural variations in automatic affective reactions or deliberative concerns of the appropriateness of one's reactions to mental illness still remains unknown. Asian Americans showed stronger negative implicit attitudes towards mental illness relative to Caucasian Americans, suggesting that cultural variation in stigma of mental illness can be observed even when concerns regarding the validity and appropriateness of one's attitudes toward mental illness are minimized. Asian Americans also explicitly endorsed greater desire for social distance from mental illness relative to Caucasian Americans (Cheon & Chiao, 2012).

Every culture in this world has its own medical system. It can be distinguished between personalistic and naturalistic ethno medical system. In a personlistic system, illness is attributed to some supernatural agent (e.g.) a deity or ancestral spirit, or a human being with special powers (e.g.) that has an intention to cause harm. In naturalistic system illness is believed to be an outcome of a disturbed equilibrium of the physical body (e.g. infection or hormones). Personlistic illness may be caused by the person disobedience, conforming not to social norms, religious beliefs or rituals whereas, naturalistic explanation assumes that illness is due to impersonal, mechanistic causes in nature that can be understand and cured by the appropriate application of scientific method (Kleinman, 1978; Littlewood, 1988).

Culture also influences on how mental illness is experienced. Culture affects mental heath by influencing the way people experience the discomfort associated with mental illness. Some cultures do not express their emotional pain overtly, and restrained themselves from upsetting though or believe in control. Cultural norms provide basis for characteristic modes of manifesting suffering. In a study Dinnel, Kleinknecht, and Tanaka-Matsumi, J. (2002) had examined two forms of social anxiety or phobia, social phobia as defined by DSM-IV and *Taijin Kyofusho* (TKS, a Japanese form of social anxiety), in relation to their respective culturally prescribed self-construal as independent and interdependent. Japanese University students and U.S. University students were administered the Social Interaction Anxiety Scale, the Social Phobia Scale, the TKS Scale, and the Self-Construal Scale. From the results of a hierarchical regression analysis, TKS symptoms are more likely to be expressed by individuals who are Japanese and individuals who construe themselves low on independence but high on interdependence. In addition, social phobia symptoms are more likely to be expressed by individuals who construe themselves low on independence but high on interdependence irrespective of culture. Asian psychiatric patients have a tendency to focus on physical discomfort while ignoring or suppressing the reporting of emotional symptoms has been a challenge for clinicians who work with this population. Many theories have been anticipated for such a phenomenon, with assumptions about Asians' relative lack of psychological mindedness and a putative deficiency of psychological descriptive terms in Asian languages. Kleinman (1988) and his colleagues demonstrated that for the majority of the Asian patients, somatic symptoms are operated as culturally sanctioned "idioms of distress," whose mechanism may thus be quite distinct from the process of somatization as commonly understood. In Hong Kong a series of studies conducted by Cheung (1982, 1985) found that although patients typically focused on their somatic complaints when visiting a physician, they were often fully aware of their emotional problems as well as stresses derived from social relationships that might be related to their emotional as well as somatic symptoms. In the same way, in a longitudinal follow-up study of Vietnamese refugees (Lin, Tazuma, & Masuda, 1979), most of those who were firstly interviewed reported only physical symptoms (Lin, Tazuma, & Masuda, 1982). Nevertheless, their response to the Cornell Medical Index showed extremely high mean psychological as well as somatic scores, indicating that when they were asked specifically, they did not have difficulty reporting psychological symptoms (Masuda, Lin & Tazuma, 1980). Other studies using a variety of self-report instruments have also supported the notion that Asians have no difficulties in identifying and reporting psychological symptoms (Chun, Enomoto & Sue, 1996; Cheung & Lau, 1980).

Culture-bound or Culture Specific Syndromes

Culture has a crucial role in the psychopathology of various psychiatric disorders. Nonetheless, some psychiatric syndromes pertain to particular cultures. Such disorders are known as culture specific or culture bound syndrome (Bhatia & Malik, 1991; Neki, 1973). *Culture-specific syndrome* or *Culture-bound syndrome* is a combination of psychiatric and somatic symptoms that are considered to be a recognizable disease only within a specific society or culture (Chhabra, Bhatia & Gupta, 2008). The "culture-bound syndromes" are a heterogenous collection of folk terms, some of which describe true syndromes, whereas others represent culturally determined notions of disease causation or idioms of distress (Levine & Gaw, 1995). Culture-bound syndromes are disorders that are thought to occur in certain cultural contexts or among particular ethnic groups. The term "culture-bound syndrome" originated from an attempt to recognize ways of describing maladies that fell outside the framework of contemporary biomedicine (Griffith, 2014). The term culture-bound syndrome was included in the fourth version of the *Diagnostic and Statistical Manual of Mental Disorders* (American Psychiatric Association, 1994) which also includes a list of the most common culture-bound conditions. Although there is not any definite diagnostic criteria which have been formulated till date, but many of the culture bound syndromes contain the features, such as, these are the diseases categorized in that culture, extensive familiarity in that culture and unknown in other cultures, such culture bound syndromes have no objectively demonstrable biochemical or organ abnormality and mostly treated by folk medicine/ traditional healers (Chhabra, Bhatia & Gupta, 2008).

In India, common culture-bound syndromes are Dhat Syndrome, Possession Syndrome, Koro, Gilhari Syndrome, Bhanmati, Compulsive spitting, culture-bound suicide (*sati, santhra*), ascetic syndrome, *Jhinjhinia* etc.

In other cultures like Korean and Korean American patients suffering from mixtures of a wide variety of somatic and emotional symptoms often label themselves as suffering from "hwa-byung," which literally means both "fire disease" and "anger disease" (Lin, 1983). *Ataque de nervios* is a popular illness category among Puerto Ricans and other Latinos (Guarnaccia, 1993). Anorexia nervosa and Bulimia nervosa, two eating disorders are more prevalent in industrialized and often Western cultures and are far more common among females than males, mirroring cross-cultural differences in the importance of thinness for women (Miller & Pumariega, 2001; Pate, Pumariega, Hester & Garner, 1992). Furthermore, eating disorders seem to have become more common among younger females during the latter half of the twentieth century, during a period when icons of American beauty (Miss America contestants and *Playboy* centrefolds) have become thinner and women's magazines have published significantly more articles on methods for weight loss (Owen & Laurel-Seller, 2000; Rubinstein & Caballero, 2000). *Taijin kyofusho* is described as a "culturally distinctive phobia in Japan" in DSM-IV. However, in the indigenous Japanese diagnostic system, depending on the content of the patients' fear that they will displease or embarrass others, *taijin kyofusho* is classified into four subtypes: *sekimen-kyofu* (the phobia of blushing), *shubo-kyofu* (the phobia of a deformed body), *jikoshisen-kyofu* (the phobia of eye-to-eye contact), and *jikoshu-kyofu* (the phobia of one's own foul body odour) (Takahaski, 1989). Koro (which is called *suk-yeong* among the Southern Chinese) is a syndrome usually found among young men of poor education and immature, dependent personality who lack confidence in their own virility and are in conflict over the expression of genital impulses, although some may show hypersexual tendencies. The presenting complaint of penile shrinkage is shown to be in fact a depersonalization of that organ, occurring in the context of acute anxiety with fears of dissolution (Yap, 1965). *Hikikomori*, a form of acute social withdrawal, is becoming a silent epidemic in Japan. As it has not been reported from other parts of the world, *hikikomori* fulfils the criteria for "a culture-bound syndrome" (Sakamoto, Martin, Kumano, Kuboki & Al-Adawi, 2005).

Dhat Syndrome in India and neighbouring countries is a clinical entity recognized both by general public as well as medical practitioners. *Dhat* derives from the Sanskrit word *dhatu* meaning 'metal', and also 'elixir' or 'constituent part of the body'. In the Western psychiatric texts Wig (1960) firstly described about *dhat* which comprises vague somatic symptoms of fatigue, weakness, anxiety, loss of appetite, guilt and sexual dysfunction attributed by the patient to loss of semen in nocturnal emissions, through urine and masturbation. Dated between the 5th millennium B.C. and the 7th century A.D. in the Ayurvedic literature the process of semen production is described as the food converts to blood, which converts to flesh, which converts to marrow, and the marrow is eventually converted into semen. It is said that it takes 40 days for 40 drops of food to be converted to one drop of blood, 40 drops of blood to one drop of flesh, and so on (Bhugra & Buchanan, 1989). *Susruta Samhita* (ancient Indian text of surgery) has described 7 *Dhatus* in the body. *Dhatus* are elixir of the body. Disturbances of it can cause physical and mental weakness. Of all seven, Semen is considered to be the most precious. *Charak Samhita* (ancient text of Indian Medicine) describes a disorder resembling *Dhat* Syndrome by the name '*Shukrameha*'. *Shukra* is the word used for sperms in Sanskrit. Another term denoting semen is '*Veerya*' which in Sanskrit means bravery, valour and strength. On the other hand its preservation will lead to health and longevity. Thus, the belief in precious and life-preserving properties of semen is deeply ingrained in Indian culture. The belief is further reinforced by traditional healers and perpetuated by friends and elders who had suffered from this syndrome. Malhotra & Wig (1975) called *dhat* a 'sex neurosis of the Orient'. This syndrome is also seen in surrounding countries like Sri Lanka (*Sukra Prameha*) (De Silva & Dissanayake, 1989), Pakistan (Khan, 2004), Bangladesh (Verma, Khaitan & Singh, 1998) and even in China (Sen-k'uri) (Wen & Wang (1980). Concomitant psychiatric morbidity like depression, somatoform disorder, anxiety disorder may be present (Dhikav *et al.*, 2008). Treatment mainly consists of dispelling of myths by psychoeducation, reassuring the patient, treating any underlying psychiatric disorder, even symptomatic relief (of severe anxiety that these patients suffer) with the help of medications in initial stages of treatment is required to gain confidence of the patient (Chhabra, Bhatia & Gupta, 2008).

Possession Syndrome diagnosable under Dissociative disorders was introduced into modern scientific literature by P.M. Yap in 1960, and was called as "possession syndrome" though the phenomenon of an individual getting possessed by god or spirit is an age old one. Possession can occur sporadically involving one individual or can occur simultaneously as an epidemic involving many people (Teja *et al.,* 1970; Varma, Srivastava & Sahay, 1970). It can be voluntary and involuntary (Carstairs & Kapur, 1976). It occurs as an organised religious phenomena in many cultures, e.g. Voodoo services in Haiti (Wittkover 1970); The prophet healing in Liberia and the candomble cult rituals in Brazil (Wittkover, 1970); The Zar ceremony in Egypt (Nelson, 1971). Witztum, Grisaru & Budowski (1996) described a cultural pattern related to altered states of consciousness, observed amongst new immigrants from Ethiopia in Israel. The belief in possession by Zar spirits is one of the most common possession phenomena in Africa and in other continents. Possession by Zar is expressed by a wide range of behaviours, such as involuntary movements (often resembling epileptiform convulsions), mutism and incomprehensible language. Possession can occur as a symptom of mental illness. This syndrome is very common in all parts of India and it has specific names in all Indian languages such as *Bharna* (Hindi), *Bhar Koreche* (Bengali), *Devadu* or *Bhutum pattukonnadi* (Telugu), *Swami* or *Peyi pudichiriki* (Tamil), *Devaru*, *Pisacha gigidide* or *maimelu bandhie* (Kannada), *Vanden per padachu* (Malayalam), *Bharwana* or *thapatna* (Marathi), *Mata arya chhe* (Gujarati), *Khedna* (Punjabi) and *Hingarnai* (Dongri) (Rao, 1978). Patient is possessed usually by 'spirit/soul' of deceased relative or a local deity. Speaks in changed tone, even gender changes occur at times if the possessing soul is of opposite sex and usually seen in rural areas or in migrants from rural areas. Majority of these patients are females who otherwise don't have any outlet to express their emotions. Treatment includes careful exploration of underlying stress which precipitated the possession attack. Also to decrease any secondary gains patient may be getting from this behaviour, antidepressant and anxiolytics are helpful in certain cases. Syndrome is seen in all parts of India and many religious shrines hold special annual festivals where hundreds of people get possessed simultaneously. These people are looked upon as special by their families and villages which reinforce the secondary gains. Chandrasheker (1989) has suggested that possession is best understood by reference to three theoretical frameworks. According to *dissociation theory* it is a hysterical state in which the Id wishes to overwhelm the Ego in a state of dissociation. *Communication theory* holds that possession is exhibited by oppressed individuals who assume a sick role in an attempt to gain attention. *Socio-cultural theory* maintains that possession is a culturally sanctioned phenomenon to which people are exposed from an early age in the expectation that they may experience it later.

Included in ICD-10 under Dissociative disorders *Sati* means self-immolation by a widow on her husband's pyre. According to Hindu mythology, *Sati*, daughter of *Daksha*, was so overcome at the by insult of her husband (Lord Shiva) by her father that she immolated herself by jumping into the *havan Kund*. Since then her name 'Sati' has come to be symptomatic of self-immolation by a widow. It was seen mostly in Upper Castes notably Brahmins and Kshatriyas. It is banned in India since 19th century.

Santhara/Sallekhana is mostly seen in Jain Community who celebrates these events as religious festivals *by* voluntarily giving up life by fasting unto death over a period of time for religious reasons to attain God/*Moksha*. Person initially takes liquids, later even refusing to take them.

Koro is a culture bound syndrome characterized by acute anxiety and fear that the genital organ would retract into the body and may even cause death. Promodu, Nair and Pushparajan (2012) conducted a study to report the mass Koro epidemic which broke out at the labour camps in Kochi, Kerala, South India during the months of August and September 2010, and described its symptomatology and identified the etiological factors of Koro syndrome. Victims belong to the floating migrant labour population from north India. Within a period of two weeks Koro epidemic spread to nearly 100 individuals in three labour camps. Illiteracy, poor living conditions, economic problems, occupational stress and separation from family were found to be the major causes. Individuals with histrionic and anxious personality traits or disorders were more likely to be affected by such conditions. Previous knowledge of the koro syndrome combined with unhealthy premorbid personality traits and life stress led to the outbreak of the epidemic. Etiology was found to be exclusively psychogenic factors (Chowdhury, Chatterjee & Pal, 1988). A massive Koro epidemic has hit India again in 2010. It affected four States, viz. Assam, Maharashtra (Mumbai), West Bengal and Tripura. This is the fifth Koro epidemic in India. One of the authors (A.N. Chowdhury) made a field trip to North East India and found that in this Koro epidemic from Assam had quite a few good number of Muslim Koro patients seen (Ghosh, Nath, Brahma, & Chowdhury, 2010).

Ascetic Syndrome was first described by Neki in 1972. This syndrome appears in adolescents and young adults and it is characterised by social withdrawal, severe sexual abstinence, practice of religious austerities, lack of concern with physical appearance and considerable loss of weight.

Out of various forms of culture-bound syndromes reported, *Dhat* syndrome was most common (76.7%), followed by possession syndrome (13.3%), Koro (5%) (Bhatia, 1999).

Conclusion

From problem identification to choice of treatment providers, the bearings of culture and context are intense across the whole help-seeking pathway. The inter-relationship of culture, mental health and medical illness should be extensively researched and understood because of deeply rooted cultural meanings of various disorders, the emotional burden caused by it and underuse of effective therapy. An examination of cross-cultural studies in mental health reveals that cultural insensitivity stems from procedural norms in the development of content validity based on experts' rational analysis of concepts, in linguistic translations that try to conform to the exact terms of standardized instruments, and in the uncritical transferring of concepts across cultures. There is a need for wide-ranging examination of existing procedural norms, with the objective of keeping such norms from suppressing, biasing, or deflecting cultural understandings (Rogler, 1999). The recent revision of the nosology of the American Psychiatric Association, DSM-5, includes a Cultural Formulation Interview that aims to help clinicians contextualize diagnostic assessment.

References

Barua, A., Jacob, G.P., Mahmood, S.S., Udupa, S., Naidu, M., Roopa, P.S., *et al.* (2007). A study on screening for psychiatric disorders in adult population. *Indian Journal of Community Medicine*, 32, 65-66.

Berry, J.W., Poortinga, Y.H., Segall, M.H., and Dasen, P.R. (1992). *Cross-cultural psychology: Research and applications*. New York: Cambridge University Press.

Bhatia, M.S. (1999). An analysis of 60 cases of culture bound syndromes. *Indian Journal of Medical Science,* 53, 149-52.

Bhatia, M.S. and Malik, S.C. (1991). Dhat syndrome—a useful diagnostic entity in Indian culture. *British Journal of Psychiatry*, 159, 691-95.

Bhugra, D. and Buchanan, A. (1989) Impotence in ancient Indian texts. *Sexual and Marital Therapy,* 4, 87-92.

Carstairs, G.M. and Kapur, R.L. (1976). *The Great Universe of Kota*. The Hogarth Press, London.

Chandrashekar, C.R. (1989). Possession syndrome in India. In Ward CA (eds.) *Altered States of Consciousness and Mental Health: a Cross-cultural Perspective*. London: Sage.

Cheon, B.K., and Chiao, J.Y. (2012). Cultural variation in implicit mental illness stigma. *Journal of Cross-Cultural Psychology*, 43(7), 1058-1062.

Cheung, F.M. (1985). An overview of psychopathology in Hong Kong with special reference to somatic presentation. In Tseng, W.S. and Wu, D. (eds.) *Chinese Culture and Mental Health*. Orlando, Fla, Academic.

Cheung, F.M., and Lau, B.W. (1982). Situational variations of help-seeking behaviour among Chinese patients. *Comprehensive Psychiatry,* 23, 252-262.

Chhabra, V., Bhatia, M.S., and Gupta, R. (2008) Cultural Bound Syndromes in India. *Delhi Psychiatry Journal,* Vol. 11 (1), 15-18.

Chowdhury, A.N., Chatterjee, A. and Pal, P. (1988). Analysis of North Bengal Koro epidemic with three years follow up. *Indian Journal of Psychiatry,* 30, 69-72.

Chun, C.A., Enomoto, K., and Sue, S. (1996). Health care issues among Asian Americans: implications of somatisation. In P.M. Kato and T. Mann (eds.) *Handbook of Diversity in Health Psychology,* New York, Plenum.

De Silva, P. and Dissanayake, S.A.W. (1989). The loss of semen syndrome in Sri Lanka. A clinical study. *Sexual and Marital Therapy*, 4,195-204.

Deswal, B.S. and Pawar, A. (2012). An Epidemiological Study of Mental Disorders at Pune, Maharashtra. *Indian Journal of Community Medicine*, 37(2), 116-121.

Dhar, G. (2013). How depressive are our elderly population? A prevalence study in a slum of West Bengal. *International Journal of Pharma and Bio Sciences*, 4, 2.

Dhikav, V., Aggarwal, N., Gupta, S., Jadhavi, R., and Singh, K. (2008). Depression in Dhat syndrome. *The Journal of Sexual Medicine*, 5(4), 841-844.

Dinnel, D.L., Kleinknecht, R.A., and Tanaka-Matsumi, J. (2002). A Cross-Cultural Comparison of Social Phobia Symptoms. *Journal of Psychopathology and Behavioural Assessment,* Vol. 24 (2), 75-84.

Eaton, W.W., and Harrison, G. (2000). Epidemiology, social deprivation, and community psychiatry. *Current Opinion in Psychiatry*, 13(2), 185-187.

Elnaggar, M.N., Moitra, P. and Rao, M.N. (1971). Mental health in an Indian rural community. *British Journal of Psychiatry,* 118, 499-503.

Ganguli, H.C. (2000). Epidemiological Findings on Prevalence of Mental Disorders in India. *Indian Journal of Psychiatry*, 42 (1), 14-20.

Ghosh, S., Nath, S., Brahma, A., and Chowdhury, A.N. (2010). *Fifth Koro epidemic in India: A review report.*

Government of India (1946). *Report of Health Survey and Development Committee* (Bhore Committee). Vol.Ill, Appendix. Government of India, New Delhi, 75.

Griffith, L. (2014). Culture-Bound Syndrome. *The Wiley Blackwell Encyclopedia of Health, Illness, Behaviour, and Society.*

Guarnaccia, P.J. (1993). Ataques de nervios in Puerto Rico: Culture-bound syndrome or popular illness? *Medical Anthropology*, 15(2), 157-170.

Hackett, R., Hackett, L., Bhakta, P., and Gowers, S. (1999). The prevalence and association of psychiatric disorder in children in Kerala, South India. *Journal of Child Psychology and Psychiatry,* 40(5): 801-807.

Herkovits, M.J. (1948). *Man and his works*. New York, A.A. Knopf.

Jané-Llopis, E., Anderson, P., Stewart-Brown, S., Weare, K., Wahlbeck, K., McDaid, D. and Litchfield, P. (2011). Reducing the silent burden of impaired mental health. *Journal of Health Communication*, 16 (sup2), 59-74.

Kar, N., Dutta, S., and Patnaik, S. (2002). Mental health in an Indian industrial population: Screening for psychiatric symptoms. *Indian Journal of Occupational Environment Medicine*, 6, 86-88.

Kar, N., Dutta, S., and Patnaik, S. (2002). Mental health in an Indian industrial population: Screening for psychiatric symptoms. *Indian Journal of Occupational Environment Medicine*, 6, 86-88.

Khan, N. (2004). Dhat syndrome in relation to demographic characteristics. *Indian Journal of Psychiatry*, 47(1), 54-57.

Kleinman, A. (1978). What kind of model for the anthropology of medical systems? *American Anthropologist*, 80(3), 661-665.

Kleinman, A. (1987). Anthropology and Psychiatry. The role of culture in cross-cultural research on illness. *The British Journal of Psychiatry,* 151(4), 447-454.

Kleinman, A. (1988). *Rethinking Psychiatry*. New York, Free Press.

Kleinman, A., Kleinman, J. (1993). Suffering and its professional transformation: Toward an ethnography of interpersonal experience. *Culture, Medicine and Psychiatry*, 15, 275-301.

Kopp, M.S., Skrabski, Á., and Szedmák, S. (2000). Psychosocial risk factors, inequality and self-rated morbidity in a changing society. *Social Science and Medicine*, 51(9), 1351-1361.

Korkeila, J. (2000). *Measuring aspects of mental health*. Stakes.

Kumar, P.K., Jayaprakash, K., Monteiro, N.P., and Bhagavath, P. (2011). Psychiatric Morbidity in Industrial Workers of South India. *Journal of Clinical Diagnosis and Research*, 5(5), 921-25.

Lehtinen, V., Riikonen, E., Lahtinen, E. (1997). *Promotion of mental health on the European agenda*. Helsinki: STAKES, National Research and Development Centre for Welfare and Health.

Leo, D.D. (2003). *The Interface of Schizophrenia, Culture and Suicide, Suicide Prevention—Meeting the Challenge Together*. Hyderabad, India. Orient Longman.

Levine, R.E., and Gaw, A.C. (1995). Culture-bound syndromes. *Psychiatric Clinics of North America*.

Lewis-Fernandez, R., Kleinman, A. (1995). Cultural psychiatry. Theoretical, clinical, and research issues. *Psychiatric Clinics of North America*,18, 433-448.

Lin, K.M. (1983). Hwa-byung: a Korean culture-bound syndrome? *American Journal of Psychiatry,* 140, 105-107.

Lin, K.M., Tazuma, L., and Masuda, M. (1979). Adaptational problems of Vietnamese refugees: Part I. health and mental health status. *Archives of General Psychiatry*, 36, 955-961,

Lin, K.M., Masuda, M., and Tazuma, L. (1982). Adaptational problems of Vietnamese refugees: part III. case studies in clinic and field: adaptive and maladaptive. *Psychiatric Journal of the University of Ottawa*, 7, 173-183.

Linton, R. (1936). *The Study of Man*. D. Appleton Century Company.

Littlewood, R. (1988). From vice to madness: the semantics of naturalistic and personalistic understandings in Trinidadian local medicine. *Social science and medicine*, 27(2), 129-148.

Madhav, M.S. (2001). Epidemiological study on prevalence of mental Disorders in India. *Indian Journal of Community Medicine*, 26 (4), 198-200.

Manoranjitham, S.D., Rajkumar, A.P., Thangadurai, P., Prasad, J., Jayakaran, R., and Jacob, K.S. (2010). Risk factors for suicide in rural south India. *British Journal of Psychiatry*, 196(1): 26-30.

Masuda, M., Lin, K.M., and Tazuma, L. (1980). Adaptational problems of Vietnamese refugees: Part II, life changes and perception of life events. *Archives of General Psychiatry,* 37, 447-450.

Math, S.B. and Srinivasaraju, R. (2010). Indian psychiatric epidemiological studies: Learning from the past. *Indian Journal of Psychiatry,* 52, 95-103.

Miller, M.N., and Pumariega, A.J. (2001). Culture and eating disorders: A historical and cross-cultural review. *Psychiatry*, 64, 93-110.

National Crime Record Bureau (2005). *Accidental Deaths and Suicides in India*. New Delhi: Ministry of Home Affairs.

Neki, J.S. (1973). Psychiatry in South East Asia. *British Journal of Psychiatry*, 123, 257-269.

Nelson, C. (1971). Self, spirit possession and world view: An illustration from Egypt. The *International Journal of Social Psychiatry*, 17, 194-209.

Owen, P.R., and Laurel-Seller, E. (2000). Weight and shape ideals: Thin is dangerously. *Journal of Applied Sociology,* 30, 979-990.

Pate, J.E., Pumariega, A.J., Hester, C., and Garner, D.M. (1992). Crosscultural patterns in eating disorders: A review. *Journal of the American Academy of Child and Adolescent Psychiatry,* 31, 802-809.

Patel, V., and Kleinman, A. (2003). Poverty and common mental disorders in developing countries. *Bulletin of the World Health Organization,* 81(8), 609-615.

Pillai, A., Andrews, T., and Patel, V. (2009). Violence, psychological distress and the risk of suicidal behaviour in young people in India. *International Journal of Epidemiology*, 38(2), 459-69.

Promodu, K., Nair, K.R. and Pushparajan, S. (2012). Koro syndrome: Mass epidemic in Kerala, India. *Indian Journal of Clinical Psychology,* 39(2), 152-156.

Putnam, R.D. (2001). *Bowling alone*. Simon and Schuster.

Rao, A.V. (1978). Some aspects of psychiatry in India. *Trans-cultural Psychiatry,* 15(1), 7-27.

Reddy, M.V., and Chandrasekar, C.R. (1998). Prevalence of mental and behavioural disorders in India: A meta-analysis. *Indian Journal of Psychiatry*, 40, 149-57.

Rogler, L.H. (1999). Methodological sources of cultural insensitivity in mental health research. *American Psychologist*, 54(6), 424.

Rubinstein, S., and Caballero, B. (2000). Is Miss America an undernourished role model? *Journal of the American Medical Association,* 283, 1569.

Rutter, M., and Nikapota, A. (2002). Culture, ethnicity, society and psychopathology. In Rutter, M., Taylor E., (editors). *Child and Adolescent Psychiatry*. 4. Vol. 16. (pp. 277-286). Oxford: Blackwell Publications.

Sakamoto, N., Martin, R.G., Kumano, H., Kuboki, T., and Al-Adawi, S. (2005). Hikikomori, is it a culture-reactive or culture-bound syndrome? Nidotherapy and a clinical vignette from Oman. *The International Journal of Psychiatry in Medicine*, 35(2), 191-98.

Sartorius, N. (1990). Preface. In: Goldberg, D., Tantam, D., eds. *The public health impact of mental disorders*. Toronto: Hogrefe and Huber.

Seby, K., Chaudhury, S., and Chakraborty, R. (2011). Prevalence of psychiatric and physical morbidity in an urban geriatric population. *Indian Journal of Psychiatry*, 53(2), 121-27.

Shaji, S., Bose, S., and Verghese, A. (2005). Prevalence of dementia in an urban population in Kerala, India. *British Journal of Psychiatry*, 186, 136-40.

Srinath, S., Girimaji, S.C., Gururaj, G., Seshadri, S., Subbakrishna, D.K., Bhola, P. *et al.* (2005). Epidemiological study of child and adolescent psychiatric disorders in urban and rural areas of Bangalore, India. *Indian Journal of Medical Research*, 122(1), 67-79.

Takahaski, T. (1989). Social phobia syndrome in Japan. *Comprehensive Psychiatry*, 30, 45-52.

Tanaka-Matsumi, J. and Chang, R. (2002). What Questions Arise when Studying Cultural Universals in Depression? Lessons from Abnormal Psychology Textbooks. *Online Readings in Psychology and Culture,* 10(2). http://dx.doi.org/10.9707/2307-0919.1079.

Tanaka-Matsumi, J. and Draguns, J.G. (1997). Culture and psychopathology. In J.W. Berry, M.H. Segall, and C. Kagitcibasi (Eds.), *Handbook of cross-cultural psychology,* Vol. 3: *Social behaviour and applications* (2nd ed.) (pp. 449-492). Boston, MA: Allyn and Bacon.

Teja, J.S., Khanna, B.S. and Subramanyam, T.B. (1970). Possession states in Indian Patients. *Indian Journal of Psychiatry*, 12, 71.

Tylor, E. (1871). *Primitive Culture.* Volume 1. London: Bradbury, Evans and Co.

Varma, L.P., Srivastava, D.K., Sahay, R.N. (1970). Possession syndrome. *Indian Journal of Psychiatry*, 12, 59.

Verma, K.K., Khaitan, B.K., and Singh, O.P. (1998). The frequency of sexual dysfunctions in patients attending a sex therapy clinic in north India. *Archives of Sexual Behaviour*, 27(3), 309-314.

Weisner, T.S. (2002). Ecocultural understanding of children's developmental pathways. *Human Development*, 45, 275-281.

Weisz, J.R., McCarty, C.A., and Valeri, S.M. (2006). Effects of psychotherapy for depression in children and adolescents: A meta-analysis. *Psychological Bulletin*, 132, 132-149.

Wen, T.K. and Wang, C.L. (1980). Shen-k'uei syndrome: a culture-specific sexual neurosis in Taiwan. In A. Kleinman and T.Y. Lin (eds.) *Normal and Abnormal Behaviour in Chinese Culture* (pp. 357-369). Dordrecht: Reidel.

Wig, N.N. (1960) Problems of the mental health in India. *Journal of Clinical and Social Psychiatry (India)*, 17, 48-53.

Wissler, C. (1923). *Man and Culture*, Crowell, New York.

Witkover, E.D. and Hsjen, R. (1965). Transcultural psychiatry. *Arch. Gen. Psychiat.*, 13, 387.

Witztum, E., Grisaru, N., and Budowski, D. (1996). The 'Zar'possession syndrome among Ethiopian immigrants to Israel: Cultural and clinical aspects. *British Journal of Medical Psychology*, 69(3), 207-225.

World Health Organization (1992). *International statistical classification of diseases and related health problems.* 10. New York: World Health Organization.

World Health Organization (WHO) (2001).*World Health Report*. Geneva, Switzerland.

WHO (2004). *The World Health Report 2004: Changing History*. Geneva: World Health Organization, 2004.

Wilkinson, R. and Marmot, M. (1998). *The solid facts: social determinants of health.* Copenhagen: World Health Organization Regional Office for Europe.

Yap, P.M. (1965). Koro—a culture-bound depersonalization syndrome. *The British Journal of Psychiatry*, 111(470), 43-50.

5

Positive Psychology and Economic Development

Reckoning Linkages, Needs and Agendas

Rajneesh Choubisa and *Tanu Shukla*

The twin fields of *Psychiatry* and *Psychology* have always dominated the field of mental health and has allured individuals and experts, irrespective of their specializations. Both these disciplines have contributed towards the flourishment of the humankind in the best possible manner and are still continuing the trend. With more advancements in the sub-fields of psychology, the recently invigorated positive psychology movement has refurbished the mental health paradigm, through which, the focus has shifted from an overtly negative (ill-being) to a more positive (well-being) one. Before the rise of the positive psychological domain, the mental health paradox with its unique laws and statutes (including its treatment outcomes) were to some extent correlated with the indicators of economic development. Nonetheless, after the advent of positive psychology, the revitalized paradigm is having a deep impact on the policy decisions for determining the happiness of nations. For instance, the concept of gross national happiness by Bhutanese nation and its inclusion in the UN resolution for measuring human and economic development is a direct implication of the concept of well-being. There are ample research experiences which have highlighted significant correlations between the notions of well-being and economic development. This chapter reviews the scientific documents on such correlations by drawing focus on the established relationships across the world in general and the Indian subcontinent in particular. Upon careful analysis, this exclusive attempt calls attention to furthering research in this area in order to critically reflect the gaps between the entwined intricacies of mental health paradox and holistic development making it a plausible research agenda.

Positive Psychology: An Introduction

Positive Psychology Movement: Historical Predecessors

The recent decade has witnessed a plethora of researches on positive psychology, which most intellectuals, practitioners and critics of contemporary times believe to be a new and forward thinking discipline. Owing to this glorified attention, the psychological constructs like good life, happiness, flourishing or fulfilled life, which apparently informs positive psychology are much in vogue. Empirically speaking, these constructs ought to have their own phenomenological roots (that can be traced back in time) for having an in-depth understanding of their underlying theoretical background. As a matter of fact, the term "*Positive Psychology*" as such first appeared in the last chapter of Maslow's book *Motivation and Personality* (1987), the title of which was, *Towards a Positive Psychology*. In that book, Maslow maintained that psychology itself does not have an accurate understanding of human potential, and that the field tends not to raise the recognizable bar high enough with respect to the maximum attainment of mental well-being. Maslow (1987) states:

> The science of psychology has been far more successful on the negative than on the positive side; it has revealed to us much about the man's shortcomings, his illnesses, his sins, but little about his potentialities, his virtues, his achievable aspirations, or his full psychological height. It is as if psychology had voluntarily restricted itself to only half its rightful jurisdiction, and that the darker, meaner half (Maslow, 1987, p. 354).

In fact Maslow's (1943) conception of self-actualization as noted down in his famous *hierarchy of needs* has also been considered very relevant to the positive psychology movement (Snyder, Rand & Sigmon, 2005). Prior to Maslow, William James (1907) contrasted the views of morbid-minded individuals with what he called healthy-minded whereby the latter's ways to a joyful and meaningful life lies in minimizing awareness of evil. James even argued that the differences between morbid-minded and healthy-minded views of life are "functions of an underlying difference of temperament and that these persons of different temperament may belong to different types of religion" (Pawelski, 2003). For many, *mind-cure*[1] that emphasized the transformational power of thought is one example of a religion that appeals to the notion of healthy-mindedness (Anker, 1999; Hale, 1971; Satter, 1999). Rathunde (2001) has eloquently argued and deliberated in his article about the "experiential turns" which had prompted the humanistic psychologists of the likes of James (1902, 1907), Maslow (1968) and Dewey (1933) to turn towards explorations of what makes life more fulfilling and flourishing. In effect, these influential thinkers have opened the windows for optimal functioning by having built precursors and antecedents of positive psychological thought. These influential philosophers or more aptly philosophical psychologists made an immense contribution to the evolution of the positive psychology movement and their thought have provided a foundational support to the field.

Talking more about the antecedents, Rogers (1961) today is remembered pre eminently for his practical guidelines on person-centred therapy (a.k.a. *Client Centered Therapy*) which has positively influenced generations of therapists (*see* Slezackova, 2013 for some latest reflections). On the other hand, his ideas possess some similarity to the foundations of positive psychology and lent parallel support to some evolutionary principles of the movement. Rogers believed that healthy development and self-actualization can be attained if one is having a continuous awareness of one's authentic desires. According to him, self-actualization is the single motivating force which drives an individual. Rogers (1961) had his own notion about the good life about which he states:

> I believe it will have become evident why, for me, adjectives such as happy, contented, blissful, enjoyable, do not seem quite appropriate to any general description of this processes. I have called the good life, even though the person in this process would experience each one of these feelings at appropriate times. But the adjectives which seem more generally fitting are adjectives such as enriching, exciting, rewarding, challenging, and meaningful. This process of the good life is not, I am convinced, a life for the faint-hearted. It involves the courage to be. It means launching oneself fully into the stream of life. Yet the deeply exciting thing about human beings is that when the individual is inwardly free, he chooses as the good life the process of becoming (Rogers, 1961, 198-199).

The field of positive psychology as it is known today had drawn Rogers's conception of the good life as an ultimate aim for individuals.

Apart from Rogers (1951), the early pioneering works by Jahoda (1958), Erikson (1963, 1982), Vaillant (1977), Deci & Ryan (1985), and Ryff & Singer (1996) to name a few on issues such as optimal experiences, mature defences, psychosocial development, adaptive self-functioning and self-determination among others have significantly accumulated the wealth of knowledge towards forming the rudiments of positive psychology. Taken together, these constructs have eventually contributed towards the evolution of positive psychology and have expedited the growth and development of the field. Moreover, despite insignificant credit, this is how the humanistic psychological viewpoint possesses intimate affinity to the conception and genesis of positive psychological thought (Taylor, 2001; Bohart & Greening, 2001).

It has also been contended that positive psychology is nothing but revamped humanistic psychology, however, the major difference between the frames of reference of both the humanistic and positive psychological thought lies in their methodological orientation. This is because the former adopted and focused more on qualitative methodology while the latter employs rigorous quantitative and reductionist methods. Many psychologists would mark the launch of positive psychology movement with the beginning of Martin Seligman's tenure as President of American Psychological Association (APA; 1998) and to the publication of an entire issue of *American Psychologist* (2000) devoted to positive psychology. By this convention, the discipline owes this nomenclature to Seligman, who has been considered as its father and pioneered the whole movement. He was fortunate that a good number of psychologists later complied and subsequently corroborated positive psychology's premise with sound experimental support. Seligman (2002) solely rejected the principal negative assumption of human nature and argued his position pretty well about the predominance of negativity. He states:

> Current dogma may say that negative motivation is fundamental to human nature and positive motivation merely derives from it, but I have nct seen a shred of evidence that compels us to believe this [the] dual-aspect view that positive and negative traits are equally authentic and fundamental is the basic motivational premise of Positive Psychology (Seligman, 2002, p. 211).

At first it seems like there are some tight spots as far as the historical evidence is concerned, but the main aim of positive psychological scholars is to define human strengths and highlight the many paths that would lead to flourishment or better lives (Aspinwall & Staudinger, 2002; Keyes & Haidt, 2003; Lopez & Snyder, 2003; Peterson & Seligman, 2004; Snyder & Lopez, 2002). In essence, positive psychology has been busy revolutionizing and reorienting psychology back to its most neglected missions of making people stronger and productive and building high human potential actual. The bottom-line rests with the fact that positive psychology was, and is concerned, not with how to transform people. For example, from –5 to –2 but with how to move them from +2 to +5 (*see* Figure 5.1). As expected, the practitioners and followers of positive psychology have put forwarded legitimate definitions in favour of positive psychology.

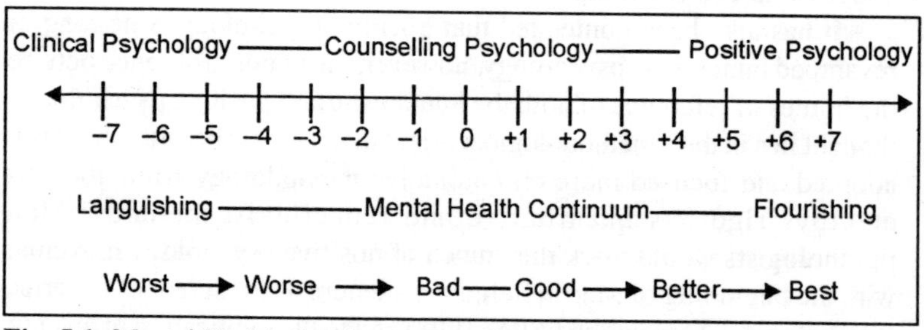

Fig. 5.1: Mental Health Continuum Paradigm*

* Mental Health Continuum is a self-constructed pictorial representation of existing definitions. Projected dimensions should not be scaled strictly as depicted. It has been added just to simply one's understanding about the discourse.

One of the most heavily cited definitions which found mention in the literature says:

> The field of positive psychology at the subjective level is about valued subjective experiences: well-being, contentment, and satisfaction (in the past); hope and optimism (for the future); and flow and happiness (in the present). At the individual level, it is about positive individual traits: the capacity for love and vocation, courage, interpersonal skill, aesthetic sensibility, perseverance, forgiveness, originality, future-mindedness, spirituality, high talent, and wisdom. At the group level, it is about the civic virtues and the institutions that move individuals towards better citizenship: responsibility, nurturance, altruism,

civility, moderation, tolerance, and work ethic (Seligman & Csikszentmihalyi, 2000).

Furthermore, it has to be necessarily summarized herein that positive psychology revitalized not only the *Aristotelian idea*[2] of a positive individual but also the view of a universal individual. Similarly, it must be noted that the positive human virtues, personal goals and personal expressions constitute the core idea of humanistic psychology which simultaneously informs positive psychology too. In spite of the fact that the positive psychology movement bears a striking resemblance in perpetual approach. It has been radically different in structure from the mind-cure of the 19th century and the mental hygiene movement of the 20th century. Thus, it may be construed that positive psychology's exclusive focus on wellness owes its history and evolutionary roots to some of the well-established schools of thought, systems and ideologies.

Having traced out the vital historical roots of positive psychology, it is time to shift our focus on its progress, development and current status with special reference to its most practical mission whereby its relationships with development can be ascertained and its scope can be further assessed.

Positive Psychology's Discourse: Current Status and Progress

Since its inception, positive psychologists have enhanced our understanding of how, why, and under what conditions positive emotions, positive character, and the institutions that enable them flourish (e.g. Cameron, Dutton, and Quinn, 2003; Easterbrook, 2003; Gardner, Csikszentmihalyi, Damon, 2001; Kahneman, Diener and Schwarz, 1999; Murray, 2003; Vaillant, 2000). Woolfolk and Wasserman (2005) have argued that, positive psychologists, all pronouncements to the contrary, value positive qualities and virtues, not for their intrinsic merit or their wholesome effects on society, but for the good feelings they induce in individuals. As envisioned by Seligman (1998b, 1998c), positive psychology had three primary goals. The first has been to delineate and measure positive traits, thereby putting the individuals in a position to begin 'building' human strengths, civic virtues, and the "good life". The second goal relates to the promotion of positive experiences and emotions. Last but not the least endeavour was to create more positive communities and institutions that would embody and promote these strengths and experiences.

These goals and related issues were taken and subsequently transformed subjectively into domains which uniquely formed the core topics that became central to the study of positive psychology. They have led to the development of certain traits (Allport, 1961)[3] that have been named *Character Strengths* in the domain of positive psychology. The development of the *Manual of the Sanities* as outlined in the *Character, strength and Virtues* (CSV) handbook marked a path breaking exploration which has challenged as well as complemented the *Diagnostic and Statistical Manual* (APA, 1994) of disorders published by the American Psychological Association (Peterson and Seligman, 2004). The *CSV* describes and classify strengths and virtues that enable human thriving. In spite of the fact, that, the character strengths and virtues have been the subject of scholarly inquiry for thousands of years, they lost flavour until recently because of their decreasing moral valence (Cawley, Martin, and Johnson, 2000; McCullough and Snyder, 2000; Sandage and Hill, 2001). A *character, strength* or *virtue* has been defined as "any psychological process that consistently enables a person to think and act so as to yield benefits to himself or herself and society" (McCullough and Snyder, 2000, 3). As a matter of fact, the character has become central to positive psychology's efforts to understand and promote human flourishing in contemporary times. With the rise of positive psychology movement, they are back into action and more so in the limelight. This action facilitates their utility and importance as essential agents for assessment, wellness promotion and enhancing well-being in diverse populations.

Nevertheless, the qualities or virtues which delineate the basic building blocks of positive psychology have been contributed and explored by Kahneman (1999) amongst many others. Other relevant constructs which found a certain mention in the PP literature, for instance range from "subjective well-being" Diener (2000); "optimal experience" Massimini & Delle-Fave (2000); "optimism" Peterson (2000); "self-determination" Ryan & Deci (2000); "happiness" Myers (2000); "wisdom" Baltes & Staudinger (2000); "mature defences" Vaillant (2000); to "social relationships" Myers (2000); Schwartz (2000) and the likes. Most of them have either been incorporated or are finding a place in the classificatory purview of positive psychology. It is also interesting to note that some virtues, which have common characteristics, have been addressed by dissimilar names and are present in varying degrees of magnitude in different cultures (Biswas-Diener, 2006). The most prominent measure described earlier called *Values in Action Inventory of Strength (VIA-IS)* which measures the signature strengths is developed, adapted and revalidated cross-culturally to assess the virtues possessed by individuals of any orientation that are dominant in one's life (e.g. Singh & Choubisa, 2009; 2010; Choubisa & Singh, 2011). Besides, other subjective and objective measurement tools from an applied perspective have also been developed to enrich the positive psychology's knowledge base.

Through these committed efforts and significant contributions from the positive psychology's proponents to make the lives of people more worthy, pleasant and meaningful, the field of positive psychology has matured with age and time. Most of the efforts are by means of enhancing the well-being (*see* Lyubomirsky, King, and Diener, 2005) of the individuals in diverse settings which bears direct implication for a country's gross happiness level. There are studies that exist which are related to classifying the strengths, effectively judging them, and efficiently inculcating the needed strengths of the individual using positive psychology based interventions (Seligman, Rashid and Parks, 2006). However, such studies are sparse because the field is still in an expansion phase and flourishing with contributors from all-around the globe. More recently, many country specific academic congregations or associations are now promoting the field in various regions of the world. It would be appropriate to say here that in order to make this field indispensable to the staunchest of the critics, educationists and practitioners, the horizontal and vertical expansion of the discipline has become an absolute necessity.

Positive Psychology: Western and Eastern Comparisons

The concurrent developments in the field of positive psychology along with the theoretical foundations have added richness to the epistemological outcomes and have provided empirical support to the area. These developments include a wide range of topics that are handled tactfully by these so called practitioners and patrons of positive psychology. The topics forming the core of research in positive psychology provide tacit evidence regarding the richness and variety of this domain. For instance, positive psychologists have been credited for their pioneering work in a wide variety of areas of interest to positive psychology, including positive prevention and therapy (Bretherton and Orner, 2004; Linley and Joseph, 2004a; Ruini and Fava, 2004; Seligman, 2005); the identification and classification of positive human qualities (Peterson and Seligman, 2004); the critique of the medical model of mental illness (Jorgensen and Nafstad, 2004; Joseph and Linley, 2004; Keyes and Lopez, 2005; Maddux, 2005;

Maddux, Snyder, and Lopez, 2004); happiness and life satisfaction (Diener, Lucas, and Oishi, 2005); joy (Robbins, 2006a); creativity (Nakamura and Csikszentmihalyi, 2003; Simonton, 2005); broaden and build theory of positive emotions (Frederickson, 2001); personal control (Thompson, 2005); hope (Snyder, Rand, and Sigmon, 2005); wisdom (Baltes, Gluck, and Kunzmann, 2005); reality negotiation (Higgins, 2005); authenticity (Harter, 2005; Swann and Pelham, 2005); humility (Tangney, 2005); positive relationships (Berscheid, 2003; Harvey, Pauwels, and Zichmund, 2005); forgiveness (McCullough and Witvliet, 2005); gratitude (Emmons and Shelton, 2005); empathy and altruism (Batson, Ahmad, Lishner, and Tsang, 2005); adaptive coping (Niederhoffer and Pennebaker, 2005; Nolen-Hoeksema and Davis, 2005); meaningfulness in life (Baumeister and Vohs, 2005); post-traumatic growth (Tedeschi and Calhoun, 2004); humour (Lefcourt, 2005); the benefits of meditation (Shapiro, Schwartz, and Santerre, 2005); healthy self-regulation (Brown and Ryan, 2004); and balanced time perspective (Boniwell and Zimbardo, 2004) to name a few.

Some of these contemporary research topics which caught public attention and brought positive psychology in the spotlight have been beautifully attended to in the millennial issue of *American Psychologist* in the year 2000. The content enrichment tradition of the same is now being carried forward with the launch of especially dedicated *Journal of Positive Psychology* inaugurated in the year 2006. With increasing focus on well-being and happiness most of the journals and books recently have rejuvenated and tremendously enriched the whole ideology and thought about positive psychology and its encompassing domains (e.g. Schui and Krampen, 2010; Brdar, 2011). Besides the journals and books, there are now available, a bunch of websites and blog posts on the subject matter of positive psychology and its applications, with a major limitation, that they do not focus on the issues from a generalized point of view. The other important limitation was the fact that a bulk of these researches is restricted only to the practices prevalent in Western societies and cultures.

On the other hand, patchy efforts have been made in some eastern cultures (specifically Indian subcontinent), though, not to the extent of theory formation or something equivalent, but towards the contextualization of some of these established constructs. There have been some original as well as replication researches in Indian settings which might be categorized as a contribution to the positive psychology's research database. Most relevant of them to name a few have been on the topics such as effects of shavasana on stress (Kumar, Kaur and Kaur,

1993); psychology of well-being (Dalal and Mishra, 2006); role of meditation in positive well-being (Nathawat, 1996); spirituality and health (Nathawat, 2000); attachment styles in coping (Narayanan and Rao, 2004; Kapanee and Rao, 2007); broaden and built theory in coping with stress (Khosla, 2006); perceived emotional intelligence and ways of coping (Shah & Thingujam, 2008); religious beliefs and psychological well-being (Joshi, Kumari and Jain, 2008); positive affect, negative affect and happiness (Singh and Jha, 2008); social intelligence and positive psychological health (Hooda, Sharma and Yadava, 2009) and *yoga* and student well-being (Jadhav and Havalappanavar, 2009) amongst similar others. The central theme in all these researches has been associated to induce positive feelings and alleviate depression in the selected participants. This advantage categorizes these researches as a potential medium in establishing the positive psychology movement as a practicing discipline in Indian context. A recent meta-analytical sort of review has criticized and highlighted available researches in India, which can be clubbed as positive psychological studies (Mehrotra, 2011).

Thus, this is how the journey of positive psychology, which began a decade ago is now making its presence felt in almost all the major world economies and has extended its wings by advancing some of the most vibrant and appealing researches in such a short period of time. The best thing is that it stili continues to do the same at a remarkable pace. Anyways, as stated previously, the most important application of positive psychology lies in its practical orientation whereby its impact on the economic development of a nation can be evaluated. This implication of PP research which facilitates and provides fruitful results in terms of enhancing a nation's happiness and making it flourish should now become the major focal point of positive psychology research in recent times. In effect, the wellness promotion agenda should realign and mould itself in such a manner that it must become synonymous with development and happiness of a nation. This significant relationship holds the key to its fate and possess the potential of becoming the practical legacy of positive psychology in the near future.

Economic Development and Mental Health

Economic Growth and Wellness

Economic growth is believed to be a significant aspect in the economic development of any country. There had been heated controversies claiming that economic growth would certainly accelerate well-being. Easterlin (who formulated the famous Easterlin paradox) studied the association between happiness and Gross Domestic Product (GDP), both across countries and within individual countries through time (1974, 1995, 2001, 2005). He concluded that there is no direct relationship between aggregate income and average happiness. It was also reported that there is a strong evidence that within countries, people are happier if they have more income. Though, these two findings contradict each other when it is said that income is a significant predictor of individual happiness, but in fact, there is no empirical linkage between the level of economic development of a society and the overall happiness of its members (*see* Biswas-Diener and Diener, 2001).

From an econometric perspective, monetary and non-monetary measures of well-being are being ideally utilized for having a deep and clear-cut understanding of well-being and related phenomena. The diverse facets of the economic development process not only helps address issues of inequality and lags in human development, but, also helps pinpoint where countries are falling behind, which once addressed, can further promote well-being. For having a detailed idea of these issues, measurement devices or instruments are normally utilized. Of the many measures available, for instance, Morris (1979) developed the Physical Quality of Life Index (PQLI) which consists of a composite index of three macroeconomic indicators of development, i.e. infant mortality, literacy and life expectancy. Even UNDP (United Nations Development Programme) in their reports has incorporated the measure of well-being in their measurement which evaluates nation's prosperity through the famous Human Development Index (HDI: UNDP, 1990). HDI indices have to take into account human capabilities (related to wellness and illness) as measured from such standardized measures in their calculation apart from the production and distribution norms of the commodities. Organization for Economic Co-operation and Development (OECD, 2006) claims that in maintaining well-being monetary issues are not mandatory but sufficient factors that play an imperative role. They constitute a significant aspect as wealthy economies sustain other conditions to promote well-being and continuing a flourishing life. Well-being will also be increased by institutions that enable citizens to feel that they control their own lives, and that investment of their time and resources will be rewarded. In turn, this will lead to higher incomes in a virtuous circle. Collectively, allied indices esse ·ially put emphasis on choices, on what individuals should have, be and do, to become capable of ascertaining their own existence.

Although from a factual viewpoint, UN General Assembly adopted a resolution entitled "Happiness: towards a holistic approach to development" which states that happiness should be a fundamental human goal and a universal aspiration. The framework highlights that Gross Domestic Product (GDP) by its nature does not reflect that goal and that unsustainable patterns of production and consumption impede sustainable development. It also states that for a more inclusive growth, equitable and balanced approach is needed to promote sustainability, eradicate poverty, and enhancement of well-being (United Nations, 2011). Human Development Report (1990) maintains that the basic objective of development is to create an enabling environment for people to live long, healthy, and creative lives. From this perspective, well-being is all about capability to function and that too function properly. To complicate the matters further, if income and resources are discarded from calculations showcasing the reflective effect on the capacity to function, the capability approach claims that they are not merely concerns to be appreciated since well-being cannot be ignored. Whatever the complicacies might seem, if we talk about the resolution, it was through this resolution that happiness was recognized as a critical variable in the economic development of any nation. As a matter of fact, the UN resolution has campaigned for reviving the old notion of subjective well-being and advocated replacing it with a more holistic measure of well-being so as to have a more precise measurement of human capabilities associated with economic development.

Furthering the credibility of the UN resolution, the Royal Government of Bhutan also undertook a landmark step towards adoption of a new global sustainability-based economic paradigm for human happiness and the well-being of all life forms. Because of their efforts, the path breaking Bhutanese conception of promoting and measuring "Gross National Happiness" (GNH) came into existence. This conception of GNH resulted in an impulsive wave of awareness about incorporating the newly invoked happiness paradigm and substituting the current dysfunctional system (where well-being was ignored) that was focusing more on the unsustainable premise of limitless growth since human capabilities were taken for granted. Some of the proponents of the GNH approach contended that while material wealth is clearly an essential precondition for poverty reduction and enhancing well-being, there is a mounting empirical evidence that economic growth alone is not a sufficient condition for building a total egalitarian society in which all citizens might have equal opportunities and capabilities to live fulfilling lives of dignity, ingenuity and happiness. In addition to these ideas, a strong support for the viewpoint that well-being is not an alternative to eradicating poverty was brought into light by the critics of this approach.

Most of the available studies on happiness and development show that the relationship between the level of absolute income and the level of happiness have a curvilinear relationship. There is a lack of proof which illustrates that the noticeable linear relationship between GDP per capita and well-being exists, because, the concept of well-being is defined subjectively rather than on an objective basis (cf. Forgeard, Jayawickreme, Kern and Seligman, 2011). Moreover, there exists a robust correlation between subjective well-being questions and more objective measures of personal well-being. It may be because the answers to subjective well-being questions have been shown to be correlated with physical evidence of affect such as smiling, laughing, heart rate measures, sociability, and electrical activity in the brain (Diener, 1984). Measures of individual happiness or life satisfaction are also correlated with other subjective assessments of well-being such as independent evaluations by friends, self-reported health, sleep quality, and personality (Diener, Lucas and Scollon, 2006; Kahneman and Krueger, 2006).

However, from a layman's point of view, the schema of a developed society is a place where people are well fed and possess access to a variety of commodities with luxurious ease and without any hardship. Therefore, in the light of the above discussion, it can be construed that to enhance income and well-being simultaneously with economic capabilities, human development should be made a prerequisite. The issue is very important for measuring development and is still tricky because a majority of existing measures are still based on indicators like, life expectancy, educational attainment and per capita income, whereas civil, political rights and well-being have yet to be enforced as tangible parameters. Over and above, these were the reasons that emerged from such meetings and it was concluded that the core goal of economic development should indeed be to maximize the happiness and well-being of current and future generations.

Well-being, Economic Development: Research Experiences and Agendas

There have been a number of cross-sectional, longitudinal researches and country level surveys which have tried to analyze the correlations between wellness indicators and economic development of nations. An ambitious project, namely World Values Survey (WVS) was conducted to rank order the most virtuous countries from amongst the chosen one's and was an attempt to highlight the value orientations of selected countries. But the sampling issues have crippled its methodology and its focus to include poorer countries resulted in unrepresentative samples and consequentially in its repeated rectifications. For instance, Argentina was included in the 1981-1984 wave, but the sample was restricted to urban areas and was not extended to turn out to be representative of the country overall till the 1999-2004 wave. Chile, China, India, Mexico, and Nigeria were included in the 1989-1993 wave. Their samples, mostly included the educated community and people staying in city areas. These limitations were even evident in the survey documentation and have been overlooked in its successive investigations. The inclusion of non-representative samples from poorer countries and involving sample from presumably richer countries (and hence likely happier individuals) resulted in selection of arguably happy respondents. This way the sampling distribution might have skewed the report in favour of richer and developed nations. Other most resolute cross-country surveys of subjective well-being come from the 2006 Gallup World Poll which was constructed to compute subjective well-being consistently across 132 countries. The survey probes into a variety of subjective well-being questions and have demonstrated a linear, logarithmic relationship between subjective well-being and GDP per capita. As is evident from such results of these surveys, because of imbuing methodology may be, the status of rich nations have got glorified unintentionally leaving the status of developing nations questionable and a matter of concern.

In addition to these cross-country surveys some within country surveys have also been reported in the literature that tries to correlate well-being with economic development. Veenhoven (1991) proposed that income has the largest effect on subjective well-being for those at the lowest economic levels. Kahneman, Krueger, Schkade, Schwarz and Stone (2006) suggests that within country comparisons overstate the true relationship between subjective well-being and income because of a "focusing illusion". The notion of focusing illusion states that people judge the standard of other's lives on few focal attributes such as personal deficits or material wealth. When people assess their life relative to others, then they only think in terms of tangible measures like income. These predispositions may have an impact on within-country comparisons. It seems likely that the bivariate well-being-GDP relationship may also reflect the control of aspects like democracy, the quality of national laws or government, health, or even favourable weather conditions. Besides, many of the identified factors raise both GDP per capita and well-being while other factors include increased savings, reduced leisure, or even increasingly materialist values that may raise GDP per capita probably at the expense of subjective well-being (Kenny, 1999).

Moreover, only per capita income does not capture all aspects of development in a holistic manner, there are other considerations that must be taken into deliberation for properly assessing the notion of development (Dasgupta, 2001). As a matter of fact, Easterlin (1974) in his analysis argued that time trends in subjective well-being undermine the view that an exclusive focus on economic growth is in the best interests of society. Though, one would consequently suppose an individual's happiness to be somewhat stable over time, research has highlighted that it is in fact not stable and accurate measurements of subjective well-being over time is difficult (Eid & Diener, 2004). Subjective well-being is a function of the individual's personality and his or her response to life actions. He also raised a question as to whether richer countries are happier countries and concluded on the basis of his findings that there exist a strong positive relationship between a country's income and the happiness of its people (Easterlin, 1995). However, Oswald (1997), while referring to income beyond the basic need fulfilment level has concluded that, "Economic progress buys only a small amount of extra happiness." Nonetheless, a typically positive happiness-income relationship turns up in international comparisons, yet, this relationship has been argued as prevailing only over low levels of GDP per capita. Once wealthy countries have satisfied basic needs, they have been described as on the " 'flat of the curve,' with additional income, buying little, if any, extra happiness" (Clark, Frijters and Shields, 2008). Deaton (2008) found that aggregate happiness rises with GDP in low-income countries, there is much less consensus on the magnitude of this relationship, or on whether a satiation point exists beyond which further increases in GDP per capita are associated with no change in aggregate happiness.

Towards a Feasible Solution: The Capability Approach

Economic transformation helps a country to adapt to eliminate unproductive regulations. The institutional instrument is a decisive constituent in transforming expansion and well-being to a more sustainable mode. The role of the government is to seek economic development so as to enlarge the 'capabilities' of individuals in the society. Noble laureate Amartya Sen asserts that the realization of human capabilities, which enlarge the range of human choices is essential for a broader notion and a holistic measure of economic well-being. Nussbaum (2000) stresses on capabilities approach which has a wider significance as a pattern of development. Nussbaum, Sen and others have presented a capability-based critique of using GDP and GNP as an indicator of well-being and quality of life (Nussbaum and Sen, 1993). Essentially, these economic measures were shaped as a basis to point to a country's economic prosperity since it is a growing economy that makes it possible to improve living standards.

With the mounting economic incorporation of countries around the world, there has been consistent stress on improving quality of life and well-being. Policies are pointing towards dipping the level of poverty and inequality of distribution against raising the quality of life in society. The new economic viewpoint has resulted in a gigantic change in the policy orientation and the main focus is on the mode of governance. Layard (2005) states that if economic growth possess a little role to improve social welfare, then it should not be a main intention of government policy. Hence, economic development is relatively a difficult aspect, but indeed the dynamics of well-being are reliant on the quality of governance and promising facets of decentralization (Layard, 1980). Good governance and state incentives (economic efficiency) are vital factors of progressing well-being of the countries. Literature suggests that for better development outcomes, the role of the democratic system and social equality is indispensable which is indeed the most intense consideration in the economic literature. The UNDP (1997) report claims that the outcome of good governance is progress that 'gives priority to poor, advances the cause of women, sustains the environment, and creates needed opportunities for employment and other livelihoods'. Hence, good governance, which is complex and inevitably demands well-being of an individual in particular and society at large should be made a focal point in the developing context to cope up with all these challenges.

In order to resolve the governance issues, there are some major proposals at the disposal of World Bank such as to construct the governance index, as described by Kaufman, Kraay, Zoido-Lobaton (1999). The World Bank's 'Quality of Growth' (2000) states that there are few aspects related to poverty outcomes as distribution, sustainability, variability, and governance surrounding the growth processes. The inference of well-being of the society shows the quality of life in a more comprehensive way and points towards the level of well-being which is essential to demonstrate the discrepancy level of economy in a highly secular country like India. Generally, GDP and GNP are being used as an approximation of well-being but this notion is also being criticized. Critics in these fields typically discuss gender inequalities, insufficient representation of the environmental costs of productions and general issues of misusing an output-based measure for unintended purposes. Capabilities approach is a strong critique of it as it emphasizes on the capacities and functioning of an individual. Development is connected to a range of indicators of life satisfaction and therefore, all of them are significant in measuring well-being. Development policies strive to create an environment for people to live long, healthy creative lives. Since, human capabilities deal with issues of egalitarianism, civic right, resourcefulness and self-right, therefore, there also exist other indices based which are based on the capabilities are also associated to well-being of an individual. This is how the capability approach apparently criticizes output-based approaches to development. Since, an agency is required to take such initiatives, the function of the state as an agency in expanding the economic well-being of the community has become promising in the contemporary age.

Emerging Research Agendas: Conclusions and Suggestions

The neoclassical economic theory assumes that individuals are rational, fully informed and seek to maximize utility. Obviously, then, the choices the individuals make, tend to maximize expected utility. The construct of happiness from an economic perspective, has long been the standard of measurement and used interchangeably with utility as well as the general welfare. Economists attempt to quantify happiness merely on the basis of measurements in consumption and profit and state that it is only the extent to which an individual's choice is satisfied. Technically, they commit an error when they conceptualize the holistic notion of well-being and happiness. In short, the economists being objective individuals consider that more educated means more healthy and high income means a high level of well-being, which is not the case. The first research agenda which comes out of these theoretical discrepancies is regarding the operationalization of the constructs that are common to all the social scientific disciplines (especially economics and psychology) but there are incidents of misunderstanding in conceptualization of those constructs (for ex., well-being). This is high time that both economists and psychologists should join hands and turn to more radical ways of thinking about and measuring utility by combining human economics and happiness psychology, so that, individual efforts can benefit from each other and that collectively, these efforts may more strongly influence international development agendas.

On a similar note, if the notion of human development index (being an authoritative measure that links happiness and development) is taken into consideration, it talks of two dimensions of human development. One focuses on the formation of human capabilities, improved health, knowledge and skills and the other stress the usage of those capabilities for productive work or leisure. It is because of the erroneous conceptualization that a reformulation of HDI is required from the standpoint of forming an alliance between happiness and development (cf. Noorbakhsh, 1998 for an earlier reformulation). As a matter of fact, the current conceptualization is concerned with the inclusion of only the first dimension while grossly undermining the second dimension. Even, the construction methodology of HDI should take both deprivation and development into consideration where the former might adopt a minimum value whereas the latter takes standard ideal values corrected to certain thresholds. Likewise, both subjective well-being and its counter measure ill-being should be used during national policies for the reason that together they provide a complete measure of the health indicator of an individual. It is because there is an insight that conventional development concepts such as GNP and Per Capita Income do not properly reflect the general well-being of the inhabitants of a nation. In order to develop real progress and sustainability and to effectively combat trends, one should aim for and develop more appropriate and inclusive indicators that truly measure the quality of life within societies and nations. This suggested reformulation puts the subjective well-being of individuals at par with the national development agenda, whereby the economics of well-being would be assessed in a more even manner. The second research agenda which comes out of the discussion on HDI is related to working on a more robust holistic indicator of development.

If the available research on positive psychology is reviewed, one thing which becomes clear is that, almost all the progress in the field of positive psychology is in a Western context. As highlighted in the preceding sections, the researches which are reviewed and the ones which are present even in an Eastern context (especially India) are pretty superfluous and talks more or less about estimation and enhancement of well-being. There is hardly any research even in Indian conditions (and to a larger extent in eastern context) that talks about or even touches on the aspects of utilization of positive psychology discourse and economic development of the society. The available results on an all exclusive economic perspective suggest that those interested in maximizing society's welfare should shift their attention from an emphasis on increasing consumption opportunities to an emphasis on increasing social contacts. When it comes to exploring the linkages between the well-being of the societies and the economic growth of those societies, the literature falls short of such research. The third and the most significant research agenda would be to carry out empirical research on the development implications of positive psychology in our societies, communities and regions. It will be through such research only that one can actually see the real utility and manifestation of positive psychology in uplifting the socio-economic status of individuals and can deliver its true goal.

In summary, we come to the conclusion that some vastly practice-oriented and applied research in the field of positive psychology along with its immediate applications in our society is the need of the hour. Only after emergence of such implications, we can be in a position to inflict the linkages which are being sought herein and ought to function properly. We also suggest that the capabilities and functionality of our citizens, society and communities bear an overt relationship with economic development since both these processes go hand in hand. As an outcome of this discussion, we finally recommend that it is high time that we should turn towards such explorations, while simultaneously keeping a check on the infinite possibilities the linkages of positive psychology and economic development has to offer. After all, its implications will bring fruitful results irrespective of the fact that the beneficiary is an individual, society, community or a nation.

Notes

1. The presidential address which James delivered to the American Philosophical Association in 1906 calls for founding of a new field of psychology that would study scientifically and apply more broadly the psychological principles underlying the success of mind-cure (*The Energies of Men*, 1907).
2. The aim of life according to Aristotle (as mentioned in Nichomachean Ethics; 1999), was eudaimonia, which is something like what Seligman (2002) meant by the term "authentic happiness".

3. Allport (1961) in a seminal definition described "character as personality evaluated and personality as character devaluated".

References

Allport, G.W. (1961). *Pattern and growth in personality.* New York: Holt, Rinehart & Wilson.

American Psychiatric Association. (1994). *Diagnostic and statistical manual of mental disorders* (4th Ed.). Washington, DC: Author.

Anker, R.M. (1999). *Self-help and popular religion in early American culture: An interpretive guide*. Westport, CT: Greenwood Press.

Aristotle. (1999). *Nichomachean Ethics* (M. Ostwald, Trans.) (Prentice Hall, Upper Saddle River, NJ).

Aspinwall, L.C., and Staudinger, U.M. (Eds.). (2003). *A psychology of human strengths.* Washington DC: American Psychological Association.

Baltes, P.B. and Staudinger, U.M. (2000). Wisdom: A metaheuristic facilitation of intrinsic motivation, social development, and well-being. *American Psychologist*, 55, 122-136.

Baltes, P.B., Gluck, J., and Kunzmann, U. (2005). Wisdom: Its structure and function in regulating successful life span development. In C.R. Snyder & S.J. Lopez (Eds.), Handbook of positive psychology (pp. 327-350). Oxford, England: Oxford University Press.

Batson, C.D., Ahmad, N., Lishner, D.A., and Tsang, J.A. (2005). Empathy and altruism. In C.R. Snyder and S.J. Lopez (Eds.), *Handbook of positive psychology* (pp. 485-498). Oxford, England: Oxford University Press.

Baumeister, R.F., and Vous, K.D. (2005). The pursuit of meaningfulness in life. In C.R. Snyder and S.J. Lopez (Eds.), *Handbook of positive psychology* (pp. 608-618). Oxford, England: Oxford University Press.

Berscheid, E. (2003). *The human's greatest strength: Other humans*. In L.G. Aspinwall and U.M. Staudinger (Eds.), A psychology of human strengths: Fundamental questions and future directions for a positive psychology (pp. 37-48). Washington, DC: APA Press.

Biswas-Diener, R. and Diener, E. (2001). Making the Best of a Bad Situation: Satisfaction in the Slums of Calcutta. *Social Indicators Research*, 55, 329-352.

Biswas-Diener, R. (2006). From the equator to the North Pole: A study of Character strengths, *Journal of Happiness Studies*, 7, 293-310.

Bohart, A.C. and Greening, T. (2001). Humanistic psychology and positive psychology. *American Psychologist*, 56, 81-82.

Boniwell, I. and Zimbardo, P. (2004). Balancing time perspective in pursuit of optimal functioning. In P.A. Linley and S. Joseph (Eds.), *Positive psychology in practice* (pp. 165-180). New Jersey: John Wiley and Sons.

Brdar, I. (Ed.) (2011). *The Human Pursuit of Well-Being: A Cross Cultural Approach.* Springer: Dordrecht. DOI: 10.1007/978-94-007-1375-8.

Bretherton, R. and Orner, R.J. (2004). Positive psychology and psychotherapy: An existential approach. In P.A. Linley and S. Joseph (Eds.), *Positive psychology in practice* (pp. 420-432). Hoboken, NJ: Wiley.

Brown, K.W., and Ryan, R.M. (2004). Fostering healthy self-regulation from within and without: A self-determination theory of perspective. In P.A. Linley and S. Joseph (Eds.), *Positive psychology in practice* (pp. 105-126). Hoboken, NJ: Wiley.

Cameron, K.S., Dutton, J.E., and Quinn, R.E. (Eds.). (2003). *Positive organizational scholarship: Foundations of a new discipline.* San Francisco: Berrett-Koehler.

Cawley, M.J., Martin, J.E., and Johnson, J.A. (2000). A virtues approach to personality. *Personality and Individual Differences*, 28, 997-1013.

Choubisa, R., and Singh. K. (2011). Psychometrics encompassing VIA-IS: A Comparative Cross-Cultural Referential Reading. *Journal of Indian Academy of Applied Psychology.* 37(2), 326-333.

Clark, A.E. and Frijters, P. and Shields. M.A. (2008). Relative income, happiness and utility: an explanation for the easterlin paradox and other puzzles. *Journal of Economic Literature,* 46 (1), 95-144.

Dalal, A. and Mishra, G. (2006). Psychology of Health and Well-Being: Some Emerging Perspectives. *Psychological Studies*, 51 (2-3), 91-104.

Dasgupta, P. (2001). *Human well-being and the natural environment.* Oxford: Oxford University Press. DOI: 10.1093/0199247889.001.0001

Deci, E.L., and Ryan, R.M. (1985). *Intrinsic motivation and self-determination in human behaviour.* New York: Plenum.

Deaton, A. (2008). Income, Health, and Well-Being around the World: Evidence from the Gallup World Poll. *Journal of Economic Perspectives*, 22(2), 53-72.

Dewey, J. (1933). *How we think.* Boston: D.C. Heath.

Diener, E. (1984). Subjective well-being. *Psychological Bulletin*, 95, 542-575.

Diener, E. (2000). Subjective well-being: The science of happiness and a proposal for a national index. *American Psychologist*, 55, 34-43.

Diener, E., Lucas, R.E., and Scollon, C.N. (2006). Beyond the hedonic treadmill: Revisions to the adaptation theory of well-being. *American Psychologist,* 61, 305-314.

Diener, E., Lucas, R.E., and Oishi, S. (2005). Subjective well-being: The science of happiness, and life satisfaction. In C.R. Snyder and S.J. Lopez (Eds.), *Handbook of positive psychology* (pp. 63-73). Oxford, England: Oxford University Press.

Easterbrook (2003). *The progress paradox: How life gets better while people feel worse.* New York: Random House.

Easterlin, R.A. (1974). Does Economic Growth Improve the Human Lot? Nations and Households in *Economic Growth: Essays in Honor of Moses Abramovitz.*

Easterlin, R.A. (1995). Will Raising the Incomes of All Increase the Happiness of All? *Journal of Economic Behaviour and Organization*. 27 (1), 35-48.

Easterlin, R.A. (2001). Income and Happiness: Towards a Unified Theory. *The Economic Journal*. 111 (473), 465-484.

Easterlin, R.A. (2005). Feeding the Illusion of Growth and Happiness: A Reply to Hagerty and Veenhoven. *Social Indicators Research*, 74(3), 429-443.

Eid, M., and Diener. E. (2004). Global Judgments of Subjective Well-Being: Situational Variability and Long-Term Stability. *Social Indicators Research* 65 (3), 245-277.

Emmons, R.A., and Shelton, C.M. (2005). Gratitude and the science of positive psychology. In C.R. Snyder and S.J. Lopez (Eds.), *Handbook of positive psychology* (pp. 459-471). Oxford, England: Oxford University Press.

Erikson, E.H. (1963). *Childhood and Society* (2nd Edition), New York: Norton.

Erikson, E.H. (1982). *The life cycle completed: A review.* New York: Norton.

Forgeard, M.J.C., Jayawickreme, E., Kern, M. and Seligman, M.E.P. (2011). Doing the right thing: Measuring well-being for public policy. *International Journal of Well-being*, *1* (1), 79-106. DOI: 10.5502/ijw.v1i1.15

Fredrickson, B.L. (2001). The role of positive emotions in positive psychology: The broaden-and-build theory of positive emotions. *American Psychologist*, 56, 218-226.

Gardner, H., Csikszentmihalyi, M., and Damon, W. (2001) *Good Work: When excellence and ethics meet*. New York: Basic Books.

Hale, N.G., Jr. (1971). *Freud and the Americans: The beginnings of psychoanalysis in the United States, 1876-1917*. New York: Oxford University Press.

Harter, S. (2005). Authenticity. In C.R. Snyder and S.J. Lopez (Eds.), *Handbook of positive psychology* (pp. 382-394). Oxford, England: Oxford University Press.

Harvey, J.H., Pauwels, B.G., and Zickmund, S. (2005). Relationship connection: The role of minding in the enhancement of closeness. In C.R. Snyder and S.J. Lopez (Eds.), *Handbook of positive psychology* (pp. 423-433). Oxford, England: Oxford University Press.

Higgins, R.L. (2005). Reality negotiation. In C.R. Snyder and S.J. Lopez (Eds.), *Handbook of positive psychology* (pp. 351-365). Oxford, England: Oxford University Press.

Hooda, D., Sharma, N.R., and Yadava, A. (2009). Social Intelligence as a predictor of Positive Psychological Health. *Journal of Indian Academy of Applied Psychology*, 35(1), 143-150.

Jadhav, S.G., and Havalappanavar, N.B. (2009). Effect of Yoga Intervention on Anxiety and Subjective well-being. *Journal of Indian Academy of Applied Psychology*, 35 (1), 27-31.

Jahoda, M. (1958). *Current Concepts of Positive Mental Health*. New York: Basic Books.

James, W. (1902). *The varieties of religious experience. A study in human nature*. New York: Longmans, Green and Co.

James, W. (1907). The Energies of Men. *The Philosophical Review,* 16 (1), 1-20.

Jorgensen, I.S., and Nafstad, H.E. (2004). Positive psychology: Historical, philosophical, and epistemological perspectives. In P.A. Linley and S. Joseph (Eds.), *Positive psychology in practice* (pp. 15-34). Hoboken, NJ: John Wiley and Sons, Inc.

Joseph, S., and Linley, P.A. (2004). Positive therapy: A positive psychological theory of therapeutic practice. In P.A. Linley and S. Joseph (Eds.), *Positive psychology in prac*tice (pp. 354-370). Hoboken, NJ: Wiley.

Joshi, S., Kumari, S., and Jain, M. (2008). Religious beliefs and its relation to psychological well-being. *Journal of Indian Academy of Applied Psychology,* 34 (2), 345-354.

Kahneman, D. (1999). Objective happiness. In D. Kahneman, E. Diener, and N. Schwartz (Eds.), *Well-being: The foundations of hedonic psychology* (pp. 3-25). New York: Russell Sage Foundation.

Kahneman, D., Diener, E., and Schwarz, N. (Eds.). (1999). *Well-being: The foundations of hedonic psychology*. New York: Russell Sage Foundation.

Kahneman, D., and Krueger, A.B. (2006). Developments in the measurement of subjective well-being. *Journal of Economic Perspectives,* 20 (1), 3-24.

Kahneman, D., Krueger A.B., Schkade, D., Schwarz, N. and Stone, A.A. (2006). Would You Be Happier If You Were Richer? A Focusing Illusion. *Science*, 312 (5782), 1908-1910.

Kapanee, A.R.M., and Rao, K. (2007). Attachment style in relation to family functioning and distress in college students. *Journal of Indian Academy of Applied Psychology,* 33 (1), 15-21.

Kaufman, A., Kraay, A., Zoido-Lobaton, P. (1999). *Governance Matters*. World Bank Policy Research Working Paper No. 2196, Available at SSRN: http://ssrn.com/abstract=188568

Kaufman, A. (2006). *Capabilities equality: basic issues and problems*, NY: Routledge.

Kenny, C. (1999). Does growth cause happiness, or does happiness cause growth? *KYKLOS*, 52, 3-26.

Keyes, C.L.M., and Haidt, J. (Eds.). (2003). Flourishing: *Positive psychology and the life well lived.* Washington, DC: American Psychological Association.

Keyes, C.L.M., and Lopez, S.J. (2005). *Toward a science of mental health: Positive directions in diagnosis and interventions.* In C.R. Snyder and S.J. Lopez (Eds.), *Handbook of positive psychology* (pp. 45-62). Oxford, England: Oxford University Press.

Khosla, M. (2006). Positive Affect and coping with stress. *Journal of Indian Academy of Applied Psychology*, 32 (3), 185-192.

Kumar, S.S., Kaur, P., and Kaur, S. (1993). Effectiveness of shavasana on depression among university students. *Indian Journal of Clinical Psychology,* 20 (2), 81-87.

Layard, R. (1980). Human satisfaction and public policy. *The Economic Journal*, 90 (360), 737-750.

Layard, R. (2005). *Happiness: lessons from a new science*. London: Penguin,

Lefcourt, H.M. (2005). *Humor.* In C.R. Snyder and S.J. Lopez (Eds.), *Handbook of positive psychology* (pp. 619-631). Oxford, England: Oxford University Press.

Linley, P.A., and Joseph, S. (2004a). Applied positive psychology: A new perspective for professional practice. In P.A. Linley and S. Joseph (Eds.), Positive psychology in practice (pp. 3-14). Hoboken, NJ: Wiley.

Lopez, S., and Snyder, C.R. (Eds.). (2003). *Positive psychological assessment: A handbook of models and measures*. Washington, DC: APA Press.

Lyubomirsky, S., King, L.A., and Diener, E. (2005). The benefits of frequent positive affect: Does happiness lead to success? *Psychological Bulletin.* 131, 803-855.

Maddux, J.E. (2005). Stopping the "madness": Positive psychology and the deconstruction of the illness ideology and the DSM. In C.R. Snyder and S.J. Lopez (Eds.), *Handbook of positive psychology* (pp. 13-25). Oxford, England: Oxford University Press.

Maddux, J.E., Snyder, C.R., and Lopez, S.J. (2004). Toward a positive clinical psychology: Deconstructing the illness ideology and constructing an ideology of human strengths and potential. In P.A. Linley and S. Joseph (Eds.), *Positive psychology in practice* (pp. 320-334). Hoboken, NJ: Wiley.

Maslow, A. (1943). A theory of human motivation, *Psychological Review*, 50, 370-396.

Maslow, A.H. (1968). *Toward a psychology of being* (2nd Ed.). New York: Van Nostrand Reinhold.

Maslow, A.H. (1987). *Motivation and personality*. New York: Harper.

Massimini, F., and Delle Fave, A. (2000). Individual development in a bio-cultural perspective. *American Psychologist*, 55, 24-33.

McCullough, M.E., and Witvliet, C.V. (2005). The psychology of forgiveness. In C.R. Snyder and S.J. Lopez (Eds.), *Handbook of positive psychology* (pp. 446-458). Oxford, England: Oxford University Press.

McCullough, M.E., and Snyder, C.R. (2000). Classical source of human strength: Revisiting an old home and building a new one. *Journal of Social and Clinical Psychology*, 19, 1-10.

Mehrotra, S. (2011). Positive Psychology Research in India: A Review and Critique. *Journal of Indian Academy of Applied Psychology*, 37 (1), 9-26.

Morris, D. (1979). *Measuring the Conditions of the World Poor, the Physical Quality of Life Index*, New York: Pergamon Press.

Murray, C. (2003). *Human accomplishment: The pursuit of excellence in the arts and sciences, 800 B.C. to 1950.* New York: Harper Collins.

Myers, D.G. (2000). The funds, friends, and faith of happy people. *American Psychologist*, 55, 56-67.

Nakamura, J., and Csikszentmihalyi, M. (2003). The motivational sources of creativity as viewed from the paradigm of positive psychology. In L.G. Aspinwall and U.M. Staudinger (Eds.), *A psychology of human strengths:*

Fundamental questions and future directions for a positive psychology (pp. 257-270). Washington, DC: APA Press.

Narayanan, G, and Rao, K. (2004). Predictor of Psychological Distress in College Students: The Role of Attachment Styles, Parental Bonding, Personality and Coping. *Indian Journal of Clinical Psychology,* 31(2), 100-105.

Nathawat, S.S. (1996). Editorial: Psychological Well-being and meditation. *Indian Journal of Clinical Psychology,* 23(2), 77-78.

Nathawat, S.S. (2000). Editorial: SQ as an indicator of Psychological well-being. *Indian Journal of Clinical Psychology*, 27(2), 159-160.

Niederhoffer, K.G, and Pennebaker, J.W. (2005). Sharing one's story: On the benefits of writing or talking about emotional experience. In C.R. Snyder and S.J. Lopez (Eds.), *Handbook of Positive Psychology* (pp. 573-583). Oxford, England: Oxford University Press.

Nolen-Hoeksema, S., and Davis, C.G. (2005). Positive responses to loss: Perceiving benefits and growth. In C.R. Snyder and S.J. Lopez (Eds.), *Handbook of Positive Psychology* (pp. 598-607). Oxford, England: Oxford University Press.

Noorbakhsh, F. (1998). A Modified Human Development Index. *World Development*, 26(3), 517-528.

Nussbaum, M.C. (2000). *Women and Human Development: The Capabilities Approach.* Cambridge: Cambridge University Press.

Nussbaum, M.C., and Sen, A. (Eds) (1993). *The Quality of Life*, Oxford: Clarendon.

OECD. (2006). "Alternative Measures of Well-being". In OECD, *Economic Policy Reforms 2006: Going for Growth*, OECD Publishing, DOI: 10.1787/growth-2006-7-en

Oswald, A.J. (1997). Happiness and economic performance. *The Economic Journal*, 107, 1815-1831.

Pawelski, O.J. (2003). William James, Positive Psychology and Healthy-Mindedness. *The Journal of Speculative Philosophy*, 17(1), 53-67.

Peterson, C. (2000). The future of optimism. *American Psychologist*, 55, 44-55.

Peterson, C., and Seligman, M.E.P. (2004). *Character Strengths and Virtues: A Handbook and Classification.* Washington, DC: American Psychological Association.

Rathunde, K. (2001). Toward a Psychology of Optimal Human Functioning: What Positive Psychology Can Learn from the Experiential Turns of James, Dewey, and Maslow. *Journal of Humanistic Psychology* 41 (1), 135-153.

Robbins, B.D. (2006a). An empirical, phenomenological study: Being joyful. In C.T. Fischer (Ed.), *Qualitative research methods for psychologists: Introduction through empirical studies* (pp. 173-211). San Diego, CA: Elsevier Academic Press.

Rogers, C. (1951). *Client-centered therapy: Its current practice, implications and theory.* London: Constable.

Rogers, C. (1961). *On becoming a person: A therapist's view of psychotherapy.* London: Constable.

Ruini, C., and Fava, G.A. (2004). Clinical applications of well-being therapy. In P.A. Linley and S. Joseph (Eds.), *Positive Psychology in Practice* (pp. 371-387). Hoboken, NJ: Wiley.

Ryan, R.M., and Deci, E.L. (2000). Self-determination theory and the facilitation of intrinsic motivation, social development, and well-being. *American Psychologist,* 55, 68-78.

Ryff, C.D., and Singer, B. (1996). The Contours of Positive Human Health. *Psychological Inquiry*, 9(1), 1-28.

Sandage, S.J., and Hill, P.C. (2001). The virtues of positive psychology: The rapprochement and challenges of an affirmative postmodern perspective. *Journal for the Theory of Social Behaviour*, 31, 241-260.

Satter, B. (1999). *Each Mind a Kingdom: American Women, Sexual Purity, and the New Thought Movement, 1875-1920.* Berkeley, CA: University of California Press.

Schui, G., and Krampen, G. (2010). Bibliometric Analyses on the Emergence and Present Growth of Positive Psychology. *Applied Psychology: Health and Well-Being*, 2(1), 52-64.

Schwartz, B. (2000). Self-determination: The tyranny of freedom. *American Psychologist*, 55, 79-88.

Seligman, M.E.P. (2002). *Authentic Happiness.* New York: Free Press.

Seligman, M.E.P. (2005). Positive psychology, positive prevention, and positive therapy. In C.R. Snyder and S.J. Lopez (Eds.), *Handbook of Positive Psychology* (pp. 3-9). Oxford, England: Oxford University Press.

Seligman, M.E.P., and Csikszentmihalyi, M. (2000). Positive psychology: An introduction. *American Psychologist,* 55, 5-14.

Seligman, M.E.P., Rashid, T., and Parks, A.C. (2006). Positive Psychotherapy. *American Psychologist*, 61, 774-788.

Seligman, M.E.P. (1998b). President's column: Positive social science. *APA Monitor*, 29(4), 1.

Seligman, M.E.P. (1998c). President's column: What is the 'good life'? *APA Monitor*, 29(10), 1.

Sen, A. (1985). *Commodities and Capabilities*. Oxford: Oxford University Press.

Sen, A. (2005). Human Rights and Capabilities. *Journal of Human Development*, 6(2), 151-166.

Shah, M., and Thingujam, N.S. (2008). Perceived emotional intelligence and ways of coping among students. *Journal of Indian Academy of Applied Psychology,* 34(1), 83-91.

Shapiro, S.L., Schwartz, G.E. R., and Santeere, C. (2005). Meditation and positive psychology. In C.R. Snyder and S.J. Lopez (Eds.), *Handbook of Positive Psychology* (pp. 632-645). Oxford, England: Oxford University Press.

Simonton, D.K. (2005). Creativity. In C.R. Snyder and S.J. Lopez (Eds.), *Handbook of Positive Psychology* (pp. 189-201). Oxford, England: Oxford University Press.

Singh, K., and Choubisa, R. (2009). Psychometric properties of Hindi translated version of Values in Action Inventory of Strengths (*VIA-IS*). *Journal of Indian Health Psychology,* 4(1), 65-76.

Singh, K., and Choubisa, R. (2010). Empirical validation of Values in Action-Inventory of Strengths (VIA-IS) in Indian context. *Psychological Studies,* 55(2), 151-158.

Singh, K., and Jha, S.D. (2008). Positive and Negative Affect, and Grit as predictors of Happiness and Life Satisfaction. *Journal of Indian Academy of Applied Psychology,* 34, 40-45.

Slezackova, A. (2013). Reflection of person-centered approach and Client-centered therapy in Positive psychology and psychotherapy. In S.K. Srivastava, N. Singh, and S. Kant (Eds), *Psychological Interventions of Mental Disorders* (pp. 294-314). New Delhi: Sarup Book Publishers. ISBN: 978-81-7625-911-8.

Snyder, C.R., and Lopez, S.J. (Eds.). (2002). *Handbook of Positive Psychology.* New York: Oxford University Press.

Snyder, C.R., Rand, K., Sigmon, D. (2005), "Hope theory: a member of the positive psychology family", in Snyder, C.R., Lopez, S. (Eds), *Handbook of Positive Psychology*, New York: Oxford University Press.

Swann, W.B., and Pelham, B.W. (2005). The truth about illusions: Authenticity and positivity in social relationships. In C.R. Snyder and S.J. Lopez (Eds.), Handbook of positive psychology (pp. 366-381). Oxford, England: Oxford University Press.

Tangney, J.P. (2005). Humility. In C.R. Snyder and S.J. Lopez (Eds.), *Handbook of positive psychology* (pp. 411-422). Oxford, England: Oxford University Press.

Taylor, E. (2001). Positive Psychology and Humanistic Psychology: A Reply to Seligman. *Journal of Humanistic Psychology,* 41(1), 13-29.

Tedeschi, R.G. and Calhoun, L.G. (2004). A clinical approach to post-traumatic growth. In P.A. Linley and S. Joseph (Eds.), *Positive psychology in practice* (pp. 405-419). Hoboken, NJ: Wiley.

Thomas, V., Dailimi, M., Dhareshwar, A., Kaufmann, D., Kishor, N., Lopez, R., and Wang, Y. (2000). *The Quality of Growth.* The World Bank. Retrieved from: http://elibrary.worldbank.org/doi/book/10.1596/0-1952-1593-1

Thompson, S.C. (2005). The role of personal control in adaptive functioning. In C.R. Snyder and S.J. Lopez (Eds.), *Handbook of positive psychology* (pp. 202-213). Oxford, England: Oxford University Press.

United Nations (2011). *Resolution 65/309 Happiness: Towards a Holistic Approach to Development.* United Nations General Assembly, Sixty-fifth Session, July 2011, New York.

United Nations Development Programme. (1990). *Human development report.* New York: Oxford University Press.

United Nations Development Programme. (1997) "UNDP and Governance: Experiences and Lessons Learned", Management Development and Governance Division, Lessons-Learned Series No. 1. Retrieved from: http:/

/portal.publicpolicy.utoronto.ca/en/StudyReports/UNDP/UNDPandGovernanceExperiencesandLessonsLearned/Pages/default.aspx.

Vaillant, G.E. (2000). Adaptive mental mechanisms: Their role in a positive psychology. *American Psychologist,* 55, 89-98.

Vaillant, G.E. (1977). *Adaptation to Life*, Boston, MA, Little, Brown.

Veenhoven, R. (1991). Is happiness relative? *Social Indicators Research,* 24, 1-34.

Woolfolk, R.L., and Wasserman, R.H. (2005). Count no one happy: Eudaimonia and positive psychology. *Journal of Theoretical and Philosophical Psychology*, 25, 81-90.

6

Well-being Among Elderly

An Indian Perspective

Mukta Rani Rastogi

Life span development approach brings forth the fact that each stage of development since birth has its own demands and pressures and at each stage one has make effects for well-being of oneself. So well-being is a major concern at all stages of development. A special attention on well-being of elderly people is due to the physical and cognitive decline in old age combined with social, financial and emotional insecurity, retirement, death of close friends and spouse, changes in living conditions, realization of one's own immorality etc.

Issue of well-being has been addressed by western psychologists in many different forms like happiness, quality of life, wellness, psychological health etc. The term well-being became popular with the work of *Deiner* (1984) as subjective well-being and personal well-being, respectively.

Indian Psychology also offers many ways to live life in a healthy manner for each stage of life span development including old age. The most despairing observation is that its teachings and traditions were translated and into Western culture and psychology but their salience is diminish accepted by us. Although in the process of inclusion by Westerners, much of their original purpose and context are stripped away but their relevance is accepted and methods are practiced. Meditation is a common practice world-wide, but the focus is on the content of meditation which is independent of the religious and philosophical context within which it was embedded historically. Vedic literature offers both an image of good life and suggestions about how to achieve it in old age. The meaning of happiness and of a balanced life and their ability to promote mental health, if embraced by elderly people, may save them from various hazards of life at this juncture.

Indian psychology does not consider well-being at surface level, focusing only on outer aspect of the person, instead it recommends to examine the basic structure of the self so that improvements and changes are built an a solid foundation that is more likely to last. Mindfulness is one such exercise both interoperated in humanistic as well as Vedantic psychology which helps in cultivating many of the personal qualities associated with well-being. Indian psychology has several schools and all schools talk about what well-being is and how to approach it. My views confuse only to ideas propagated in *triguna* theory as stated in *Gita* and vedantic of self.

The predominant feature of well-being noted in Indian thoughts is its holistic view, which has now been well admitted by Western thinkers also. The current model of health or wellness pursues this holistic motion as depicted in Elisabeth Kubler-Ross model of well-being.

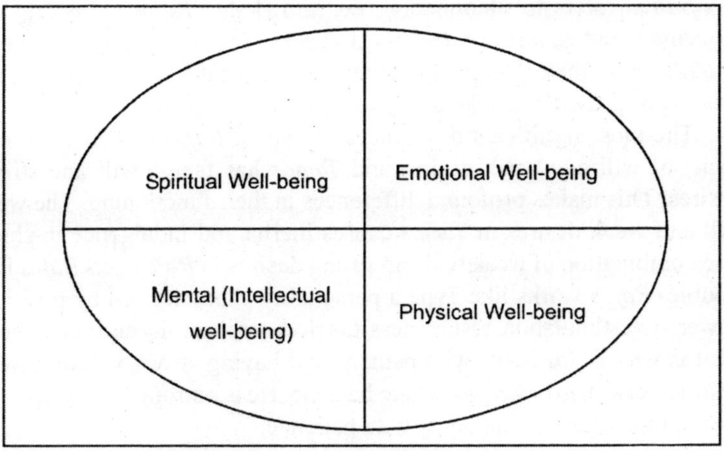

Fig. 6.1: Kubler-Ross model of well-being

The model has three implications. First, by well-being implies balance or harmony of all aspects of human condition. Secondly, each component holds specific dominance at all phases of individual's growth cycle. Thirdly, they are so interwoven that it is not possible to divide them.

According to Vedantic view, psychology is the study of whole person and therefore, it concerns with all aspects of human life, taking the person in totality. For example, Patanjali's *Yoga* deals the person at all his levels (physical, emotional, mental and spiritual), it connects body and mind and self (*Aatma*) and *parmatma*.

Daliahawa and H.C. Sutler (1998) say that the very purpose of our life is to seek well-being which can be achieved through Training the mind. Training the mind does not refer to only one's cognitive ability or intellect includes feelings, heart and mind. It is a function of how we perceive our situation or how satisfied we are with what we have. This outlook, if well cultivated in elderly may promote their well-being, Triguna theory suggests very strongly how to develop this mind set.

Triguna Theory and Well-being: According to *Samkhya* the three constituents of *Prakriti* including human beings are *Sattva, Rajas* and *Tamas*. These are present in all human beings but in varying degrees, causing individual differences and their changed dominance from one occasion to the other accounts for intra-individual differences. The evolution from *Tamas* to *Sattva* through, *Rajas* is a process of growth leading to human being. But evolution is a choice made by human and that is why we all are not engaged in achieving well-being.

Sattva refers to illumination, i.e. knowledge *Rajas* to 'energy' or movement and *Tamas* to '*nirha*' or darkness. The two Important aspects of *triguna* are their interplay and transformation, the latter facilitates the process of growth and take us to well-being (Ishwaran, 1997).

The most significant differences in *Sattva*, *Rajas* and *Tamas* are in terms of will and weak desires and *Tamas* has feeble will and strong desires. This makes profound differences in their functioning. The weak will and weak desires in *Tamas* causes inerha and indulgence in sleep. The combination of weak will and strong desires in *Rajas* gets *Rajas* into trouble. *Rajas* works like Type a personality characterized by position, power, overstimulation, restlessness, hurriedness, hostility and resentment. That is why *Rajas* binds with pain. *Sattva* having strong will and weak desires works hard when work is to be done. He is a strong headed person, moves to the goal unshakingly with patience.

According to Bhawuk (2008) cognition, emotion and behaviour all the three are anchored in desires. It is through perception, person thinks of an object (cognition) and constant thinking leads to attachment which culminates into the desire for that object (emotion). This has impact on our behavioural intensions and future behaviour. Thus an individual is directed towards goal through thoughts, attachment and desires when desired goals are not met, the person is unhappy, i.e. anger is generated. When desired goals are attained the individual wants more and greed is generated. Thus desires are the culture of both anger and greed. *Gita* says that we can go beyond desires or we may conquer desires by regulating our senses.

Further, desires may be both positive and negative. Elderly people should go for positive desires = desire for happiness, for peace, for more harmonious world. These desires are personally and socially useful. Elderly people may create such desires by embracing sattva which will promote their well-being. They may practice *Karma Yoga*, the path of work (or doing one's prescribed duties) as recommended by *Gita* as an intervention to avoid the unhappiness resulting from pursuing desires. This is done through *Manan* (self-reflection) and *Chintan* (contemplation). These two are essential for any spiritual path.

Karma Yoga asks for engaging in prescribed duties without attaching oneself with the fruits of efforts. Thus, one can break the chain of cognition, emotion and behaviour anchored in desires. This brings the state of equanimity of mind.

Senses in a *Satvik* person are controlled to the extent that neither pleasure nor pain stimulates him. When one can withdraw power from senses or will (that is what we do in meditation), the scarcely effort. One has gone beyond *gunas*, beyond all human conditioning, beyond human limitations. He is alike to friend and foe which has nothing to do with being indifferent. It is showing goodwill, patience, forgiveness, understanding not only to those we like or when it is convenient but always to everyone and for ever.

In old age we generally tend to focus on what we lack in our physical and mental decline. By adopting *Sattvik* attitude, they need to focus on positive side of life. Elderly people, after retirement and completing maximum responsibilities of their life by this of their life, they may make efforts afresh to give a new orientation, a new shape to their life focusing a *sattva gana*. This may help them immensely to promote and enhance their well-being. They need to shift their attention from achieving 'what they want' to appreciate 'what they have'.

Self and Well-Being: The control themes of *Vedanta* are consciousness and self. Self refers to *Atma* and is claimed to be identical with ubiquities. *Brahman* and is usually characterized by the terms Being, Consciousness and Bliss.

True self reveals in the fifth sheath of person, i.e. *Jiva*. Five sheaths are nested in one another known as—

1. *Annamaya Kosh*, the outermost layer.
2. *Pranamaya Kosh*, which involves breathing.
3. *Manomaya Kosh*, which involves sense organs and their functions (mind).

4. *Vigyanamaya Kosh* refers tointellect involving ideas, concepts which are use to know the world.
5. *Anandmaya Kosh* reflects bliss, the characteristics of true self.

Vedanta accepts only the self—as subject to be true self, dismissing the identification of the self with any object as ultimately deceptive. Self as subject is a consciousness based construct. Self as an object is a manifestation of ego and is an aspect of mind. Since *Atman* is similar to *parmatman*, it becomes the duty of human beings to cultivate in themselves divine like qualities which would subsequently bring well-being not only at personal level but at transpersonal level. What one needs to do for it? He is required to remind himself all the time that I am divine like and I should act divine like. This will enable him to approach divinity. The more are does it, greater will be well-being.

Human beings fail to understand true self and its limitlessness because of three misbeliefs about themselves. These three limitations are sorrow, mortality and ignorance. If we are limited by nature, we should not shive against limitations which we generally do. And these limitations should have been acceptable to us (Dayanand, 1991).

According to *Gita* knower and known cannot be the same. We know we are hurt, we feel jealous, we experience pain. Since we know our sorrow we cannot be sorrow. Similarly, only when we confuse body with self we associate mortality with the self. Lord Krishna says,

देहिनोऽस्मिन् यथा देहे कौमारं यौवनं जरा।
तथा देहान्तरप्राप्तिर्धीरस्तत्र न मुह्यति।।

Just as the self embodied in this body must pass through childhood, youth and old age, so it will assume another body (at death) with reference to that the wise do not come to grief. All agents of destruction are incapable of destroying *I-awareness* which is explicitely described in the following *shloka*:

नैनं छिन्दन्ति शस्त्राणि, नैनं दहति पावकः।
न चैनं क्लेदयन्त्यापो न शोषयति मारुतः।।
(Weapon cannot cut it, fire cannot burn it, water cannot wet it, even wind cannot dry it).

We are aware of our ignorance too. So we cannot be ignorant. In all our pursuits we seek freedom from these limitations as these are not our true nature. We are aware of these limitations (known) there the knower the self is different from the known. When these limitations are overcome, we tend not to explore happiness in outside world. No particular object can provide happiness. It is the self which is the source of happiness. It is manifested only in a satisfied mind, a mind that desires nothing. According to Swami Dayanand, "A person who understands that the self is the source of all happiness will be free from all desires".

Thus the main thrust of development of personality according to *Vedanta* is towards realization of the true self (i.e. the devine) which is all pervading, indescribable and impersonal. The course of development of personality is charted along a successive transcendence from the empirical to spiritual pot in other words from phenominal to nominal.

Aids for Self Realization: Four Methods of *Advait Vedanta* are suggested as the aids of self-realization.

These are as follows:

1. Making a wise discrimination between the permanent and the impermanent with regard to the self.
2. Detatchment from the gains of either this or the other worldly life.
3. Development of the following:
   - (i) *Sama*: It refers to control of mind so that mind may rest firmly on a single object.
   - (ii) *Dama*: Which means withdrawal of senses from the objects of pleasure.
   - (iii) *Uparati*: It cannot prevent the mind from being controlled by external objects.
   - (iv) *Titiksha*: It is endurance of hardships without lamenting or becoming anxious.
   - (v) *Shraddha*: It refers to faith in the reality of teachings of the scriptures and the advice of a capable teacher.
   - (vi) *Samadhan*: Fully resting the mind as the formless *Brahman* without being enticed by desires.
4. Desire for liberating oneself from egoism and the perpetual chain of actions and their consequences.
5. With the vast and varied experiences of life and maturity of adulthood, elderly persons may assure themselves of the worth and salience of acquiring these six values which would assist them to attain well-being in their life. The above method may be considered as a form of applied psychology as it helps in changing the human condition from a less desirable to a more desirable state.

References

Bhawuk, Dharm, P.S. (2008): Anchoring cognition, Emotion and Behaviour in desire: A model from the *Bhagvad Gita*. In Rao R., Paranjpe, A.C. and Dalal, A.K., *Indian Psychology.* New Delhi: Foundation Books.

Dalai Lama, H.H. and Cutler, H.C. (1991). *The Art of Happiness: A Handbook for Living.* London: Coronet Books, Hodder and Stoughtan.

Dayanand, S. (1991). *The Teaching of Bhagwat Gita*. New Delhi: Vision Books.

Deiner, E. (1984). *Subjective Well-being. Psychological Bulletin*, 95, 542-575.

Easwaran, E., *The Bhagwat Gita for Daily Living*, Vols. 1, 2 and 3. Jaico Pub.

Kubler-Ross, E. (1981). *Keynote Address*, American Holistic Health Association Annual Conference Lacrosse, WI, 1981.

Ryff, C.D. (1989): Happiness is everything or what is it? Explorations of Meaning of Psychological Well-being. *Journal of Personality and Social Psychology*, 5, 7, 1069-1081.

The Complete Works of Swami Vivekanand. (1989). Vol. II, Mayawati Memorial Edition, Advait Ashrama, Calcutta.

7

Mental Health of Orphans

Swaran Lata, Varsha Rani and *Shikha Verma*

Orphans are the socially deprived and most vulnerable groups of children in the society. In orphanages, they experience psychological and social challenges, several mental health problems like anxiety, depression, emotional and behavioural disorders and institutionalization in long term. All this leads to the development of psychologically impaired and economically unproductive adults. Limited attention has been paid to their psychosocial and developmental needs. The present article aims to throw light on the mental health status of orphans in terms of social change, emotional, behavioural and psychosocial problems and their outcomes.

Mental health is an essential part of health and more than the mere lack of mental disorders. It is about enhancing competencies of individuals and communities and enabling them to achieve their self-determined goals (World Health Organization, 1999), as a state of well-being whereby individuals recognize their abilities, are able to cope with the normal stresses of life, work productively and fruitfully, and make a contribution to their communities (World Health Organisation, 2003). Concepts of mental health includes subjective well-being, perceived self-efficacy, autonomy, competence, intergenerational dependence and recognition of the ability to realize one's intellectual and emotional potential.

Mental health problems have a significant impact on functioning and well-being for people of all ages, including adolescents and children. It is a resource for living to thrive and essential for optimal human development and functioning across life span. Surveys reveal that today more children and young people experience mental health problems as compared to 30 years ago. 20 per cent of children and young people experience psychological problems (Mental Health Foundation, 1999; World Federation for Mental Health, 2003). Research from National Statistics (2000) found that 10 per cent of 5 to 15 years old had a mental disorder in groups of 5 to 10 years old: 10 per cent of boys and 6 per cent of girls had a mental disorder, in groups of 11 to 15 years old, 13 per cent of boys and 10 per cent of girls had a mental disorder.

Determinants of Child Mental Health: Risk and Protection

The determinants of child mental health can be explained in terms of the concepts of risk and protective factors. Risk factors are those factors which increase the likelihood of negative mental health outcomes in a child whereas protective factors promote positive mental health outcomes in a child. These risk and protective factors combine to determine a child's vulnerability to develop mental illness.

There is general agreement in the literature that the greater the number of risk factors a child is subject to, the more likely she is to suffer mental health problems (Zeanah, Boris, and Larrieu, 1997). It is unlikely that exposure to a single risk factor significantly compromises a child's future mental health outcomes, while concurrent exposure to multiple risk factors in combination is clearly associated with increased likelihood for mental health problems (e.g., Sameroff, Bartko, Baldwin, Baldwin, and Seifer, 1998). Exposure to particular risk factors (e.g. single parenthood) increases a child's risk of being exposed to additional risk factors (e.g. poverty) (Ruchkin, Gilliam, and Mayes, 2008).

Multiple protective factors can "directly reduce the effects of risk, enhance competence, or immunize an individual against adversity" (Zeanah and Zeanah, 2001). Different protective factors can combine to promote mental health and the effects of these protective factors often endure throughout the lifespan, helping to combat various individual and environmental challenges throughout development (Sameroff, 2000). The simple fact that some children demonstrate socio-emotional resilience in the face of multiple serious risk factors highlights the importance of protective factors (Werner, 2000).

Risk Factors for Mental Health of Children

During the past decades, a number of risk factors have been identified that place children at increased risk for psychopathology. Coie *et al.* (1993) grouped empirically derived, generic risk factors into the following seven individual and environmental domains:

1. **Constitutional handicaps:** Prenatal complications,

neurochemical imbalance, organic handicaps, and sensory disabilities.

2. **Skill development delays**: Low intelligence, social incompetence, attention deficits, reading disabilities, and poor work skills and habits.
3. **Emotional difficulties:** Apathy or emotional blunting, emotional immaturity, low self-esteem, and emotional disregulation.
4. **Family circumstances:** Low social class, mental illness in the family, large family size, child abuse, stressful life events, family disorganization, communication deviance, family conflict, and poor bonding to parents.
5. **Interpersonal problems:** Peer rejection, alienation, and isolation.
6. **School problems:** Scholastic demoralization and school failure.
7. **Ecological risks:** Neighbourhood disorganization, extreme poverty, racial injustice, and unemployment.

Protective Factors for Mental Health of Children

Protective factors are variables that reduce the likelihood of maladaptive outcomes under conditions of risk. For a good mental health, it is essential for children to be in good physical health, eating a balanced diet (Levy *et al.*, 2009) and doing regular exercises (Lachman and Agrigoroaei, 2010). Brown and Siegel (1988) conducted a longitudinal study to see if adolescents who exercised were better able to cope with stress and avoid illness than those who did not. Results indicated that the negative impact of stressful life events on health declined as exercise levels increased (Taylor, 2010). Researchers have examined the effect of aerobic exercise on psychological states such as mood, anxiety, depression and tension and have a beneficial role of exercise on both mental and physical health (Taylor, 2010). According to Margoob, M.A. (2006), a positive social orientation and clear standards of behaviour are protective factors which a family provides against the development of psychiatric symptoms. Along with them some other factors like feeling loved, trusted, understood, valued, safe, hopeful, optimistic, being able to learn, having opportunities to succeed, accepting and recognizing their abilities and capabilities, having a sense of belonging in their family, school and community, having the strength to cope when something goes wrong (resilience) and the ability to solve problems are also important (Ungar, M., 2004). Family and friends play a crucial role in providing encouragement for achieving health goals.

Although less is known about protective factors and their operation (Rutter, 1985; Kazdin, 1991; Luthar, 1993), at least three broad domains of protective factors have been identified.

1. **Characteristics of the individual:** Cognitive skills, social-cognitive skills, temperamental characteristics, and social skills (Luthar and Zigler, 1992).
2. **The quality of the child's interactions with the environment:** Secure attachments to parents (Morissett, Barnard, Greenberg, Booth and Speiker, 1990) and attachments to peers or other adults who engage in positive health behaviours and have pro-social values.
3. **Aspects of the mesosystem and exosystem:** School-home relations, quality schools, and regulatory activities.

Coie *et al.* (1993) suggested that protective factors may work in one or more of the following four ways: directly decrease dysfunction; interact with risk factors to lower their effects; disrupt the mediational chain by which risk leads to disorder; or prevent the initial occurrence of risk factors.

Orphanage—The Breeding Ground of Mental Health Problems

Children placed in orphanage settings at a young age and for long periods of time are at greatly increased risks for development of serious psychopathology later in life. An orphanage is often examined through problematic psychosocial function of children (Hersor, 1980). Anna Freud (1973) concluded from several case studies that institutionalized children are doomed to fail psychologically because of maternal deprivation despite of good physical and social care (Freud, Solint and Goldstein, 1973). Bowlby (1995) also reported that maternal deprivation was the central issue causing psychological damage to orphanage children. Goodwin (1994) argues that any amount of orphanage experience is harmful; the damage is greatest during the first year of life and increases dramatically with length of stay in an institution. Children institutional cares are extremely vulnerable to psychological problem and institutionalization in long term and in early childhood increases the likelihood that they will grow into psychologically impaired and economically unproductive adult (Flank, Klass, Earls and Eisenburg, 1996-1997). According to Margoob, M.A. (2006) children who grow up in orphanages or foster care usually have no social connections, and these children are at a disadvantage for completing high school, going to college (Olley, 2008), or getting job opportunities all of which may be contributing factors in predisposing a child to psychopathology. Getachew, H. (2011) explained that living with non-relatives was identified as a risk factor for more mental health problems. Children living in orphanages are one of the most vulnerable groups of children in the society. Losing one's parents in childhood is one of the biggest emotional loss and undergoes a lot of trauma of coping with life. They experience risk problems ranging from pain of watching their parents suffer and die, worry about their future, fear of being infected, discrimination, less opportunity of education, changing homes several times, lack of adult love, guidance and protection, teasing, isolation, gossip, neglect and abuse. They experience normal stresses, avoidance, internalizing problems and fatalism, stigmatization and behavioural disturbances. These problems lead to a feeling of shame, withdrawal, self-blame, depression, grief, sadness, fear, anxiety and suicidal ideation. They commonly show signs of lack of self-confidence and low self-esteem. They live in a state of repeated neglect, abuse, fear, increased workload and social isolation. All this negatively influence the current and future mental health of orphans. Hence, a safe new home that they can trust is not by itself sufficient to repair the damage imposed by abnormal early stress on the developing nervous system (Hughes, 1999). Thus, children in foster care have a disproportionately high prevalence of mental health disorders (Halfron, Zepeda and Inkelas, 2002) and studies have indicated that between 50 and 80 per cent of children in foster care suffer from moderate to severe mental health problems (DosReis, Zito, Safer and Soeken, 2001; Simms, Dubowitz and Szilagyi, 2000). A study on Eritrean orphanages found children experiencing mood disturbances, language delays and disturbed social interaction with peers, and concluded that orphanages are necessarily the breeding grounds of psychopathological problems (Wolff and Fesseha, 1998). Thus orphans are exposed to several risk factors which adversely affect their mental health.

Bayumova, S. (2001) further zooms the picture of orphans in her essay about the children and programmes in the orphanage. She enlisted the following characteristics of orphans:

Physical Condition

- 63 per cent exhibit delayed physical development (low weight, stunted growth, hormonal imbalance).

- 70 per cent have chronic illnesses of the digestive and/or respiratory systems.
- 80 per cent indicate drug dependency (substance abuse, smoking, alcohol, etc.).

Psychological Condition

- 50 per cent have been diagnosed with delayed psychological development.
- 70 per cent display accentuated personality characteristics that manifest themselves as negative attitudes towards oral norms, absence of self-esteem, and/or difficulties in socializing.
- 85 per cent exhibit clear motivational deficits: educational motivation has not been formed; very low level in the development of personal will and self-control; easily influenced.
- 90 per cent manifest emotional characteristics through an elevated propensity for conflict, often accompanied by aggression, or the uncontrolled use of foul language; a generally emotional, unstable demeanour.
- 4 per cent adolescents exhibit psychopathic tendencies.
- 42 per cent exhibit borderline delinquent behaviour, characterized by a strongly pronounced negative attitude, as well as negative reaction towards demands or teachers.
- 60 per cent demonstrate antisocial behaviour.

Risk Factors for Mental Health Problems of Orphans

Psychosocial Problems

Orphan children are socially deprived and at higher risk of developing psychological (Wild, 2002) and psychosocial problems. Psychosocial distress is very common in orphans and may result in increased insecurity, which contributes to major impairments to their cognitive, social and moral functioning (Pharoah, 2004), aggression, helplessness, sadness, depression, negative self-concept, disciplinary or behavioural problems (Nyamukapa *et al.*, 2008), lack of ability to explore and make choices. They tend to encounter higher emotional distress, hopelessness, and frustration (Mbozi, Debit, and Munyati, 2006), sexual abuse (Pridmore and Yates, 2005) especially girls, and social discrimination (Cluver, Gardner and Operario, 2008; Nyblade, Pande, Mathur, MacQuarrie, Kidd, and Banteyerga, 2003) and exploitation (The Coordination of Humanitarian Affairs, 2003). Orphaned children receive less food, denied school fees, forced to do more work and bear sexual abuse in their new households silently because they have nowhere else to turn for shelter or protection (Human Rights, 2002). They are distressed by their new circumstance of looking after themselves, bearing care-giving responsibility for their younger ones, sibling separation, loss of friends, and problem of concentrating in school. Being cared by someone other than a parent, child labour, physical abuse, stigma and discrimination, and inadequate care leads to greater psychosocial problems (Nyamukapa *et al.*, 2008), lack of positive emotional care and empathy develops antisocial behaviours in them. Orphanhood also adversely affects the academic performance of the orphans. Teachers have reported that they find orphans day-dreaming, coming to school infrequently, arriving at school unprepared and late, or being non-responsive in the classroom. Ironically, teachers remain ignorant of the cause of the children's distress and are not sympathetic regarding it. Lata and Shukla (2012) found inadequate psycho-social environment of the orphanage with low level of togetherness among the orphan girls. They were not supportive, involved and helping. They were self-contained, shy and inhibited. Some girls were very aggressive, hostile and quarrelsome. They got less opportunity for personal growth because of strict and rigid rules of the orphanage. The psycho-social environment of the orphanage appeared like a conflict oriented and distressed family pattern. The orphans had low cohesion, expressiveness, independence, intellectual-recreational orientation and high conflict and control. Lata and Verma (2013) found low psychosocial adjustment of orphans as compared to non-orphans. They had low home, health, social, emotional and school adjustment as compared to non-orphans. After adjusting these experiences, the statistical associations between orphanhood and psychological distress disappeared or weakened, suggesting that they contribute to the higher levels of distress observed in orphans (Nyamukapa *et al.*, 2008). Naqshbandi *et al.* (2012) found that there were many psychological/adjustmental problems with the orphans living in orphanage of Kashmir.

Emotional Problems

Orphan children's minds are always occupied by the negative emotions, and they have the risk of growing up with unresolved negative emotions which are often expressed with anger and depression (Brodzinsky *et al.*

1986). They lack required support, encouragement to express their emotions and guidance to deal with grief and other emotional difficulties. Studies of childhood parental loss suggest that orphans tend to experience social depression (Furukawa, Yokouchi, Hirai, Kitamura, and Takahashi, 1999), personality disorders (Paris, Zweig-Frank, and Guzder, 1994) anxiety and insomnia (Tweed, Schoenbach, George, and Blazer, 1989). Gregory *et al.* (1958 and 1965) and Worden (1996) reported that the psychological disorders were often found in the bereaved children as depression, delinquency, antisocial personality, psychoneurosis (anxiety), and even overt psychotic disorders. Other researchers have reported similar findings elsewhere (Hunter and Williamson, 1997). According to Sengendo and Nambi (1997), orphans experience emotional problems due to several reasons. First, there is a lack of adequate information on the nature and magnitude of the problem; secondly, there is a cultural belief that children do not have emotional problems and, therefore, there is a lack of attention from adults. Thirdly, since psychological problems are not always obvious, many adults in charge of orphans are not able to identify them. The irony is that when the problem may have been identified; there is a lack of knowledge of how to handle it appropriately. In many cases orphans are punished for showing their negative emotions, thereby adding to their pain. In orphanages, there is an obvious lack of appropriate training of staff in identifying psychological and social problems and therefore, offering individual or group attention. Worldwide, studies have consistently shown orphans to have higher rates of emotional and behavioural problems than non-orphans. Van Eerdewegh and colleagues (1982) did a follow up study on 105 children aged from 2-17 years who had lost a parent and noted that by 1 month, 77 per cent of the bereaved children showed symptoms of depressive disorder as compared to 34 per cent in the control group. In addition to symptoms of depression, they also noted these children to have poor school performance and bed-wetting. By one year, however, there was a lessening of the depressive symptoms and the associated bed wetting although the disinterest in school continued. Lata and Verma (2013) found that orphan children witnessed greater health problems like depression, anxiety, somatic symptoms and social dysfunction than non-orphans.

A study conducted by Irudayasamy (2006) showed that orphan children face many psychological disorders. At the age when they need support from their parents and siblings to cope up with physical and emotional development, they are prone to psychological disorders. Chan *et al.* (2006) conducted a study on psychiatric disorders and problems of children in orphanages of Kashmir. An orphanage for young women in Srinagar was surveyed by psychiatrists using DSM-IV guidelines to evaluate children for psychopathology. Children were in the age group of 5 to 12 years. Post-stress traumatic disorder (PSTD) was the commonest psychiatric disorder (40.62%) easily attributable to the prevailing mass trauma state of almost two decades. The next commonest diagnoses were major depressive disorder (MDD) with 25 per cent and conversion disorder with 12.5 per cent. The report says that there is a general agreement among researchers that children placed in special home settings at a young age and for long periods of time are at an increased rate of developing serious psychopathology later in life.

Behavioural Problems

Orphans in institutional care have more behavioural problems, such as aggressive behaviour and have higher levels of depression and anxiety, compared to children that are reared in a family environment (Trout, A.L., 2009; Vorria, P., 2003; Johnson, R., 2006). They are observed to be more depressed, anxious, and less optimistic and displayed angry feelings and disruptive behaviours compared to other children, (Segendo and Nambi, 1997; Atwine *et al.*, 2005; Nyamukapa *et al.*, 2008). The depression that orphans and vulnerable children experience interferes with all aspects of their lives and lead to energy loss, sadness, weight changes, feeling of worthlessness, difficulty in sleeping or oversleeping, loss of interest in social activities and suicidal thoughts or thoughts about death (Foster and Williamson, 2000). Existing studies of children's reactions suggest that they tend to show internalizing rather than externalizing symptoms in response to such impacts—depression, anxiety and withdrawal—as opposed to aggression and other forms of antisocial behaviour (Forehand, Steele, Armistead, Morse, Simon and Clarke, 1998; Makame, Ari and Grantham-McGregor, 2002; Sengendo and Nambi, 1997). Lata and Shukla (2011), analysis of social skills of young orphaned girls, revealed that they lacked the skill of handling frustration, embarrassment, anger and decision-making.

Among the behavioural problems associated with early institutional privation are inattention and hyperactivity, externalizing and internalizing problems, social and peer difficulties, and autistic-like features. A review of the literature indicates that early institutional rearing has been associated with both externalizing (Hoksbergen, Rijk, van Dijkum and Ter Laak, 2004) and internalizing problems. Children in orphanages showed the same delayed physical and behavioural development as children from globally deficient orphanages (St. Petersburg-USA Orphanage Research Team, 2005; in press). Across studies, it has been consistently found that the more time children spent in an orphanage the higher their rates of externalizing, internalizing, attention, social, and thought problems (Ames, 1997; Fisher *et al.*, 1997; Groza and Ryan, 2002; Gunnar *et al.*, 2007; Hoksbergen *et al.*, 2004; Kreppner *et al.*, 2001; Le Mare and Audet, 2002; Marcovitch *et al.*, 1997, Verhulst *et al.*, 1992). Dunn *et al.* (1991) reported that orphaned children had a tendency to acquire juvenile delinquent traits such as petty theft, poor socialization and rebelliousness.

Dealing with Social Change

Death of parents introduces a major change in the life of a child. This change may involve moving from a middle or upper-class urban home to a poor rural relative's home, separation from siblings or forced to live on their own, constituting child-headed families. All these changes easily affect not only the physical, but also the psychological well-being of a child. Many children find it difficult to adapt to these new changes. According to Minde (1988), it is not the social change that causes psychological problems rather it is the failure of the individual to adapt to social change also. Social change, bereavement and the resultant need to adapt to new demands and constraints to life creates stress which appear in symptoms of confusion, anxiety, depression and behavioural disorders such as disobedience and learning problems. Frustrated, fearful, and depressed children fail to concentrate and perform badly in class. Failure by the school, caregivers and the home systems to recognize these symptoms and address them aggravates the child's psychological problems. Such situational factors are very commonly seen in orphans and adversely influence their mental health.

Children who are orphans due to death of parent are less likely to be employed, as they have a lower chance of completing basic and secondary education. Without education and skills training, they are more likely to fall deeper into the cycle of poverty and engage in high-risk behaviour. Ultimately, this affects dealing with social change. The economic challenges of orphans occur in stages. They begin to fear for their future, wonder who will care for them, and worry about how they will be able to stay in school. Children are often pulled out of school. At this stage, the quality of child-rearing is compromised, and many important lessons on life skills and self-sufficiency are not taught, mostly because the parent(s) is too ill to transfer the knowledge. After one parent dies, most children continue to live with the surviving parent or a relative, but they often slide more deeply into poverty. For some, the next stage begins when they find themselves the heads of households. A young adolescent may be responsible for many siblings, some of whom may be infants. Children who are the heads of households are in a difficult position not only because they must now support their siblings with little to no education and/or employable skills, but also because they most likely have limited resources. In many cases much of the family's possessions may have been sold to care for the sick. Large numbers of orphans find themselves in homes that cannot afford to pay school expenses and drop out to work in the household, fields, or on the street. Young children with minimal education or employable skills can be found doing work such as shining shoes, begging for money in the streets, bartending, selling food, and most often in the case of girls, becoming domestic workers (Salaam, T., 2005).

Cognitive and Intellectual Impairment

Orphans are consistently reported to have problems in the area of attention (Andresen *et al.*, 1992; Groza and Ileana, 1996; Marcovitch, Cesaroni, Roberts, and Swanson, 1995; Stevens *et al.*, 2007; Verhulst *et al.*, 1990b). The more time a child spends in an orphanage, the more profound the cognitive and intellectual impairment. For every year that a child spends in an institution, his cognitive development is delayed by about six months. Some of this damage is observable at the biological level. Total brain volume is significantly negatively correlated with time spent in an institution. The hippocampus in particular shows markedly decreased volume, which is due to overproduction of cortisol a hormone released in stressful situations. Repeated release of cortisol in stressful situations destroys the hippocampus, which is central in learning and memory. Damage is not limited to the hippocampus, however; Functional Magnetic Resonance Imaging (FMRI) of formerly institutionalized children have revealed that the prefrontal cortex tends to be both immature and reduced in volume, which leads to problems with impulse control and decision making (Aslanian, 2006; Frederici, 2007).

Child neglect and child abuse are chronic societal problems. However, the impact of childhood social deprivation on brain function in humans has been largely unexamined. Studies of children following removal from the orphanages and adoption by families in the United Kingdom and North

America revealed the presence of cognitive, social, and physical deficits (Ames, 1997; Rutter, 1998). At the time of adoption, the majority of the children showed cognitive performance in the mental retardation range based upon parent report on the Denver scale (Rutter, 1998). Longitudinal studies have demonstrated that these children showed considerable recovery by 4 years (Ames, 1997; Rutter, 1998), but that deficits remaining at 4 years were also present at 6 years of age (O'Connor and Rutter, 2000). Interestingly, behavioural abnormalities reported in these children are qualitatively similar to some seen in socially deprived non-human primates (Suomi, 1997). Motor stereotypies and self-stimulatory behaviours were observed, and indiscriminately friendly behaviour and insecure attachment were measured (Chisholm *et al.,* 1995).

Locus of Control of Orphans

The concept of locus of control provides a picture of the psychological situation of the orphans and the challenges it poses. It is used to show the relationship between the environment and individuals' assessment of their ability to deal with it and to adjust behaviour. Most orphans are at risk of being confronted by powerful cumulative and often negative social changes in their lives over which they have no personal control. Experiences in continuously adverse circumstances do not make life appear to be subject to control through one's own efforts (Lefcourt, 1976). Perceived lack of control produces a feeling of helplessness and loss of hope, and diminishes an individual's will power (Richter, 1959; Overmier and Seligman, 1967; Lefcourt, 1976). Death of parents makes children vulnerable and predisposes them to physical and psychological risks over which they have no control. The feeling of helplessness is very costly in terms of psychological well-being and may be reflected in lack of concern, involvement and vitality in social and school activities. Emotionally, it is indicated by sadness and depression. Sengendo and Nambi (1997) presented selected statistical evidence as children who headed their families were more externally oriented than those who lived with widowed mothers. Similarly, the child-headed families were more external than orphans living with grandparents. This is expected since being left all alone in the world is more depressing than being left in the hands of a mother or a grandparent. There is a need for increased intervention through therapeutic programmes for children living without adult care. Orphans with the surviving relatives have something from their past to cling to, while those without any surviving relative are left at the mercy of the environment. Hence the higher degree of externality is found among the child-headed families.

Conclusion

The present review exposes on the basis empirical researches done in this area that the orphans experience several risk factors to mental health and are vulnerable to mental illness due to increase in their emotional, behavioural and psychosocial problems. The government and community interventions need to be initiated to enhance the protective factors which lower the incidence of mental health risks. The orphanages should also start mental health enhancement and mental health problems prevention programmes for the betterment of the orphans. Finally, it should be realized that awareness of mental health problems among orphans at all levels should be built up. Responsible and cooperative attitudes of all members of society can make a big difference in improving their lives and in developing them into psychologically and economically productive adults.

References

Ames, E. (1997). *The Development of Romanian Orphanage Children Adopted to Canada* (Final Report to the National Welfare Grants Program: Human Resources Development Canada). Burnaby, British Columbia: Simon Fraser University.

Andresen, I.L. (1992). Behavioural and school adjustment of 12-13-year-old internationally adopted children in Norway: A research note. *Journal of Child Psychology and Psychiatry*, 33(2), 427-439.

Aslanian, S. (2006). *Researchers still learning from Romania's orphans*. Retrieved from http://www.npr.org/templates/story/story.php?storyId=6089477

Atwine, B., Cantor-Graae, E. and Bajunirwe, F. (2005). Psychological distress among AIDS orphans in rural Uganda. *Social Science and Medicine*, 61, 555-564.

Bayumova, S. (2001). *Friends of Russian Orphanage-Supporting Yaroslavl's children.* http://www.russianorphans.org/orphans_pyatyorka_essay.htm.

Bowlby, J. (1995). *Maternal care and mental health*, Geneva, WHO.

Brodzinsky, D.M., Gormly, A.V. and Ambron, S.R. (1986). *Lifespan Human Development* (3rd.) New York: CBS College Publishing.

Brown, J.D. and Siegal, J.M. (1988). Exercise as a buffer of life stress: A prospective study of adolescent health. *Health Psychology*, 7, 341-353.

Chan, A.A.L., Busam, K.J., Benvenuto-Andrade, C., Scope, A., Gil, M.,

Marghoob, A.A. and Halpern, A.C. (2006). Reflectance confocal microscopy of pigmented basal cell carcinoma. *J. Am. Acad. Dermatol*, 54(4): 638-643.

Chisholm, K., Carter, M.C., Ames, E.W., and Morison, S.J. (1995). Attachment security and indiscriminately friendly behaviour in children adopted from Romanian orphanages. *Dev. Psychopathol.* 7: 283-294.

Cluver, L., Gardner, F. and Operario, D. (2008). Effects of stigma and other community factors on the mental health of AIDS-orphaned children. *Journal of Adolescent Health,* 42, 410-417.

Coie, J.D., Watt, N.F., West. S.G., Hawkins, J.D., Asarnow, J.R., Markman, H.J., Ramey, S.L., Shure, M.B., and Long, B. (1993). The science of prevention: A conceptual framework and some directions for a national research programme. *American Psychologist*, 48, 1013-1022.

Donovan, J.E., Jessor, R., and Costa, F.M. (1988). Syndrome of problem behaviour in adolescence; A replication. *Journal of Consulting and Clinical Psychology*, 56, 762-765.

DosReis, S., Zito, J.M., Safer, D.J. and Soeken, K.L. (2001). Mental health services for youths in foster care and disables youth. *Am. J. Public Health*, 91(7): 1094-1099.

Dryfoos, J.G. (1990). *Adolescents at risk: Prevalence and Prevention*. New York: Oxford University Press.

Dunn, A., Hunter, S., Nabongo, C., Ssekiwanuka, J. (1991). Enumeration and Needs.

Fisher, L., Ames, E.W., Chisholm, K. and Savoie, L. (1997). Problems reported by parents of Romanian orphans adapted to British Columbia. *International Journal of Behavioural Development,* 20(1), 67-82.

Flank, D., Klass, P., Earls, F. and Eisenburg, L. (1996). Infant and young children in orphanages. *One view from pediatrics and child psychiatry*, 97 (4): 569-578.

Forehand, R., Steele, R., Armistead, L., Morse, E., Simon, P. and Clark, L. (1998). The Family Health Project: Psychosocial adjustment of children whose mothers are HIV infected. *Journal of Consulting and Clinical Psychology*, 66, 3, 513-520.

Foster, G. and Williamson, A. (2000). Review of the current literature on the impact of HIV/AIDS on Children in Sub-Saharan Africa. *AIDS*, 4 (4), 275-284.

Frederici, R. (2007). The neuropsychology of bonding and attachment disorders. Retrieved from http://www.rainbowkids.com/expertarticledetails.aspx?id=57

Freud, A., Solint, A. and Goldstein, H. (1973). *Beyond the best interest of the child*, London: Andre Deutsch.

Furukawa, T., Yokouchi, T., Hirai, T., Kitamura, T. and Takahashi, K. (1999). Parental loss in childhood and social support in adulthood among psychiatric patients. *Journal of Psychiatric Research,* 33, 165-169.

Getachew, H., Ambaw, F., Abebe, L., Kasahun, W. (2011). Psychological distress and its predictors in AIDS orphan adolescents in Addis Ababa city: A comparative survey. *J. Health Dev.,* 25(2): 135-142.

Goodwin, D.K. (1994). *No ordinary Times*, p. 416, Simon and Schuster, N.Y.

Gregory, I. (1958). Studies of Parental Deprivation in Psychiatric Patients. *American Journal of Psychiatry*, 115: 432-442.

Gregory, I. (1965). Anterospective Data following Childhood Loss of a Parent I and II. *Archives of General Psychiatry,* 13: 99-109, 110-120.

Groza, V. and Ryan, S.D. (2002). Pre-adoption stress and its association with child behaviour in domestic special needs, and international adoptions. *Psychoneuroendocrinology*, 27(1/2), 181-198.

Groze, V. and Ileana, D. (1996). A follow-up study of adopted children from Romania. *Child and Adolescent Social Work Journal*, 13(6), 541-565.

Gunnar, M.R. and Quevedo, K. (2007). The neurobiology of stress and development. *Annual Review of Psychology*, 58, 145-173.

Halfron, N., Zepeda, A. and Inkelas, M. (2002). *Mental health services for children in foster care*. UCLA Center for Healthier Children, Families and Communities, Los Angeles.

Hersor, L. (1980). The Seventh Jack Tizard Memorial Lecture: Aspects of Adoption. *J. Child Psychol Psychiatry*, 31(4): 493- 510.

Hoksbergen, R., Rijk, K., van Dijkum, C. and ter Laak, J. (2004). Adoption of Romanian children in the Netherlands: Behaviour problems and parenting burden of upbringing for adoptive parents. *Developmental and Behavioural Pediatrics*, 25(3), 175-180.

Hughes, D.A. (1999). *Building the bonds of attachment: awakening love in deeply troubled children*. Jason Aronson, London.

Human Rights Watch (2001), "In the Shadow of Death: HIV/AIDS and Children's Rights in Kenya, *Human Rights Watch Publications,* Vol. 13, No. 4(A), 17. [http://www.hrw.org/reports/2001/kenya/].

Hunter, S. and Williamson, J. (1997). *Children on the Brink: Strategies to Support Children Isolated* by HIV/ AIDS. USAID.

Irudayasamy, P. (2006). *Institute of research and development and rural poor*.

Johnson R., Browne K., and Hamilton-Giachritsis C. (2006). "Young children in institutional care at risk of harm," *Trauma, Violence, and Abuse*, Vol. 7, No. 1, 34-60.

Kazdin, A.E. (1991). *Prevention of conduct disorder. The prevention of mental disorders: Progress, problems, and prospects*. Washington, DC: National Institute of Mental Health.

Kreppner, J.M., O'Connor, T.G. and Rutter, M. (2001). Can inattention/over activity be an institutional deprivation syndrome? *Journal of Abnormal Child Psychology*, 29, 513-528.

Lachman, M.E. and Agrigoroaei, S. (2010). Promoting functional health in midlife and old age: Long-term protective effects of control beliefs, social support, and physical exercise. *PLoS ONE, 5*(10), e13297. doi:10.1371/journal.pone.0013297.

Lata, S. and Shukla, A. (2011). Social Skills Deficits in Young Orphan Girls. *Gorakhpur Social Scientist*, 2, 1, 42-50.

Lata, S. and Shukla, A. (2012). Psychosocial Environment of the Orphanage, *United Journal of Awadh Scholars*, 6, 2, 38-45.

Lata, S. and Verma, S. (2013). General Health and Psychosocial Adjustment of Orphan and Non-Orphan Children, *Indian Journal of Psychology*, Indian Psychological Association, Special Issue, 61-71.

Le Mare, L. and Audet, K. (2002). *Attention abilities of Romanian orphans ten years after being adopted to Canada*. Poster presented at the International Society for the Study of Behavioural Development, Ottawa, Ontario.

Lefcourt, H.M. (1976). *Locus of Control: Current Trends in Theory and Research*. Hillsdale: Lawrence Erlbaum Associates.

Luthar, S.S. and Zigler, E. (1992). Intelligence and social competence among high-risk adolescents. *Development and Psychopathology*, 4, 287-299.

Luthar, S.S. (1993). Annotation: Methodological and conceptual issues in research on childhood resilience. *Journal of Child Psychology and Psychiatry and Allied Disciplines*, 34, 441-452.

Makame, V., Ani, C. and Grantham-McGregor, S. (2002). Psychological well-being of orphans in Dar El Salaam, Tanzania. *Acta Paediatrica,* 91(4), 459-465.

Marcovitch, S., Cesaroni, L., Roberts, W. and Swanson, C. (1995). Romanian adoption: Parents' dreams, nightmares, and realities. *Child Welfare*, 74, 993-1017.

Marcovitch, S., Goldberg, S., Gold, A., Washington, J., Wasson, C., Krekewich, K., *et al.* (1997). Determinants of behavioural problems in Romanian children adopted in Ontario. *International Journal of Behavioural Development*, 20(1), 3-16.

Margoob, M.A, Rather, Y.H., Khan, A.Y., Singh, G.P., Malik, Y.A., Firdosi, M.M., and Ahmad, S.A. (2006). Psychiatric disorders among children living in orphanages—Experience from Kashmir. *JK-Practitioner*. 13 (Suppl. 1): S53-S55

Mbozi, P.S., Debit, M.B. and Munyati, S. (Eds), (2006). Psychosocial conditions of orphans and McKenzie R, 'Neglected solutions, orphanages may be preferable over foster families', *National Review*, 18, 1-5.

Mental Health Foundation (1999). *Bright futures*. London: MHF. www.mentalhealth.org.uk

Minde, K. (1988). The effects of social change on the behaviour and academic performance of school age children. Unpublished paper.

Morissett, C.E., Barnard, K.E., Greenberg, M.T., Booth, C.L. and Spieker, S.J. (1990). Environmental influences on early language development: The context of social risk. *Development and Psychopathology*, 2, 127-149.

Naqshbandi, M.M., Sehgal, R., Hassan, F. (2012). Orphans in orphanages of Kashmir "and their Psychological problems". *International NGO Journal,* 7(3), 55-63.

National Statistician Welcomes Statistics and Registration Service Bill (2000) news release from ONS website.

Nyamukapa, C., Gregson, S., Lopman, B., Saito, S., Watts, H., Monasch, R. and Jukes, MC. (2008). HIV-associated orphanhood and children's psychosocial distress: Theoretical framework tested with data from Zimbabwe. *Amercian Journal of Public Health*, 98, 133-141.

Nyblade, L., Pande, R., Mathur, S., MacQuarrie, K., Kidd, R. and Banteyerga, H. (2003). *Disentangling HIV and AIDS stigma in Ethiopia, Tanzania and Zambia*. Available at <http://www.icrw.org/docs/stigmareport093003.pdf>.

O'Connor, T.G. and Rutter, M. (2000). Attachment disorder behaviour following early severe deprivation: Extension and longitudinal follow-up. *J. Am. Acad. Child. Adolesc. Psychiatry* 39: 703-712.

Olley, B.O. (2008). Health and Behavioural Problems of Children Orphaned by AIDS as Reported by their Caregivers in Abuja, Nigeria. *Nigerian Journal of Psychiatry*, 6 (2) 20: 70-75.

Overmier, J.B. and Seligman, M.E.P. (1967). Effects of inescapable shock upon subsequent escape and avoidance responding. *Journal of Comparative and Physiological Psychology*, 63:23-33.

Paris, J., Zweig-Frank, H. and Guzder, J. (1994). Risk factors for borderline personality in male outpatients. *Journal of Nervous and Mental Disease*, 182, 375-380.

Pharaoh, R. (2004). *A Generation at Risk? HIV/AIDS, vulnerable children and security in Southern Africa*. Pretoria: Institute for Security Studies.

Pridmore, P. and Yates, C. (2005). Combating AIDS in South Africa and Mozambique: the role of open, distance, and flexible learning (ODFL). *Comparative Education Review*, 49(4), 490-511.

Richter, C.P.I. (1959). The phenomenon of unexplained sudden death in animals and man. In *The Meaning of Death*, (ed.) H. Feifel. New York: McGraw-Hill.

Ruchkin, V., Gilliam, W. and Mayes, L. (2008). Developmental pathway modelling in considering behaviour problems in young Russian children. *Child Psychiatry and Human Development*, 39, 49-66.

Rutter, M. (1985). Resilience in the face of adversity: Protective factors and resistance to psychiatric disorder. *British Journal of Psychiatry*, 147, 598-611.

Rutter, M. (1998). Developmental catch-up, and deficit, following adoption after severe global early privation. English and Romanian Adoptees (ERA) Study Team. *J. Child Psychol. Psychiatry*, 39: 465-476.

Salaam, T. (2005). *AIDS Orphans and Vulnerable Children (OVC): Problems, Responses, and Issues for Congress*. CRS Report for Congress Received through the CRS Web. Congressional Research Service, The Library of Congress.

Sameroff, A. (2000). Developmental systems and psychopathology. *Development and Psychopathology*, 12, 297-312.

Sameroff, A., Bartko, W., Baldwin, A., Baldwin, C. and Seifer, R. (1998). Family and social influences on the development of child competence. In M. Lewis & C. Feiring (Eds.), *Families, risk, and competence*. Mahwah, New Jersey: Lawrence Erlbaum Associates.

Sengendo, J. and Nambi, J. (1997). The psychological effect of orphanhood: A study of orphans in Rakai district. *Health Transition Review*, 7 (Suppl), 105-124.

Simms, M.D., Dubowitz. H. and Szilagyi, M.A. (2000). Health care needs for children in the foster care system. *Pediatrics*, 106 (4): 909-918.

St. Petersburg-USA Orphanage Research Team. (2005). Characteristics of children, caregivers, and orphanages for young children in St. Petersburg, Russian Federation. *Journal of Applied Developmental Psychology:* Child Abandonment, Special Issue. Vulnerable children in two Zimbabwean Districts. HSRC Press, Cape Town, South Africa.

Stevens, S.E., Sonuga-Barke, E.S., Kreppner, J.M., Beckett, C., Castle, J., Colvert, E., Groothues, C., Hawkins, A. and Rutter, M. (2007). Inattention/ overactivity following early severe institutional deprivation: Presentation and associations in early adolescence. *Journal of Abnormal Child Psychology.*

Suffering in Silence: The Links between Human Rights Abuses and HIV Transmission to Girls in Zambia, a Human Rights Watch report released in November 2002, discusses the sexual vulnerabilities of young girls, [http://www.hrw.org/reports/2003/zambia/zambia1202.pdf].

Suomi, S.J. (1997). Early determinants of behaviour: Evidence from primate studies. *Br. Med. Bull.* 53: 170-184.

The Effects of Institutionalization on Children available at http://haberdasher.hubpages.com/hub/The-Effects-of-Institutionalization-on-Children.

The World Federation for Mental Health (2003). World Mental Health Day: Emotional and behavioural disorders of children and adolescents. USA: WFfMH.

Trout, A.L., Casey, K., Chmelka, M.B., DeSalvo, C., Reid, R. and Epstein, M.H. (2009). "Overlooked: children with disabilities in residential care," *Child Welfare*, 88, 2, 111-136.

Tweed, J.L., Schoenbach, V.J., George, L.K. and Blazer, D.G. (1989). The effects of childhood parental death and divorce on six-month history of anxiety disorders. *British Journal of Psychiatry,* 154, 823-828.

Tyrer, R. (2010). *Psychological distress amongst orphaned, neglected and formet street children in institutional care home in Arusha*, Tanzania. University of Lincoln. 1-39.

UN Office for the Coordination of Humanitarian Affairs, "Botswana: AIDS Orphans Exploited," October 8, 2003, [http://www.irinnews.org/AIDSreport.asp?ReportID=1477].

Ungar, M., Brown, M., Liebenberg, L., Othman, R., Kwong, W.M., Armstrong, M. and Gilgun, J. (2004) 'Unique pathways to resi ›nce across cultures', *Adolescence*, 42 (166), 287-310.

Van Eerdewegh, M.M., M.D. Bieri, R.H., Parrilla and Clayton, P.J. (1982). The Bereaved Child. *British Journal of Psychiatry*, 140, 23-29.

Verhulst, F.C., Althaus, M. and Versluis-den Bieman, H.J. (1990b). Problem behaviour in international adoptees: II. Age at placement. *Journal of the American Academy of Child and Adolescent Psychiatry,* 29(1), 104-111.

Verhulst, F.C., Althaus, M. and Versluis-den Bieman, H.J. (1992). Damaging backgrounds: Later adjustment of international adoptees. *Journal of the American Academy of Child and Adolescent Psychiatry,* 31(3), 518-524.

Werner, E. (2000). Protective factors and individual resilience. In J. Shonkoff & S. Meisels (Eds.), *Handbook of Early Childhood Intervention, 2nd Edition* (pp. 115-132). NY: Cambridge University Press.

Wild, J. (2002). The psychological adjustment of children orphaned by AIDS, Southern African. *Journal of Child and Adolescent Mental Health,* 13, pp. 3-22.

Wolff, P.H. and Fesseha, G. (1998). The orphans of eritrea: are orphanages part of the problem or part of the solution. *Am. J. of Psychiatry,* 155(10): 1319-1324.

Worden, J.W. (1996). *Children and Grief: When a Parent Dies*. N.Y.: The Guilford Press, 10012.

World Health Organization (1999). *Strengthening Mental Health Promotion* accessed 14/08/2003 from www.who.int/inf-fs/en/fact220.html

World Health Organization (2003). *Investing in mental health Geneva: World Health Organization* http://www.who.int/mental health/media/investing_mnh.pdf

Zeanah, C. and Zeanah, P. (2001). Towards a definition of infant mental health. *Zero To Three,* 22, 13-20.

Zeanah, C., Boris, N., and Larrieu, J. (1997). Infant development and developmental risk: A review of the past 10 years. *Journal of the American Academy of Child and Adolescent Psychiatry,* 36, 165-178.

8

Common Mental Disorders and Etiology in Childhood and Adolescence

Neelam Verma

Child psychiatry has been the focus of interest since decades in the field of mental health. This discipline has progressed rapidly in past some years and significant work is being done by the clinicians and the young researchers to make improvements in the current available literature and more importantly availing the society by using best treatment modalities. Usually child and adolescent psychopathology can be detected by observing one's overt behaviours, emotional states, and quality of interpersonal relations along with adequate use of cognitive functions. If any of the area attracts the attention of family members and teachers, it calls for a professional help; especially, when the observed behaviours interfere with the development of one or more areas like peer relationships, parental contact, school performance, classroom behaviours, emotional control, appearance in the community, good utilization of leisure time and sense of identity.

Childhood and adolescent mental health issues manifest widely ranging from emotional, behavioural and thinking difficulties; however, they broadly fall in to the two major categories, i.e. internalizing and externalizing problems. Both the terms symbolically represent the manifestation of symptoms in a particular disorder. The internalizing problems are usually related to the factors where symptoms are exhibited in terms of emotional, thinking and somatic difficulties. On the other hand externalizing problems usually represent marked behavioural problems like excessive aggression, hyperactivity, delinquency and other conduct issues. There is possibility of children showing both the patterns simultaneously and carry out the symptoms till adulthood in some form or the other.

Disorders of psychological development usually have an onset during infancy or childhood and they possess delay or impairment in functional developments related to central nervous system and other biological maturation processes. Most of the cases show functional impairments like language, visuo-spatial skills and motor coordination. Usually the history of delays and impairments is evident in early years. This category of disorders includes:

- Specific Developmental Disorder of Speech and Language;
- Specific Developmental Disorder of Scholastic Skills;
- Specific Developmental Disorder of Motor Functions;
- Mixed Specific Developmental Disorder;
- Pervasive Developmental Disorders;
- Other Disorders of Psychological Development; and
- Unspecified Disorder of Psychological Development.

Behavioural and emotional disorder with onset usually occurring in childhood and adolescence are mainly characterized by manifestation of symptoms that are purely behavioural and emotional in nature. This category includes:

- Hyperkinetic Disorder;
- Conduct Disorder;
- Mixed Disorder of Conduct and Emotions;
- Emotional Disorder with Onset Specific to Childhood;
- Disorder of Social Functioning and Onset Specific to Childhood and Adolescence;
- Tic Disorders;
- Other Behavioural and Emotional Disorders with Onset Usually Occurring Childhood and Adolescence; and
- Mental Disorders Not Otherwise Specified.

Above classification of disorders based on ICD-10 criteria differs slightly from DSM-IV criteria of childhood and adolescent disorders. DSM-IV classifies these disorders as disorders usually first diagnosed in infancy, childhood and adolescence; however, it is not necessary that the disorders classified here must be diagnosed in this age only and also apart from these disorders no other disorder can be diagnosed at the specified age. Disorders usually diagnosed in adulthood may occur at this age and disorder usually occurring in childhood may remain undetected till adulthood. As per DSM-IV classification this category includes:

- Mental Retardation;
- Learning Disorders;
- Motor Skills Disorder;
- Communication Disorder;
- Pervasive Developmental Disorder;
- Attention Deficit and Disruptive Behaviour Disorder Involving Conduct and Oppositional Defiant Disorder;
- Feeding and Eating Disorder of Infancy and Childhood;
- Tic Disorder;
- Elimination Disorder; and
- Other Disorders of Infancy, Childhood or Adolescence including Separation Anxiety Disorder.

There is a wide range of psychiatric disorders that has specific onset during childhood and adolescence. The labelling of disorders differs in ICD and DSM classification systems; however, the manifestation of symptoms is far more common in both. In this chapter, only the major disorders will be discussed along with their etiological factors that contribute to the specific clinical condition. The inclusion of specific disorders here is based on their reporting frequencies in clinical set-ups, i.e. only the major disorders have been included here in this chapter. For better understanding of readers all the risk factors of such conditions have been accommodated in the following table:

Personal Risk Factors	*Primary Environmental/ Familial Risk Factors*	*Cultural/Societal Risk Factors*
• Genetic Vulnerability • Developmental Delays • Medical Illness • Neurological conditions • Scholastic failure/ Underachievement • Learning disabilities • Temperamental issues • Low Self-esteem	• Single parenting • Parental separation/ divorce • Faulty child rearing practices • Family breakdown • Child abuse (physical, sexual, emotional) • Family member with psychiatric or terminal illness • Death of loved one leading to grief and bereavement	• Lack of social support • Low socio-economic status • Homelessness • Natural Disasters • Racial Discrimination • Lack of facilities for basic needs • Bullying behaviour of peers

Learning Disorders

Inclusion of learning disorders has been a controversial issue between the psychiatric stream and those working as speech-language pathologists and educational therapists. According to the educational therapists and speech-language pathologists, these disorders should not be included in the classification system of clinical disorders as they do not contain actual psychiatric syndrome. However, the representation of such disorders is compatible with the underlying general definition of DSM-IV, i.e. "*a clinically significant behavioural or psychological syndrome or pattern that occurs in an individual and that is associated with present distress ...or disability...or with a significantly increased risk of suffering.*" According to this explanation learning disorders are very much associated with the disability, distress and increase risk of suffering, thus have been included in the current classification system.

Learning disabilities possesses disturbance in the normal pattern of skill acquisition evident from early developmental stages. These disorders are a consequence of abnormalities in cognitive processing largely derived from some kind of biological disturbance. The presentation of learning disorders involve impaired reading skills, writing difficulties with problems in written expression, inability to understand mathematical basics and difficult to comprehend the read material. It is essential to know that diagnosis of learning disability is made only when there is absence of or the condition is not associated with any significant intellectual deficit, lack of stimulation and opportunity to learn and any kind of brain trauma or neurological disease. To make a diagnosis of learning disability it is essential that—

- Specific scholastic skill must possess significant degree of impairment, i.e. deterioration of at least two grades below of current academic level.
- The impairment should not be solely explained by the mental retardation.
- The impairment must be developmental, i.e. presence of poor performance in early academic years.
- There should be absence of any external factors that can explain the academic difficulties and poor scholastic performance.

Learning disabilities are often associated with other clinical conditions and co-morbidity exists with Attention Deficit Hyperactivity

Disorder (ADHD), Conduct Disorder, Depressive Disorder, and Anxiety Disorder. Individuals with learning disorders may suffer from low self-esteem/confidence and poor social skills leading to maladjustment in personal, academic and social areas. Learning disorders are classified in the following categories:

Specific Reading Disorder

Reading disorder is specifically related to impairment in reading skills characterized by slow rate of reading, hesitations, wrong pronunciations, inaccurate phrasing, ignoring punctuations, and reversals of words in sentences or of letters within words. In addition, they may have poor comprehension characterized by inability to recall facts of the text read and use of previous experience or knowledge as background information. Children with reading disorder exhibit problem in word recognition; however, the pattern to recognize a word is far more common in both types of children, i.e. those who suffer from reading disorder and those who are normal readers. Both of them primarily rely upon phonological cues and contextual information to detect the word and it increases the possibility of struggling with the recognition of low frequency words.

Reading disorder is often found to be associated with conditions mostly related to other categories of learning disorders itself and speech and language disorders. In addition, some of the cognitive skills may also be impaired like attention, memory, visuo-spatial skills etc.

Specific Disorder of Arithmetic Skills or Mathematics Disorder

This disorder involves impairment of arithmetical or mathematical skills with no connection to mental retardation, inadequate schooling or inadequate teaching methods, visual or auditory impairment, neurological illness or psychiatric co-morbidity. The onset of problem is not decided; however, most of the cases are detected in late years of schooling as they manage to perform in early schooling years but fail to perform on graded difficulty tasks. Most of the symptoms of this disorder fall into four major clusters:

1. The **Linguistic Symptoms** include difficulty in understanding and naming mathematical terms, procedural or operational difficulties while solving the problems and decoding mathematical symbols.

2. The **Perceptual Symptoms** include difficulty to recognize mathematical signs and symbols along with impaired skill to identify numbers. It also includes difficulty to organize objects in a cluster along with impaired ability of aligning and ordering strings of numbers.
3. The **Mathematical Symptoms** are characterized by inability to learn, memorize and follow mathematical operations resulting in poor performance while doing basic arithmetical tasks. Learning the multiplication tables is usually a hard task for such individuals and they mostly develop an elaborative method to avoid multiplications. Since the methods are elaborative they involve more steps and increase the likelihood of committing more errors.
4. The **Attentional Symptoms** of this disorder majorly involve errors characterized by omissions of digits and mathematical symbols while solving mathematical problems. There may also be errors related to copying numbers and forgetting the carried numbers while performing sums.

Disorder of Written Expression

This disorder have been frequently found to be associated with other disorders of language and learning and majorly exhibit signs of poorly structured sentences characterized by spelling mistakes, wrong use of grammatical rules and punctuation errors. The disorder causes significant impairment in scholastic performance of the individual which is not attributed to any neurological/psychiatric condition, visual or hearing impairment, mental retardation and lack of stimulation at home and school. The most characteristic features of this disorder are impairment in the ability to compose written text. This may include grammatical mistakes, inability to write down correct spellings of the words, excessively poor and slow handwriting, significant punctuation errors along with wrong capitalizations. Written expression may be poor in terms of thematic presentation of the text.

Usually, the grammatical and syntactical errors in the written text of such individuals involve wrong choice of words, omission of important words that add to the meaning and syntactic quality of sentence, wrong order of word presentation in a sentence, incorrect use of verbs or pronoun and they might end up the sentence with an inappropriate word. The major writing mechanics, i.e. punctuation and capitalization may appear faulty in writings. Poor handwriting with excessive crudeness in formation of alphabets is another sign of this disorder. It does not include messy writing rather a combination of letter formations that are difficult to decode, inversion and rotation of letters, mixture of different styles of writing like block or cursive and inappropriate mixture of capital and small letters. Poor composition of text while writing imaginary stories is also an essential feature of this disorder characterized by two major components, one is inadequate development of story components such as theme, character, scene setting etc. and other is poor cohesion such as transitional errors in dramatic scenes and abrupt ending of the story.

Specific Spelling Disorder

The main feature of the disorder possesses significant impairment in the development of spelling skills. In this disorder, the ability to write a word with correct spelling and spell it out verbally both are impaired and errors may be noted in both the conditions. The condition may be caused by difficulty to use phonetic cues adequately. To be diagnosed in this specific category the performance on individually administered test of spelling should be below the expected level. Also the condition should not be a result of mental retardation, visual acuity problem, hearing problem, any neurological or psychiatric condition and inadequate teaching or lack of stimulation in school. Those having symptoms of reading and writing disorder should not be categorized under this category; this category solely belongs to impairment in development of spelling skills.

In some cases, symptoms of all types of learning disorders may be present and it may be difficult for the examiner to differentiate or categorize the symptoms in one single disorder. Diagnosis of this disorder may be adequately done by using individual tests and their comparative score on each domain.

Etiology of Learning Disorders: Etiology of learning disorders is again a controversial issue and the factors that cause the condition are still not well defined. Most of the researchers have identified the correlational factors rather than the causal factors.

Etiology of Reading Disorders: It has been described as neurobiological disorder that seems to have a genetic origin. It is found that those having reading disorder have difficulty in phonetic understanding of the words or have difficulty to process sounds. Since the condition is associated with language the MRI findings have suggested disturbed temporal lobe functioning. Genetic factors have been found to have a strong relation with development of this disorder and those with the family history of this disorder in first degree relatives are at greater risk. Particular chromosomes could be identified in the studies that contribute to the ability to decode sounds, identify words; phonological awareness etc. Positive correlation has been found between reading disorder and left handedness, left-handedness and mixed laterality. Neuropsychological assessment findings have revealed significant deficits in working memory of such children. The prenatal period also has an impact on this condition as any history of infection during pregnancy like influenza or alcohol induced fetal damage has been found to have a strong relation to this condition. Many co-morbid conditions have been found to be correlated with reading disorder such as cerebral palsy, epileptic children with normal IQ and neurological conditions like lesion in left occipital lobe leading to visual field blindness.

Etiology of Mathematics Disorder: Like reading disorder this condition is likely to be less correlated with the genetic factors. They rather seem to be correlated with the neurological processing and environmental factors. Research findings have suggested that the amount and quality of stimulation and instructions plays an important role in development of arithmetic skills. The neurological findings suggested deficit in occipital lobe of right cerebral hemisphere that are responsible for information processing of visual spatial stimuli and also major part of mathematical skills. Generally, the cause of mathematics disorder is explained as a multi-factorial thing which combines maturational, emotional and cognitive factors together responsible for the condition.

Etiology of Writing Disorder: The etiology of writing disorder supports the causal factors of reading disorder and strongly relates to genetic factors. Findings have supported the importance of genetic loading and deficit in use of language components adequately.

Pervasive Developmental Disorders (PDD)

Pervasive Developmental Disorders are mainly a composite of impairments in individual's developmental areas and the impairments are distinctly deviant to the developmental age of the individual. The composite of such disorders involves impairment in reciprocity in interactive skills, communication disturbances or lack of communication skills and behaviours associated with unusual interests, activities and stereotypical behaviours. The description of categories of this disorder is as follows:

Autistic Disorder: Autistic Disorder is often called as ***Early Infantile Autism, Childhood Autism or Kanner's Autism***. It is a condition characterized by three major symptoms or essential conditions:

1. **Significant Impairment in Social Interactions or Poor Interactional Skills:** This condition involves inability to use social cues while interacting with others and inability to use non-verbal behaviours that improve quality of social interactions like eye to eye contact, facial expressions, gestures and posture etc. due to the same impairments such individuals are unable to make peer groups as compared to other children of similar age group. Social reciprocity may be lacking in such individuals and they may not enjoy active participation in social activity or games played by other children. Usually they enjoy self play and solitary activities. There may be inability to judge emotional states of others and they may not react on emotional reactions of others.
2. **Qualitative Impairment in Communication Skills:** This condition is associated with late or less development of language and speech functions. Those who use language for communication may exhibit specific ways of using it like idiosyncratic language with stereotyped and repetitive patterns. Tone of voice may be monotonous and grammatical structure of language may be immature specific to age. There may be repetitive use of certain words of phrases regardless of context and it may appear inappropriate in a situation. Similar to the production of language, understanding of the language is also impaired. Usually such individuals have poor comprehension or may have delayed response for verbal instructions. Usually the games enjoyed by normal children are typically performed in mechanical ways without any enjoyment by such individuals.
3. **Stereotyped and Restricted Patterns of Behaviour along with Unusual Interests and Activities:** These individuals are usually rigid in following routines. There may be difficulty in adjusting with changed routines. Overall the flexibility to adapt changes is missing and they are preoccupied with one or more interests or restricted patterns of behaviours. Rigidity may be evident while following a route and difficulty to change it. Some stereotyped body movements are other typical symptoms of this condition and may be exhibited as clapping, rocking, dipping, and walking

on tip of toes, odd body postures, frequent finger flicking or hand flapping. They may also enjoy specific movements like spinning of wheels or liking for toys having wheels or any other movement with rapidity. Typical ways of seeing the objects may be seen or there may be interest in seeing specific parts of objects rather than the whole. In some cases, attachment with inanimate objects may be seen or they might be fond of them.

In ICD-10 the disorder has been labelled as **Childhood Autism**. Symptoms of autism are evident or detected under the age of three years. In some cases there may be normal development of language but deterioration is reported within three years. In some cases the condition may be evident only after the mentioned age and also the three major components of autism may be missing. Usually those with profound mental retardation have less scope to exhibit such symptoms due to poor functioning. Since the condition is little different from Autistic disorder; thus labelled as **Atypical Autism**.

Rett's Disorder: The condition is termed as Rett's Syndrome in ICD-10 which is mainly characterized by normal development in the prenatal and perinatal period. Individuals with this disorder achieve normal psychomotor growth till the first five years of life. Usually the head circumference is within the normal limit at the time of birth; however, there is evident deceleration in head growth between the ages of 5 to 48 months. Similarly, the acquired hand movement skills are deteriorated and subsequently the individual develops stereotyped hand movements such as wringing, stereotypical wetting of hands with saliva, hyperventilation, inability to achieve or maintain bladder control, excessive drooling etc. Loss of interest in social environment is evident under the first five years; however, it may develop later in life. There may be presence of "social smile"; however, the social interaction is often lacking. Significant disturbances in psychomotor coordination and gait-trunk movement are evident along with impaired development of both receptive and expressive language. The condition lasts through out the life and usually the deterioration in acquired skills is progressive and persistent. Development of epileptic attacks may be seen in majority of cases before the age of 8 years. The condition differs from autism in terms of absence of self-injurious and stereotypical behaviours along with rare preoccupations with routines.

Childhood Disintegrative Disorder: The Childhood Disintegrative Disorder is mainly characterized by normal development till the age of two years and marked deterioration in acquired skills after this age (under the age of three years). In this disorder, the development related to verbal and non-verbal communication, social relationships, play behaviours, bowel-bladder control and motor skills etc. are found to be normal till two years of age. Apparently there is marked regression in the mentioned acquired skills. Often there may be a period of irritability, over activity and vague illness. The condition is highly regressive and most people are left with severe to profound retardation. In some cases the condition may appear like dementia in adults; however, there is clear demarcation in both the conditions based on the absence of organic disorder or damage and possibility of some degree of recovery in deteriorated skills.

Asperger's Disorder: The condition is essentially characterized by significant impairments in social interactional skills and development of repetitive, restricted behaviours with unusual interests and activities. The condition differs from autism in terms of development of language functions. The condition possesses no significant delays in acquisition of language functions and cognitive development. The impairments in social interactions are so gross that they interfere with the socio-occupational functioning of the individual. It may create problems in establishing social relations or peer group. Younger individuals may have little or no interest in developing friendships whereas older individuals with this condition may find it difficult to understand social cues. The presentation of symptoms in Asperger's disorder is far more common as in autistic disorder; however, the condition differs from it in terms of absence of delay in the development of speech functions and use of language. Cognitive functions are usually normal; however, mild retardation in intellectual functioning may be present. There may be strong command on vocabulary with good verbal ability and not so good performance abilities.

Etiology of Pervasive Developmental Disorders

The etiology of pervasive developmental disorders is still in the process of identification and no such evidences have been given that explain the actual causal factors which lead to the condition. With less evidences researchers have explained the causes using various theoretical models as follows:

Biological Theories: Some disturbance in the central nervous system that contributes to the condition of PDDs. Overall the genetic factors, perinatal factors, models of neuro anatomy and neurochemical hypothesis has been a part of biological factors and most of the researches have been based on the mentioned factors. Twin studies of autistic children have shown a higher rate of possibility of the disorder in monozygotic twins as compared to dizygotic twins. The studies have also shown some correlation of autistic children with fragile X syndrome. Siblings of such children who born after the disabled child are at risk of developing symptoms of this disorder majorly the cognitive deficits. The perinatal factors included the period of pregnancy where the findings suggested that fetal distress and use of inappropriate medications by mother can adversely affect the condition. The models of neuroanatomy have explained specific areas of brain dysfunctions found to be correlated with pervasive developmental disorders, mainly autism. The language abnormalities have been found to be associated with impairment in left hemisphere. The neurochemeical hypothesis has shown importance of some neuro-chemicals like dopamine, serotonin and endogenous opioids. The disturbance in the secretion and functioning of these neuron chemicals might be related with the pervasive developmental disorders. It has been found that those with history of viral infections like congenital rubella or any other infection in the postnatal period are at risk of the disorder.

Psychosocial Theories: The psychosocial theories and models suggested concept of "emotional refrigeration". The concept explains inadequate parenting in terms of lack of emotional expression such as lack of responsiveness, warmth, affectionate unresponsiveness while interacting with the child.

Cognitive Theories: The cognitive theories support the presence of cognitive deficits that may account for the condition. Major work in the field has been done on autistic children and researchers have found that children with this condition have difficulty in encoding, sequencing and abstract abilities. Lack of understanding of social cues leads to difficulty in social responsiveness and they seem to possess a condition of mind blind. Subsequently, they face difficulty to form cognitive representations of mental states. Since these children have unusual interest and do not participate in activities requiring joint attention they do not process the information related to emotion and its correlation to facial expression resulting in inappropriate or no response for emotional stimulus. Findings have also suggested deficit in episodic autobiographical memory of such individuals and they face difficulty correlating the events with themselves. Information input difficulties may lead to poor problem solving skills and also correlates to lack of central coherence. They seem to have a bottom up processing of information rather than using top-down information processing.

All the theories and explanations of etiology of pervasive developmental disorders have given the correlation factors of the condition rather than the actual causal factors.

Attention Deficit Hyperactivity Disorder (ADHD)

Attention deficit/hyperactivity disorder is mainly characterized by three major symptoms that are known as the triad of ADHD. The triad comprises clustering of three main components or symptoms of this disorder, i.e. (a) inattention, (b) hyperactivity, and (c) impulsivity.

In ADHD the behaviours are severe in nature and the frequency of such behaviours is quite higher than other children of comparable age group. The behaviours are so persistent and difficult to manage as they are displayed not only in the home environment but also in school settings and neighbourhood. The symptoms are so prominent to influence the socio-occupational functioning of the child and lead to impairment in developmental areas. Most of the symptoms are detected in the early years of schooling when children fail to perform well in the academics due to interference caused by symptoms, yet they are assumed to be present before the age of seven years. It is important here to understand the components of this disorder separately and the description is given below:

Inattention: Inattention can interfere with the functioning mainly concerned with the school work and home assignments. Children with ADHD may fail to give attention to smaller details of any task and may commit careless mistakes, their work is found to be messy with lot of errors in the writings, they find it difficult to persist with the task till the end of it even in the play activities, they keep shifting their activities and appear indulged in their own thoughts and most of the times leave tasks unaccomplished, they often do not follow the commands adequately due to poor attention and as a result fail to finish home assignments, play group activities or other duties.

Attention problems may be accompanied by difficulty to focus or sustained attention. In case of difficulty with sustained attention planning and organizing activities may be poor. They might find it unpleasant to participate in tasks requiring sustained mental activities or abilities. Such individuals are easily distracted by irrelevant external stimuli (like background conversations, others passing through the room or somebody talking outside the room, etc.) that are usually ignored by other healthy individuals. They may find it difficult to carry out social conversations as they do not listen to others carefully, and they might shift the topics of discussion during conversation as they don't pay attention on the ongoing topic. Children suffering from ADHD often exhibit behaviours lead by forgetfulness like not carrying notebooks according to schedule, forgetting to bring their lunch boxes, forgetting test schedules and not bringing necessary stationary material etc. the diagnosis should be made only in the case when the impairments are not accountable by understanding difficulty to follow instructions or any oppositional attitudes.

Hyperactivity: Hyperactivity in the disorder is mainly concerned with performing overactive behaviours at inappropriate places. It may be driven by a motor activity or excessive talking. This particular symptom may vary in young children, toddlers and preschooler. Usually most of the children of early school years show difficulty sitting in classroom for long time and may indulge in playing and talking to other children but in less frequency. Whereas in children with significant hyperactive component frequent fidgeting behaviours are seen. They find it difficult to remain seated, difficulty in playing quietly or engaging in any other constructive activity. These children are observed to be always on the go like jumping, running all over the place, climbing at inappropriate places and taking frequent seat breaks. When instructed strictly to sit quiet, they exhibit frequent fidgeting with objects, tapping and flapping hands or legs, squirming etc. when hyperactivity persists till adolescence or adulthood, it may be manifested in the form of restlessness and difficulty to perform tasks requiring sustained mental abilities.

Impulsivity: Such individuals are markedly impatient to wait for their turns whether it is required in play activities, other day-to-day activities or in conversations. In social conversations they find themselves unable to wait for their turn to give answer and they may start talking before the other person finishes the question. While playing activities they may keep touching the things kept around, snatching and grabbing toys of other children. Behaviours are manifested in day-to-day activities that may lead to accidents like touching hot pots, putting finger in the running fan, touching electric appliances passing current, running all over the place and slipping on the floor, climbing on things that are dangerous etc. Usually the behaviours are performed without knowing the potential dangerous result of the activity.

Etiology of ADHD

The research findings have suggested correlates of genetic,

neurobiological and neurochemical basis for ADHD; however, no researches have proved that the identified factors lead to development of ADHD.

Genetic Factors: The twin studies have indicated high concordance rate in monozygotic twins as compared to dizygotic twins. The possibility of genetic loading is also high in the first degree relatives. It has been found in the family studies that children with ADHD may have a parental history of alcohol use disorder and anti-social personality disorder; therefore, they have high chances of developing conduct problems in childhood.

Neurological and Neurochemical Factors: It has been found that in prenatal period children with ADHD has subtle damage to central nervous system. The brain damage caused by this condition may be a result of infection, inflammation, trauma etc. it has been noted that children with ADHD exhibit soft neurological signs at increased rate as compared to those in the normal population. The neurotransmitter hypothesis has explained the condition on the basis of dysfunction in the adrenergic and dopaminergic system.

Neuro-physiological Factors: These factors are the conditions related to sequence of maturation and growth. Those who have maturation delays exhibit symptoms of ADHD that normalizes after some time. The findings have supported increased beta band percentage and decreased delta band percentage to be an important contributor of this condition identified by EEG reports. PET results have explained the condition on the basis of lower cerebral blood flow and metabolic rates in frontal lobe areas of children with ADHD.

Environmental/Acquired Factors: Variety of brain insults such as perinatal and neonatal hypoxia and other obstetrical trauma have been found to be associated with risk of developing ADHD. The most subtle type of brain insult has been hypothesized caused by dietary influences named as "Dietary Deficiency Hypothesis". The hypothesis states that the individuals with ADHD have a constitutional need for increased doses of vitamins than the identified recommended allowance.

Psycho-Social Factors: These factors support the fact that those who have been living in the institutions have poor attention span and overactive. The symptoms result from prolonged conditions of emotional deprivation which may cause stressful life situations, anxiety etc. that may be controlled when the deprivation is removed either by keeping them in foster care or by adoption. Predisposing factors or temperamental characteristics may also be a contributing factor for this condition. Studies indicated that children who had maternal deprivation showed more hyperactive behaviours.

Interactive Additive Model

The need for this model rose because of no factual evidences of etiology of this disorder. The model explains that how the symptoms of ADHD exacerbate by stress, unstructured situations and complex demands of performance at home. The model explains that the children or individuals with genetic predispositions are susceptible to the stressors, on the contrary, those with the extreme genetic loading are likely to exhibit the symptoms/disorder in more supportive situations or environment. The valuable part of the model is that it promotes comprehensive formulation of the disorder thus a comprehensive treatment plan for rehabilitation.

Conduct Disorder

Conduct disorder is essentially featured by repetitive and persistent behavioural patterns violating basic rights of others and rules of age appropriate societal norms. The dissocial, defiant and aggressive tendencies are so prominent that they differ from the ordinary mischief and rebellion tendencies shown by children and adolescents. The behaviours may be manifested towards humans or animals. Conduct behaviours may be sub-grouped into the following four categories:

1. **Aggressive Conduct** is mainly characterized by performing or threats of performing physical harm towards people or animals. Such children or adolescents may react aggressively on others. Their tendencies often lead to intimidating, bullying and threatening behaviours. They appear physically cruel towards people or animals by stealing precious belongings of others like snatching chain or purse, armed robbery etc. and performing serious physical assaults, for example hitting them by using knife, brick, glass or any other kind of weapon.
2. **Non-Aggressive Conduct** is mainly characterized by the acts or behaviours that are harmful but does not involve any physical aggression towards people or animals. It involves damaging the belongings of others. It may involve serious damage or loss of property in terms of car smashing, breaking windows, school vandalism and fire setting.
3. **Theft or Deceitfulness** involves stealing by forcefully breaking in to someone's home, building or car. They often lie to avoid obligations and observed often be indulged in shoplifting behaviours.

4. **Serious Violation of Age Appropriate Societal Rules** involve going for night outs despite of familial prohibitions, frequent tendency to run away from home, truancy from school or being absent from duties without any genuine reason.

When the symptoms are present prior to the age of 10 years the disorder is likely to have "**Childhood Onset Type**" whereas the absence of symptoms prior to age ten years yet evident in the adolescence is said to have an "**Adolescent Onset Type**". In some cases the age of onset may not be identified or difficult to establish. For such cases the onset is said to be "**Unspecified**".

Individuals with conduct disorder seem lacking in empathizing with others and their emotions and feelings. They may have a tendency to blame others in order to cover-up their own faults. Their temperament may be characterized by low frustration tolerance, irritability, and impulsivity and anger outbursts. Individuals with this disorder often indulge in early sexual activities and substance taking behaviours. Children and adolescents often face rustication from school due to violation of rules made by school authorities. In extreme cases, suicidal ideation, suicidal attempts and complete suicide occur at the higher than the expected rate.

Oppositional Defiant Disorder

This disorder is essentially featured by recurrent patterns of negativistic and oppositional behaviours towards others especially authorities in the form of stubbornness, disobedience, arguing tendency, deliberate avoidance of commands or directions and annoying others. This disorder usually does not contain serious physical violence; however, it can be seen occasionally in extreme conditions. Usually the symptoms are present in conditions confined to home and people the individual is familiar with, so the oppositional behaviours may not be evident during clinical observation or interview. The disorder is often seen in children below the age of 9-10 years. The behaviours are characterized by marked temper tantrums, low frustration tolerance, deliberately annoying others by not following instructions or avoiding commands, blaming others for their own faults, sensitive to criticism, being resentful and vindictive. These individuals not only annoy others but they themselves are annoyed easily by others and initiate confrontations with highly argumentative behaviours, rudeness and resistance to authority.

The key to distinguish oppositional defiant disorder from conduct disorder is absence of behaviours characterized by violation of legal rules and threatening basic rights of others. The disorder excludes features like theft, cruelty, assault and serious physical harm to others.

Etiology of Conduct Disorder

Etiology of conduct disorder cannot be explained with a single factor, it involves variety of factors that contribute to the condition.

Familial Factors: Studies have indicated that children brought in the harsh and punitive family environment are more likely to exhibit conduct symptoms. The notion explains that verbal and physical aggression of parents of other family members may be associated with child's maladaptive aggressive behaviours. Usually the chaotic family environment, parental separation or divorce, poor interaction among family members etc. have been identified as the risk factors of conduct problems in children. Parental psychopathology such as alcoholism, chronic mental illness, psychopathy or anti-social behaviours/personality has also been identified as a contributing factor to this disorder. Children rose in negligent environment, affectional deprivation and lack of family support are at higher risk of developing such behaviours. Learning theories have explained that lack of discipline and poor limit setting behaviours may increase the risk of developing such behaviours.

Socio-Cultural Factors: It has been found that children being raised in the urban society exhibit more conduct or disruptive behaviours possibly due to increased rate of alcohol use. The socio-economical background may also be a contributing factor for this condition such as unemployed parents, poor social networking, lack of support from the community etc.

Psychoanalytic Factors: These factors are based on the Psychoanalytic perspectives of human behaviours. It is explained that children with conduct disorder unconsciously exhibit their parent's hostility in their own behaviours. Exposure to harsh and punitive behaviour of parents leads to poor modulation of affects and emotions resulting in anger outbursts, frustration and irritation. Dissatisfaction of their own emotional needs and wishes leads to less developed empathy and sense of relatedness with others.

Neurobiological and Neurological Factors: These factors explain the etiology based on neurochemical causes of the conduct behaviours. According to these factors the conduct behaviours result from high level of serotonin in blood and low level of plasma dopamine that converts dopamine into norepinephrine. Resting patterns of EEG and activation of aggressive behaviours has been found to be associated with each other as frontal resting brain electrical activity has been hypothesized to reflect the ability for emotional regulation.

Maltreatment and Abuse

It is well established that individuals exposed to violence in any form, i.e. physical, verbal or emotional develop a tendency to behave aggressively over the period of time. Studies have also indicated that children who witness abuse of their mothers behave aggressively in later situations. In severe cases abused and maltreated children and adolescents seem to be hyper-vigilant and they perceive benign situations as directly threatening and response in highly violent manner and they are likely violating rights of others.

Tic Disorder

Tic is basically an involuntary, recurrent and non-rhythmic motor movement or vocalizations presented in rapid form that tends to be irresistible but can be suppressed in some situations. There can be two major types of tics:

1. **Motor Tics:** Motor tics usually involve rapid movement of body parts or motor muscle groups.
2. **Vocal Tics:** Vocal tics are generally related to unusual vocalizations.

Both motor and vocal tics can be either simple or complex.

1. **Simple Motor or Vocal Tics:** Those involving only few muscles or simple sounds and persist only for few milliseconds.
2. **Complex Motor or Vocal Tics:** Those involving multiple muscle groups and multiple vocalizations together and last for seconds or may be longer than that.

Examples of ***simple motor tics*** are rapid blinking of eyes, shoulder shrugging, neck jerking, nose wrinkling, facial grimacing and abdominal tensing. ***Simple vocal tics*** can be observed as frequent and rapid throat clearing, grunting, chirping, sniffing, snorting and hissing. Similarly,

complex motor tics include behaviours like jumping, stomping, pressing, repeatedly smelling objects, deep knee bends, retracing steps while walking. There can be presence of "Dystonic tics", i.e. holding unusual postures like holding a particular body part in a particular tensed position. At times some sexual or obscene gestures can also be present as tics that are known as "Copropraxia". When imitation of someone else's movement is done rapidly and immediately involuntarily the condition is termed as "Echopraxia". ***Complex vocal tics*** on the other hand involve sudden and spontaneous expression of single word or phrases. There can be speech blocking, sudden changes in pitch or tone of voice that are meaningless to the context. One may repeat one's own words or sounds which are known as "Palilalia". If repetition of word or phrases is done of last heard word or sound only, then the condition is said to be "Echolalia". At times there may be presentation of obscene and socially unaccepted words of phrases where it is termed as "Coprolalia".

Usually the tics are involuntary in nature; however can be suppressed on occasions for varying periods of time. Most of the individual are not aware of their tics, yet they feel a sensation when a tic is about to occur. In such conditions they may feel it as between voluntary or involuntary act. The time where they notice the occurrences of tic is usually anxiety inducing and performing a tic behaviour usually gives a sense of relief. The frequency of tics is generally continuous and they are often emitted in bouts of one or several tics. Tics can increase in frequency when get severe and may be performed forcefully to achieve the condition of relief. Tics are usually absent during sleep; however, in some cases they may appear in sleep also. Generally, the impact of tics is negative as they might create a shameful or awkward condition when performed in social situations and simultaneously influence the self-esteem also.

Tourett's Disorder: Tourett's disorder or Tourett's syndrome is a condition characterized by multiple motor tics and one or more vocal tics that are present recurrently throughout the day for one year and remission in condition for not more than three months in-between this period. Usually the condition is evident before the age of 18 years and the tics are not correlated with the physiological effect of any substance or neurological condition. The frequency, severity and location of tics changes over the period of time and tics (either simple or complex) may affect any of the body part, i.e. face, head, neck etc. Usually the condition starts with eye blinking or single tic and may involve other parts of the face or body. Sometimes, the condition may start with multiple tics at a time. Tics may persist lifelong; however, in most cases the severity diminishes in adolescence or adulthood. On the other hand, tics may get worsen in the adulthood.

Chronic Motor or Vocal Tics: This condition is characterized by presence of motor or vocal tics; however, the absence of their simultaneous presence is the characteristic feature in this disorder. The condition is diagnosed only when there is a specific type of tic present, either motor or vocal. The condition differs from Tourett's Disorder as it lacks simultaneous presence of both types of tics. Apart from this, overall presentation of the disorder is far more similar to tourett's disorder; however, the severity of disorder and associated functional impairments are less. If the individual showing these symptoms has ever been detected to have tourett's disorder, condition of chronic vocal or motor tics cannot be diagnosed.

Transient Tic Disorder: The presentation of transient tic disorder is common to the presentation of tic disorder and Tourett's disorder; however, the condition differs from both of them in terms of persistency of symptoms of tics. In transient tic disorder single or multiple motor or vocal tics occurs rapidly many times a day for about a period of one month but not more than one consecutive year. This condition is only diagnosed if the quality and representation of tics does not match with any of the other mentioned category of this disorder.

If tics are the prominent characteristic behaviour but do not meet any of the mentioned guidelines, it can be kept in the category of "Tic Disorder Not Otherwise Specified".

Etiology of Tics

Genetic Factors: Various studies conducted in this field have supported the genetic causes for these disorders. Twin studies identified high concordance rate among monozygotic as compared to dizygotic twins. Studies also supported the fact that tics disorders may appear in children having parents with history of this disorder. The risk of developing this disorder is found to be higher in the first degree relatives of such persons. Condition of ADHD has been found to be highly associated with Tourett's syndrome and in many cases they have been found to be co-existing.

Neuro-Chemical and Neuro-Anatomical Factors: The studies have indicated that pharmacological agents antagonizing dopamine suppress tics and those agents increasing central dopaminergic activity exacerbate tics. The association between tics and neurotransmitters is complex and yet to be explored. These individuals have deficits in the neural density of neuronal and non-neuronal cells. Abnormalities in basal ganglia have been found to be associated with many movement disorders. Tics may be caused by the same condition and dysfunction in basal ganglia's major fibre pathways. Some researchers have proposed dopaminergic dysfunction to be a cause of this disorder and others have concluded that the biochemical structure of the limbic forebrain have connection to Tourett's syndrome.

Neuro-endocrine and Immunological Factors: Studies indicated that levels of antibodies and elevated titers of circulating antibodies bindings to the serotonergic receptors have relation to this condition. Increased prevalence of tics among males might be related to exposure of developing male CNS (Central Nervous System) to increased level of dihydrotestosterone or other gender related factors. Streptococcal infection; an autoimmune process has been found to be a potential mechanism for Tourett's disorder.

Prenatal Factors: Mothers of children with Tics disorder may face complications during pregnancy. Weight of the infant has also been found to be associated with the disorder. Studies have also indicated correlation between stresses in the mother; severe nausea and vomiting in the first trimester of pregnancy and severity of tics. On the other hand, some of the studies failed to prove any such evidences.

Psychological Factors: Tics somehow have been identified to have a strong relation with stresses. Some teachers and parents seem to misunderstand the displaying of tic behaviours and they forcefully try to suppress these behaviours by punishing the child. The punishment and associated humiliation most of the times exaggerate the symptoms/tics. Sometimes, the exaggeration can further lead to stresses and this vicious cycle can demoralize the child in societal situations.

Elimination Disorders

Elimination disorders are mainly characterized by mostly involuntary and in some cases voluntary passage of feces and urine at inappropriate places which is not caused by or a resultant condition of any physiological/ medical condition like gastrointestinal diseases, urinary tract infections or seizures. The disorder involves following two major categories:

Enuresis

Enuresis is the condition characterized by repeated voiding of urine either during night or day hours in bed or clothes. Like encopresis, the passage of urine is usually involuntary but in some cases may be voluntary. In most cases there is a prior condition of achieving adequate bladder control; however, other cases may lack the acquisition of this skill. Cases presented with symptoms of this disorder without achieving age appropriate bladder control are categorized as having ***primary enuresis***. On the other hand, those with adequate achievement of bladder control and later developing the symptoms are categorized under ***secondary enuresis***. Usually the feature should be present at the age where continence or adequate bladder control is expected (usually 5 years) and the passage of urine is not due to the result of any substance effect or general medical condition. There are two major subtypes of this disorder:

> ***Nocturnal Enuresis***: This condition is described as voiding of urine only during the night hours or during night time sleep and also the most common condition of this disorder. Usually passage of urine takes place during REM sleep.
>
> ***Diurnal Enuresis***: This is a totally reversed condition of the above mentioned as it involves voiding of urine during waking hours. This condition may be exhibited in two forms:
>
> 1. *Urge Incontinence*: This condition is characterized by voiding of urine characterized by sudden urge to pass urine.
> 2. *Voiding Postponement*: This condition is essentially featured by consciously deferring the micturition until incontinence results. Sometimes, it may be due to reluctance to use toilet, preoccupation with school or play activity etc.

Nocturnal and Diurnal Enuresis: This condition is characterized by presentation of symptoms as combination of both above mentioned types.

Usually children with this disorder often suffer from low self-esteem due to shameful conditions at home, school and other social situations. At times they may also face harsh and punitive behaviour of their caregivers. Most of the children with this disorder achieve continence till adolescence; however, some may carry over the problem till adulthood.

Encopresis

The essential feature of this disorder is repeated passage of feces either voluntary or involuntary at inadequate places. In most cases the behaviour is involuntary; however, it may be voluntary in some cases. The condition does not have any direct physiological association and is not caused by due to effects of drugs or laxatives; however, constipation may or may not be present as a factor in this disorder. When the passage of feces involuntary it is associated with constipation, retention along with subsequent overflow. Some cases may involve smearing of feces over the body and other external environment. The condition sometimes may be associated with organic conditions such as anal fissure, gastrointestinal infection etc. This disorder has two subtypes:

> ***With Constipation and Overflow Incontinence*:** This condition is characterized by evidence of constipation in physical examination.
> ***Without Constipation and Overflow Incontinence*:** This condition is characterized by absence of constipation either in the physical examination or in the history.

The disorder may arise in different ways or due to different reasons:

1. Inadequate/lack of toilet training or appropriate response to toilet training with history of failure to acquire bowel control.
2. There may be reluctance or failure to confirm to social norms in defecating at appropriate places despite of normal physiological control over defecation.
3. Excessive retention and withholding of feces leading to impaction, with secondary overflow and de-positioning of feces at inappropriate places.

Etiology of Enuresis

Genetic Factors: Genetic factors have been found to play an important role in enuresis. Studies have indicated high concordance rate among monozygotic twins as compared to dizygotic twins. Longitudinal studies have shown developmental delays to be associated with enuresis; however, they have not proven to be a causal factor for this condition. Most findings support the fact that children are at higher risk of developing the condition if their father had a history of enuresis in childhood.

Biological Factors: Studies have indicated that individuals with enuresis have normal anatomical structure of bladder; yet they feel the need to urinate with less urine in the bladder. Other studies have advocated occurrence of nocturnal enuresis due to lower than expected levels of nighttime antidiuretic hormone when bladder is full. It may lead to increased output of urine as compared to expected. Some studies indicated that sleep stages may be associated with the condition; however, further researches discarded this finding and it was found that bed-wetting appears randomly.

Psycho-social Factors: Researches indicated that those who have been exposed to stressful conditions at home or at school may experience enuresis at increased rate. The psycho-social factors may be related to anxiety provoked by birth of a younger sibling and perceived lack of status or affection by the family members. Hospitalization of very young children is also a stressful condition for them and it has been found to be associated with developing bed-wetting. Some children start wetting their beds when they start schooling. It may be accompanied by fearful thoughts about school or stress related to the new condition. Familial conflicts and parental issues may also contribute to the condition.

Etiology of Encopresis

Psychodynamic Factors: It has been found that psychological factors contribute to this condition and are governed by the tendencies of parents regarding showing affection and nurturance and parenting patterns. Researches indicated that children with distant father and a neurotic mother along with inadequate or harsh toilet training are likely to be at risk of developing this problem. Many times even with those who sometime achieved bowel control the fecal soiling occurs as a result of anxiety induced by new born sibling, changes in the environmental conditions like parental divorce, separation, dislocation of home, change of school etc. some evidences report that it is a reaction to avoid pain of bowel control.

Familial and Societal Factors: Maternal hostility has been found to be associated with encopresis. Researches indicate that children brought in the harsh and punitive parenting are at greater risk of developing this condition. Children being bullied in school may also exhibit the symptoms. It has been found in studies that children with history of sexual abuse are likely to develop encopresis.

Anxiety Related Disorders

Only the major disorders of this category have been included here.

Separation Anxiety Disorder

The main characteristic feature of this disorder is excessive anxiety displayed by a child in conditions of separation from home or primary attachment figure. Significant distress may occur before or during the separation mainly governed by the thoughts of unavailability of care giver in needful situations. Anticipation of separation may cause nightmares or other somatic or physical symptoms in the child such as stomachache, multiple pain symptoms, sleep disturbances etc. The anxiety symptoms in this condition are so intense that they create almost a panic like condition and child may resists going to school due to the same reason. Resistance is evident not only for school going behaviour but also for playing activities performed outside home or being alone at home (any area of the home) itself. The symptoms are present in the absence of attachment figure even if the other family members are present. Children with this disorder suffer from highly distressful conditions with anticipation of harm to the attachment figure or with themselves followed by not being together ever with that figure. In cases where the individual is supposed to live outside home due to educational reasons, homesickness may take place and the distress may be displayed in forms of excessive anger outbursts and in some cases as withdrawal and solitary behaviours. The condition leads to significant impairments in child's socio-occupational functioning and may lead to maladjustment in various areas of life like academic, social and peer group. Usually the condition is detected under the age of 18 years and is not associated with any other co-morbid condition like pervasive developmental disorder or schizophrenia.

Reactive Attachment Disorder of Infancy or Early Childhood

This disorder is characterized by impairments in social interaction patterns that are associated with emotional disturbances and reactions to environmental changes. The poor interaction patterns are found to be associated with the characteristic problems in social relatedness. The condition may exhibit two different forms and child's behaviours are governed by the predominant form of the condition:

1. **Inhibited Type:** Children with this form display behaviours characterized by hyper vigilance, ambivalent and contradictory responses in social situations. For example, there may be a mixed reaction of avoidance and resistance for the caregiver.

2. **Disinhibited Type:** This form of the disorder is characterized by diffused attachment patterns subsequently failure to exhibit adequate selective attachment. In later ages, the exhibition of symptoms may include attention seeking and indiscriminately friendly behaviours. Selective attachments may be developed on further stages; however, poor peer interactions are not rare. The condition may result from frequent changes in primary caregivers and subsequently the lack of opportunity to develop selective attachment patterns.

Many children may show different patterns of attachment to primary caregivers or attachment figure and significant insecurity in selective attachment towards anyone of the parents, yet the condition should not be confused with the disorder based on its persistency and associated difficulties in growth and development of the child. The disorder is characterized by abnormal or unusual insecurity which is uncommon in other children of similar ages. Such children lack social responsiveness and may exhibit apathy, fearfulness and frozen watchfulness.

Many times the features of this disorder may appear as in pervasive developmental disorder; however, there is clear demarcation between the two conditions.

1. Children with this disorder have normal capacity for social reciprocity which is absent in PDD.
2. Remission of symptoms is possible if child is kept in favourable conditions like adequate rearing environment and responsive care giving.
3. Language development may not be adequate; yet the typical communication disturbances of autism are absent.
4. Repetitive and stereotypical behaviours are not a part of this disorder.

The disorder has been found to be associated with faulty child rearing practices and in some cases due to child abuse and child neglect.

Etiology of Reactive Attachment Disorder

Variety of familial factors has been found to be associated with the etiology of reactive attachment disorder. Inadequate parenting in some cases due to premature parenthood and inability to identify or react appropriately towards child's needs does play an important role for this condition. Any form of child maltreatment, abuse, neglect or ignorance of emotional needs may have an important role. Many times parent's own parenting may affect the care giving behaviour such as parental psychopathology, deprivation from attachment figures during childhood, poor upbringing or insecure attachment. Researchers have also indicated the influence of frequent changing of caregivers, multiple lengthy hospitalizations etc. Overall, the researches have supported the importance of parent-child ties and quality of bonding.

Etiology of Separation Anxiety Disorder

Genetic Factors: It has been found that those with panic disorder and agoraphobia have a higher risk of offspring with separation anxiety. Researches indicated towards inherited predisposition of anxiety that triggers as high level of arousal, emotional reactivity along with sorts of negativity in thoughts and emotions increasing the risk of anxiety disorders.

Social Factors: These factors are largely related to observation and modelling at home or of significant others. It has been found to be highly correlated with anxious parenting characterized by overprotection, exaggerated presentation of social situations involving uncertainty or novelty correlating them with the expected danger. If children observe anxious responses of parents in a particular situation they learn them and implement in the same manner. The explanation supports the fact that anxious parenting may cause anxiety disturbances in children; yet the genetic predisposition have an important role in the condition. Many times the changes in life circumstances may also influence the condition. There is possibility of occurrence or exaggeration of symptoms in conditions of first visit to school, change in neighbourhood, death of loved one or significant other.

Substance Abuse among Adolescents

Substance taking behaviours have been found to be a major issue among adolescents. Usually those with familial conflicts, lack of parental supervision, peer pressure or bad company are likely to perform these behaviours; however, these are not the only contributing factors of substance taking behaviours among this population. Type of substance being consumed, pattern of intake and time spend in substance taking behaviour have been found to be common issues related to this problem. Consumption of alcohol and tobacco has been found to be the common among adolescents; however, use of other substances like marijuana, nicotine, cocaine, heroin, inhalants or a combination of some particular drugs is not rare. Individuals with this condition may significantly exhibit conduct and oppositional symptoms. The condition when becomes severe causes significant decline in socio-occupational functioning resulting in maladjustment at home, school and other social situations. The condition also leads to significant physical losses resulting in poor health and subsequently affecting the overall functioning of the individual.

Substance taking behaviour goes through different phases before reaching to the ultimate problematic condition that is difficult to manage and may induce other physical or psychological illnesses. Various categories of substance related disorder are as follows:

- **Substance Dependence:** The condition of dependence is characterized by cognitive, behavioural and physiological symptoms leading to the decline of daily functioning, yet the person is unable to control the use of substance being taken. Persistent intake of substance results in tolerance where a person re-applies the doses in order to achieve intended satisfaction which is not being obtained with the use of prior doses. In absence of adequate amount of intake person may exhibit withdrawal symptoms like restlessness, tremors etc. the behaviour may turn to compulsive drug taking when it does not produces intended results. Individuals with substance dependence usually fail to control or resist substance taking behaviours and their productivity and efficiency may reduce. They may also reduce social interactions and get-togethers.
- **Substance Abuse:** Use and abuse are two different behaviours in substance related problems. Usually the use may not be harmful for many people, however, the condition of abuse tends to result in significant disturbances in personal, social and occupational life. The condition explains much more severe condition as continuing substance taking behaviour in situations of physical dangers, impairment in academic functioning, frequent failures, legal problems and disturbed inter-personal relations. Despite of all the mentioned difficulties the individual fails to decrease or stop the intake of substances and maladaptive patterns of substance intake leads to significant distress.

- **Substance Intoxication:** Many times, substances may induce a reversible effect on the user. The condition causes significant changes in behavioural and psychological functioning that are maladaptive in nature. Difference in the substance consumed results in different substance-specific syndromes/symptoms.
- **Substance Withdrawal:** The condition of withdrawal results by cessation or reduction in prolonged use of substance or the significant reduction in amount of substance.

Etiology of Substance Abuse among Adolescents

Genetic Causes: The concordance rate for monozygotic twins is high than dizygotic twins and they have a higher chance of adapting alcoholic behaviours. Researches also indicated that the rate is even higher for the male monozygotic twins. Other researches that have coined a neurobiological perspective of substance abuse have explained the reinforcing effects of substance being taken and continuing the intake in order to maintain the reinforcements. The studies explained the causes due to which a person continues to consume substance rather than giving a certain reason that which particular condition will definitely lead to consume substance in future. Important implications are related to functioning of dopamine and amygdale. Most researches that reported reinforcing impact of substances explained the behaviour as learning and conditioning between substance consumptions and its association with positive results such as enhanced mood state, lowering of stress levels etc. On the other hand the withdrawal effects of substance have been explained as related to the negative reinforcement.

Psycho-Social Factors: The studies conducted in families have advocated that the children being raised in an environment with minimal parental supervision and monitoring are at higher risk of developing such problems. Also, modelling has been found to be a contributing factor to this condition. Children with alcoholic parent have been found to be at greater risk to develop substance abuse in future. Many times, especially among adolescents, substance consuming behaviour may result from peer pressure, perceived status symbol, bullying by others leading to maladaptive behaviour in form of alcohol consumption etc. Researchers have shown that those with history of anti-social behaviour in father have high chances of alcohol consumption at early stages of life.

Psychopathological Factors: Researchers have explored that substance abuse rates are higher among relatives of children with depression and bipolar disorder. Antisocial behaviours, conduct disorder and substance abuse have been found to be linked with each other. Association of psychiatric disorders and poly substance use has been found to be evident. Surveys conducted on adolescents have shown higher rates of mood disorder among those consuming substances. The rate is not avoidable among those with disruptive behaviour and personality disorders.

Psychodynamic Factors: This perspective explains substance taking behaviours as a dominant need to search for pleasure which may result from affective dysregulation. Some researches viewed it as an inability to manage painful affects like anger, anxiety and guilt. The motivational source for substance consumption in initial phase has been found as underlying pathological factor and also some users may use it as a self-medication. For example, opioids help in controlling anger, alcohol helps to control panic and smoking may be used to control symptoms of depression.

References

Americal Psychiatric Association. (2000). *Diagnostic and Statistical Manual of Mental Disorders* (4th ed., text rev.). Washington, DC: Author.

Kaplan, H.I., Sadock, B.J. (2007). *Comprehensive Textbook of Psychiatry*. 6th ed. Vol. 2. Wolters Kluwer, Lippincott Williams and Wilkins.

Kauffman, J.M. (2001). *Characteristics of Emotional and Behavioural Disorders of Children and Youth*. 7th ed., New Jersy Columbus, Ohio. Upper Saddle River: Merrill Prentice Hall.

Larry, B., Silver, M.D. (2008). *Attention Deficit/Hyperactivity Disorder; A clinical Guide to Diagnosis and Treatment for Health and Mental Health professionals*. 3rd ed. American Psychiatric Publishing. Inc. Washington, DC, London, England.

Linehan, M.M. (1993). *Cognitive-behavioural treatment of borderline personality disorder*. New York: Guilford Press.

O'Carroll, P.W., Mercy, J.A., and Steward, J.A. (1988). CDC recommendations for a community plan for the prevention and containment of suicide clusters. *Morbidity and Mortality Weekly Report,* 37(5-6), 1-12.

Sadock, B.J., Sadock, A.S., Ruiz, P. (2009). *Comprehensive Textbook of Psychiatry*. 9th ed. Vol. 2. Wolters Kluwer, Lippincott Williams and Wilkins.

Sadock, B.J., Sadock, V.A. (2007). *Synopsis of Psychiatr,. Behavioural Sciences, Clinical Psychiatry*. 10th ed. Lippincott Williams and Wilkins—a Wolters Kluwer Business 530 Walnut Street, Philadelphia, PA 19106-3621 USA.

Shneidman, E.S. (1996). *The suicidal mind*. New York: Oxford University Press.

Silverman, M.M., Berman, A.L., Sanddal, N.D., O'Carroll, P.W., and Joiner, T.E. (2007a). Rebuilding the Tower of Babel: A revised nomenclature for the study of suicide and suicidal behaviours, Part 1: Background, rationale, and methodology. *Suicide and Life—Threatening Behaviour,* 37, 248-263.

Silverman, M.M., Berman, A.L., Sanddal, N.D., O'Carroll, P.W., and Joiner, T.E. (2007b). Rebuilding the Tower of Babel: A revised nomenclature for the study of suicide and suicidal behaviours, Part 2: Suicide-related ideations, communications, and behaviours. *Suicide and Life—Threatening Behaviour,* 37, 264-277.

Viskochil, J. *School Refusal Behaviour from Terminology to Treatment*, University of Utah. (year could not be found)

Wade, N.L. (1987). Suicide as resolution of separation-individuation among adolescent girls. *Adolescence,* 22, 169-177.

Wagner, B.M. (2009). *Suicide Behaviour in children and adolescents.* Yale University Press. New Haven and London.

9

Mental Health in Adolescents

Problems and Challenges

Rupali Srivastava

The present age is the age of challenge. There are lots of crises in modern society. Despite the increasing demands of technology for more highly trained citizens and accumulation of knowledge, something more is required of education than the development of intellect. Society has a dire need for competent, self-respecting. Schools can no longer evaluate the effects of education by what a person knows, but it must be concerned also with what he is.

The word 'mental' means 'of the mind'. It describes our thoughts, feelings and understanding of our self and the world around us. The word 'health' generally describes the working order of our body and mind. So when we talk about 'mental health', we are referring to the working order of our mind. Mental health can be conceptualized as a state of well-being in which the individual realizes his or her own abilities, can cope with the normal stresses of life, can work productively and fruitfully and is able to make a contribution to his or her community. In the positive sense, mental health is the foundation for well-being and effective functioning for an individual and for a community. This core concept of mental health is the foundation for well-being and effective functioning for an individual and for a community. In this positive sense, mental health is the foundation for well-being and effective functioning for an individual and for a community. This core concept of mental health is consist with its wide and varied interpretation across cultures.

Mental health is defined by the W.H.O. as 'a state of well-being in which the individual realizes his or her own abilities, can cope with the normal stresses of life, can work productively and fruitfully and is able to make a contribution to his or her community. Chauhan (1987) defines mental health as a condition that permits the maximum development of physical, intellectual and emotional status of the individual, so that he can contribute maximum to the welfare of the society and can realize his ideas/aims in life. Encyclopaedia of Applied Ethics (1988) writes that it is very difficult to define mental health in clear and universal way. Mental health is not synonymous with pleasure. Knowledge, absence of illness or disease, thought, it includes the capacity of all these. A man's mental health depends on where he or she lives, the sort of society he or she lives, live in and his or her gender, race or age. Bhagi and Sharma (1992) refers mental health to a state of mind characterized by emotional well-being relative freedom from anxiety and disabling symptoms, a capacity to establish constructive relationships and cope with ordinary demands and stresses of life. Menninger (1945) defined mental health as the adjustment of human beings to the world and to each other with a maximum of effectiveness and happiness. It is the ability to maintain an even temper, an alert intelligence, socially considerate behaviour and a happy disposition. Mental health can be described as absence of symptoms of maladjustment, be they mild or severe. Mentally healthy person is free from all types of maladjustment (Klein, 1956). Jahoda (1958) has said that aspects of attitudes towards self growth and development, self-actualization, integration of personality and mastery of the environment must be considered in judging whether a person is mentally healthy or not. Bhatia (1982) considers mental health as the ability to balance feelings, desires, ambitions and ideals in one's daily living. It means the ability to face and accept the realities of life.

Mental Health and Mental Illness

The 1999 Surgeon General's Report on Mental Health defined mental health as "successful performance of mental function, resulting in productive activities, fulfilling relationships with other people, and the ability to change and to cope with adversity." According to United States, Department of Health and Human Services (1999), mental illness refers to diagnosable mental disorders that are characterized by alterations in thinking, mood, or behaviour (or a combination thereof) associated with distress and/or impaired functioning. A 2004 report by the World Health Organization (WHO) includes a similar distinction between mental health and mental illness. With children this includes a wide range of emotional and behaviour problems that in lay term may not be considered mental or psychiatric disorders. Here, the terms emotional, behavioural, and mental disorders are used interchangeably.

Common Mental Health Disorders

Depression

Depression refers to a wide range of mental health problems characterized by the absence of a positive effect (a loss of interest and enjoyment in ordinary things and experiences), low mood and a range of associated emotional, cognitive, physical and behavioural symptoms. Distinguishing the mood changes between clinically significant degrees of depression (for example, major depression) and those occurring 'normally' remains problematic and it is best to consider the symptoms of depression as occurring on a continuum of severity (Lewinsohn *et al.*, 2000). Commonly, mood and effect in a major depressive illness are unreactive to circumstance remaining low throughout the course of each day, although for some people mood varies diurnally, with gradual improvement throughout the day only to return to a low mood on waking. In other cases a person's mood may be reactive to positive experiences and events, although these elevations in mood are not sustained with depressive feelings often quickly re-emerging (Andrews and Jenkins, 1999). Behavioural and physical symptoms typically include tearfulness, irritability, social withdrawal, an exacerbation of pre-existing pains, and pains secondary to increased muscle tension (Gerber *et al.*, 1992). A lack of libido, fatigue and diminished activity are also common, although agitation and marked anxiety can frequently occur. Typically there is reduced sleep and lowered appetite (sometimes leading to significant weight loss), but some people sleep more than usual and have an increase in appetite. A loss of interest and enjoyment in everyday life, and feelings of guilt, worthlessness and deserved punishment are common, as are lowered self-esteem, loss of confidence, feelings of helplessness, suicidal ideation and attempts at self-harm or suicide. Cognitive changes include poor concentration and reduced attention, pessimistic and recurrently negative thoughts about oneself, one's past and the future, mental slowing and rumination (Cassano and Fava, 2002).

Generalized Anxiety Disorder

The essential feature of GAD is excessive anxiety and worry (apprehensive expectation), occurring on more days than not for a period of at least 6 months, about a number of events or activities. The person with GAD finds it difficult to control the anxiety and worry, which is often accompanied by restlessness, being easily fatigued, having difficulty concentrating, irritability, muscle tension and disturbed sleep (Brown *et al.*, 2001). The focus of the anxiety and worry in GAD is not confined to features of another disorder, for example having panic attacks (as in panic disorder) or being embarrassed in public (as in social anxiety disorder). Some people with GAD may become excessively apprehensive about the outcome of routine activities, in particular those associated with the health of or separation from loved ones. Some people often anticipate a catastrophic outcome from a mild physical symptom or a side effect of medication. Demoralisation is said to be a common consequence, with many individuals becoming discouraged, ashamed and unhappy about the difficulties of carrying out their normal routines. GAD is often comorbid with depression and this can make accurate diagnosis problematic (Wittchen *et al.*, 2002).

Panic Disorder

People with panic disorder report intermittent apprehension, and panic attacks (attacks of sudden short-lived anxiety) in relation to particular situations or spontaneous panic attacks, with no apparent cause. They often take action to avoid being in particular situations in order to prevent those feelings, which may develop into agoraphobia (Breier *et al.*, 1986). The frequency and severity of panic attacks varies widely. Situational triggers for panic attacks can be external (for example, a phobic object or situation) or internal (physiological arousal). A panic attack may be unexpected (spontaneous or uncued), that is, one that an individual does not immediately associate with a situational trigger. The essential feature of agoraphobia is anxiety about being in places or situations from which escape might be difficult, embarrassing or in which help may not be available in the event of having a panic attack. This anxiety is said to typically lead to a pervasive avoidance of a variety of situations that may include: being alone outside the home or being home alone; being in a crowd of people; travelling by car or bus; being in a particular place, such as on a bridge or in a lift.

Obsessive-Compulsive Disorder

OCD is characterised by the presence of either obsessions or compulsions, but commonly both. An obsession is defined as an unwanted intrusive thought, image or urge that repeatedly enters the person's mind. Obsessions are distressing, but are acknowledged as originating in the person's mind and not imposed by an external agency. They are usually regarded by the individual as unreasonable or excessive. Common obsessions in OCD include contamination from dirt, germs, viruses, body fluids and so on, fear of harm (for example, that door locks are not safe), excessive concern with order or symmetry, obsessions with the body or physical symptoms, religious, sacrilegious or blasphemous thoughts, sexual thoughts (for example, of being a paedophile or a homosexual), an urge to hoard useless or worn out possessions, or thoughts of violence or aggression (for example, stabbing one's baby) (Lochner and Stein, 2003). Compulsions are repetitive behaviours or mental acts that the person feels driven to perform. A compulsion can either be overt and observable by others, or a covert mental act that cannot be observed. Covert compulsions are generally more difficult to resist or monitor than overt ones because they can be performed anywhere without others knowing and are easier to perform. Common compulsions include checking (for example, gas taps), cleaning, washing, repeating, mental compulsions (for example, repeating special words or prayers in a set manner), ordering, symmetry or exactness, hoarding/collecting and counting (Foa *et al.*, 1995). The most frequent presentations are checking and cleaning, and these are the most easily recognized because they are on a continuum with everyday behaviour. A compulsion is not in itself pleasurable, which differentiates it from impulsive acts such as shopping or gambling, which are associated with immediate gratification.

Post-Traumatic Stress Disorder

Post-Traumatic Stress Disorder (PTSD) often develops in response to one or more traumatic events such as deliberate acts of interpersonal violence, severe accidents, disasters or military action. Those at risk of PTSD include survivors of war and torture, of accidents and disasters, and of violent crime (for example, physical and sexual assaults, sexual abuse, bombings and riots), refugees, women who have experienced traumatic childbirth, people diagnosed with a life-threatening illness, and members of the armed forces, police and other emergency personnel (Foa *et al.*, 2008). The most characteristic symptoms of PTSD are re-experiencing symptoms. People with PTSD involuntarily re-experience aspects of the traumatic event in a vivid and distressing way. Symptoms include flashbacks in which the person acts or feels as if the event is recurring; nightmares; and repetitive and distressing intrusive images or other sensory impressions from the event. Reminders of the traumatic event arouse intense distress and/or physiological reactions. As a result, hypervigilance for threat, exaggerated startle responses, irritability, difficulty in concentrating, sleep problems and avoidance of trauma reminders are other core symptoms. However, people with PTSD also describe symptoms of emotional numbing. These include inability to have any feelings, feeling detached from other people, giving up previously significant activities and amnesia for significant parts of the event.

Social Anxiety Disorder

Social anxiety disorder, also referred to as social phobia, is characterised by an intense fear in social situations that results in considerable distress and in turn impacts on a person's ability to function effectively in aspects of their daily life. Central to the disorder is a fear of being judged by others and of being embarrassed or humiliated. This leads to the avoidance of a number of social situations and often impacts significantly on educational and vocational performance. The fears can be triggered by the actual or imagined scrutiny from others. The disorder often begins in early adolescence, and although an individual may recognise the problem as outside of normal experience, many do not seek help (Liebowitz *et al.*, 1985). Social anxiety disorder is characterised by a range of physical symptoms including excessive blushing, sweating, trembling, palpitations and nausea. Panic attacks are common, as is the development of depressive symptoms as the problem becomes chronic. Alcohol or drug misuse can develop because people use these substances in an attempt to cope with the disturbing and disabling symptoms. It is also often comorbid with other disorders such as depression (Kessler *et al.*, 1999).

Specific Phobias

A specific phobia is an unwarranted, extreme and persistent fear of a specific object or situation that is out of proportion to the actual danger or threat (Humphris *et al.*, 1995). The fear and anxiety occur immediately upon encountering the feared object or situation and tend to lead to avoidance or extreme discomfort. The person with a specific phobia recognises that the fear is excessive, unwarranted or out of proportion to the actual risk. Specific phobias result in significant interference with the activities of daily life; they are usually grouped under a number of subtypes including animal, natural environment, blood-injection-injury and situational.

Prevalence Rate of Mental Health Problems

Estimates of the prevalence of common mental health disorders vary considerably depending on where and when surveys are carried out, and the period over which prevalence is measured. The 2007 Office for National Statistics (ONS) household survey of adult psychiatric morbidity in England found that 16.2 per cent of adults aged 16 to 64 years met the diagnostic criteria for at least one disorder in the week prior to interview (McManus *et al.*, 2009). In the three ONS surveys carried out so far, the proportion of adults meeting the criteria for at least one disorder increased between 1993 and 2000 but did not change between 2000 and 2007 (15.5% in 1993, 17.5% in 2000 and 17.6% in 2007). The largest increase in the rate of disorders found between 1993 and 2007 was in women aged 45 to 64 years, among whom the rate went up by about one-fifth (McManus *et al.*, 2009). More than half of the adults identified with a common mental health disorder in the ONS survey presented with a mixed anxiety and depressive disorder (9% in the past week). The 1-week prevalence for the other common mental health disorders were 4.4 per cent for GAD, 2.3 per cent for a depressive episode, 1.4 per cent for phobia, 1.1 per cent for OCD and 1.1 per cent for panic disorder (McManus *et al.*, 2009). In the US, Kessler and colleagues conducted the National Comorbidity Survey, a representative household interview survey of 9,282 adults aged 18 years and over, to estimate the lifetime (Kessler *et al.*, 2005a) and 12-month (Kessler *et al.*, 2005b) prevalence rates of mental disorders classified using the Diagnostic and Statistical Manual of Mental Disorders (4th text-revision version; DSM-IV-TR) of the American Psychiatric Association (APA, 2000). Of the 12-month cases in the US National Comorbidity Survey, 22.3 per cent were classified as serious, 37.3 per cent as moderate and 40.4 per cent as mild. Fifty five per cent carried only a single diagnosis, 22 per cent two diagnoses and 23 per cent three or more diagnoses. Latent class analysis identified three highly comorbid classes representing 7 per cent of the population, and the authors concluded that, although mental disorders are widespread, serious cases are concentrated among a relatively small proportion of people with high comorbidity (Kessler *et al.*, 2005b).

Mental Health in India

Mental health planners in India have from time to time estimated the prevalence of mental disorders in the country. The data helps in understanding the status of mental health in the country and in planning for prevention and treatment of disorders. The Bhore Committee (Government of India, 1946) extrapolated from rates in U.K. and U.S.A. and concluded that mental patients requiring hospitalization in India be taken as 2 per 1000. Again in 1966, the Mental Health Advisory Committee of the Government of India suggested a probable prevalence of mental illness of 20 per 1000 population in general, 18 per 1000 for semi-rural and 14 per 1000 for rural (Elnaggar *et al.*,1971). In the age group 0-5 years, maximum number of children (33%) had diagnosis of hyperkinetic syndrome. According to Mental Health Research (2005) in India, the common diagnoses in age group 6-11 years were hysterical neurosis, hyperkinetic syndrome, and conduct disorders. The common disorders in age group 12-16 years were: psychosis, hysterical neurosis, and conduct disorders. Psychoses and conduct disorder cases were significantly more among males while hysterical neurosis cases were more common among female children. Mild mental retardation was present in 22 per cent children in 0-5 years age group, 19 per cent children in 6-11 years age, and among 6 per cent children of 12-16 years age group among those attending the psychiatric clinics/child guidance clinic.

Mental Health and Adolescents

Adolescence is a time of great change and transition, when youth are starting to make decisions about career paths, further schooling, and living on their own. Parents, practitioners, and policymakers are recognizing the importance of young people's mental health. Youth with better mental health are physically healthier, demonstrate more socially positive behaviours and engage in fewer risky behaviours (Resnick, 2000). Conversely, youth with mental health problems, such as depression, are more likely to engage in health risk behaviours (Brooks, Harris and Thrall, 2002). Furthermore, youth's mental health problems pose a significant financial and social burden on families and society in terms of distress, cost of treatment, and disability (Saunders, 2003; Busch and Barry, 2007,

Merikangas, Ames and Lihong, 2007). Most mental health problems diagnosed in adulthood begin in adolescence. Half of lifetime diagnosable mental health disorders start by age 14; this number increases to three-fourths by age 24 (Kessler, Berglund and Demler, 2005).The ability to manage mental health problems, including substance use issues and learning disorders, can affect adult functioning in areas such as social relationships and participation in the workforce.

Studies Related with Mental Health and Adolescents in India

Mental health is about how a person thinks, feels, and acts when faced with life's situations. Mental health is how people look at themselves, their lives, and the other people in their lives; evaluate their challenges and problems; and explore choices. This includes handling stress, relating to other people, and making decisions. Mentally healthy children and adolescents enjoy a positive quality of life; function well at home, in school, and in their communities; and are free of disabling symptoms of psychopathology (Hoagwood *et al.*, 1996).

Shylaja and Raj (1994) conducted a study to test whether there will be significant difference among alcohol and drug addicts and non-addicts on mental health status and value variables. Sample consisted of 30 alcohol addicts, 15 drug addicts and 30 non-addict males with age range of 15 to 20 years. Mental health status scale by Giressan and Sananda Raj (1988) and value scale developed by Thankam (1968) were administered. The results showed a significant difference between non-addicts and addicts, where non-addicts had better mental health. Moreover no significant difference was found between alcohol addicts and drug addicts.

Studies Related to Mental Health, Age and Gender

Sharma (1979) focused on self-concept, level of aspiration and mental health as factors in academic achievement. A sample of 1060 students selected randomly from X, XI and XII grades of schools of Uttar Pradesh was studied. Piers-Harris children's self-concept scale, Ansari and Ansari's LA coding test, Asthana's adjustment inventory to measure the mental health and personal data schedule were used for data collection. The results reported that boys and girls had better mental health during early adolescence (13 years); while boys in late adolescence showed better mental health than girls.

Mortimer *et al.* (1992) examined the relationship between early work experience and adolescent mental health and behavioural adjustment. The data was obtained from 1,001 ninth graders. Information about current jobs, attributes of work was examined in relation to dimensions of mental health (self-esteem and self-derogation, depressive effect and well-being, and internal and external control orientations) and indicators of behavioural adjustment (smoking, alcohol use, and problem behaviour in school). Boys and girls appear to experience psychological benefits when they perceive their jobs as providing skills that will be useful to them in the future However, boys who report more stress at work also manifest more depressive affect, more self-derogation, less internality, and a more external control orientation. For girls, the level of integration of school and work had pervasive associations with the psychological outcomes.

Anand (1999) conducted a study on mental health of 370 students of IX, X, XI and XII grades. Mental Health Scale developed by the author was used to measure the mental health. He reported no significant impact of gender and class on the mental health.

Nanda (2001) studied the mental health of high school students. The sample consisted of 1579 students from 86 schools covering Cuttack district, Orissa. Mental Health Scale developed by Nanda (1989) along with the interview schedules for parents, teachers and head masters was administered. The results revealed that female students were found to have better mental health than male students. While comparing male and female students in urban, rural and *ashram* schools separately it was found that male and female students in urban and *ashram* schools had similar mental health, whereas female students had better mental health than male students in rural schools. Rask *et al.* (2002) conducted a study on adolescent subjective well-being and realized values, and examined the relationships between socio-demographic variables, realized values and subjective well-being from the adolescent perspective. Adolescent subjective well-being was conceptualized by means of four different dimensions: satisfaction, ill-being, knowledge and activities related to well-being. The values were operationalized by eight core ideas from which principal components analysis identified 10 factors representing the realized values. Data was gained by self-report questionnaires from 245 adolescents from 7th and 9th grades, with a mean age of 14 years, in 13 secondary schools in southern Finland. The data were analysed statistically. The results revealed that most of the respondents were satisfied with life. However, one out of 10 did not experience the joy of life. There was no statistically significant difference in global satisfaction between girls and boys. Total ill-being among the adolescents was rare, but one out of four participants had fairly often worried about money and 17 per cent were frequently unusually tired. Girls and pupils from the 9th class experienced more ill-being than boys and pupils from the 7th class. The findings suggest that certain values such as personal equilibrium, safe family relations, and family type are predictors of adolescent global subjective well-being. They concluded that while assessing and promoting adolescent well-being it is important to pay special attention to the realization of values in life and not merely to appreciation of things. Implications for practice include the need to create opportunities for the realization of values when adolescents require health care services.

Ojha (2002) compared the social anxiety and mental health of normal and physically challenged adolescents. The sample constituted of 60 subjects (15 orthopaedically challenged males, 15 orthopaedically challenged females and matched control group of normal adolescents) randomly selected from different colleges located in Varanasi. Social anxiety scale (Sheikh and Kaushik, 1989) and Mental Health Inventory (Jagadish and Srivastava, 1983) was administered individually to measure the anxiety and mental health respectively. Social anxiety was observed significantly high in orthopaedically challenged group, where females were found to be more anxious. With regard to mental health, normal group and orthopaedically challenged group showed no significant difference.

Studies Related to Mental Health and Socio-economic Status

The results of the study conducted by Ray and Yadav (1993) on 251 boys and 250 girls from grades nine to twelfth of two urban and two rural higher secondary schools revealed that mental health and socio-economic status were positively and significantly correlated.

Similarly, Shek (2002) examined the association between family functioning and adolescent adjustment in 1,519 Chinese adolescents using an indigenously developed measure of family functioning. Results showed that family functioning was significantly related to measures of adolescent psychological well-being (existential well-being, life satisfaction, self-esteem, sense of mastery, general psychiatric morbidity), school adjustment (perceived academic performance, satisfaction with academic performance, and school conduct), and problem behaviour (delinquent and substance abuse behaviour). Family functioning was generally more strongly related to measures of adjustment for adolescents with economic disadvantage than for adolescents without economic disadvantage.

Gulati and Dutta (2004) conducted a study on the mental health profile of 245 rural adolescents (12 to 16 years) drawn from persistent poor but intact families of Ludhiana district. Socio-economic status scale (Pareek & Trivedi, 1964) and child behaviour checklist (Achenbach and Edelbrock, 1990) were used for data collection. Results indicated that despite economic diversity and the presence of other risk conditions, majority of the adolescents were found to be performing within normal status of mental health without any manifest conduct disorders and also the effect of gender was found to be non-significant. The results revealed that the dominant problem in males was delinquency and in females were anxiety and depression.

Rahi *et al.* (2005) studied the association of psychopathology with demographic, developmental and social factors on 620 children from an urban slum of Miraj (Maharashtra). Childhood psychopathology measurement schedule (CPMS) developed and standardized by Malhotra *et al.* (1988) was used to measure the magnitude of probable psychopathology and a schedule to record the demographic, developmental and social factors of the children. They reported that males were significantly affected more than the females and the prevalence increased significantly as the socio-economic status lowered. The studies revealed that socio-economic status has greater impact on mental health of adolescents, lower socio-economic status lower the mental health of the adolescent.

Studies Related to Mental Health and Residential Area

The place one has been brought up may have an impact on the make up of the person. The personality differs for a person from rural background with a person with urban background in same environment.

Jha (2005) examined the impact of the social residential areas with gender on mental health problem on 110 secondary school children of age (11-17 years). Langner's (1962) mental health scale was used to identify the mental health problem. The study revealed that rural children faced more problems than urban children, especially girls. This is in congruency with Nanda (2001) who reported that urban students had better mental health than the rural students.The studies revealed that urban area mental health, but cannot be generalized.

Studies Related to Mental Health and Home Environment

Home is the first and primary society an individual is exposed. It builds up one's personality.

Dhoundiyal (1984) studied on 276 emotionally disturbed adolescents, who were identified from randomly selected rural and urban intermediate colleges with the help of emotional disturbance inventory developed by Rawal (1983). Home environment was measured by Home Environment Scale developed by Rawal (1983). The results revealed that the quality of home environment is a significant factor in determining emotional disturbance among adolescents. Also the study revealed that over-protection of parent's facilitated emotional disturbance among adolescents.

Ensminger *et al.* (2003) examined the relationship of mothers' symptoms of depression and anxiety reported during their offspring's childhood and adolescence on depressive disorder and educational achievement of their adult children. The data was collected from a longitudinal cohort study of first graders from Woodlawn, Chicago, followed from age 6 to 32 years (N = 879). Adult children's depression and educational attainment are regressed on earlier self-reports of mothers' psychological distress. Results reported that daughters of mothers with persistent maternal psychological distress had two and a half times the risk of lifetime depressive disorder, but no increased risk of high school dropout. For sons, mothers' psychological distress was not related to depression but was related to poorer educational attainment. They concluded mothers' depressed feelings during the child-rearing years relate to their children's depression and educational attainment as measured in adulthood. The patterns differ for sons and daughters.

Dwairy (2004) also supported the earlier study, where the researcher examined the parental styles and psychosocial adjustment of adolescents and the relationship between them in gifted as compared to non-gifted Arab adolescents. The Parental Authority Questionnaire, Child Attitude Towards Parents, Lipsitt's Self-Concept Scale for Children, Rosenberg Self-Esteem Scale, and the Psychological State Scale were administered to 118 gifted and 115 non-gifted Arab adolescents in Israel. Results indicated that parents of gifted adolescents tend to be more authoritative and less authoritarian than parents of non-gifted adolescents. The attitudes of the gifted adolescents towards their parents were more positive than those of the non-gifted adolescents. The gifted displayed higher self-esteem and fewer identity disorders, phobias, and conduct disorders than the non-gifted adolescents. The authoritative parental style correlates positively with the mental health of both gifted and non-gifted adolescents, while the authoritarian parenting style impacts negatively on the mental health of the gifted, but not of the non-gifted adolescents. The study results indicated that the authoritarian parenting style is a crucial factor that influences the well-being of gifted children and may affect their psychological adjustment.

Abu-Rayya (2006) explored the relationship between ethnic identity, ego identity and psychological well-being among mixed-ethnic adolescents with European mothers and Arab fathers in Israel. The sample of 127 mixed-ethnic adolescents (13 to 18 years) were instructed to respond to a modified version of Phinney's (1992) Multi-group ethnic identity measure (MEIM), Bennion and Adam's (1986) ego identity measure (EOM-EIS) and Ryff's (1999) psychological well-being scale. It was found that Arab and European ethnic identities, composed of ethnic behaviours, affirmation and belonging and achievement of a sense of oneself as part of an ethnic group, were significantly positively correlated with participants' psychological well-being. Findings revealed positive and significant relationship between Arab and European ethnic identity and psychological well-being for the mixed-ethnic adolescents. The results also suggested that ego identity status was significantly associated with the psychological well-being of mixed-ethnic adolescents.

Studies Related to School and Mental Health

Next to the home, an individual gets in contact with the school and spend most of the time at school especially till adolescents.

Srivastava *et al.* (1999) studied the mental health of 80 students studying in 11th and 12th standard from English medium and Hindi medium schools located at Haridwar. Mithila Mental Health Status Inventory (MMHSI) developed by Kumar and Thakur was used to measure the mental health of the students. The results showed that Hindi medium students had better mental health in comparison to English medium students. The authors also reported that symptoms of ego-centrism and emotional instability in English medium students were high in comparison to Hindi medium students. They suggested that parents and teachers should content-operate each other in solving the problems of educational medium among college students.

Reddy *et al.* (2002) studied 720 school-going children of 9th and 10th grades drawn randomly from private and public schools in and around Chittoor district of Andhra Pradesh. The aim was to find out the effect of co-education on mental health of the students. Mental health status inventory developed by Manjuvani (1989) was used to assess the mental health. Results revealed that there was a significant impact of the type of school on mental health status of both boys and girls. The students of co-educational schools were mentally healthier when compared to the students of non-co-educational schools.

Ostberg (2003) focused on social relations in school classes and their importance for mental well-being in middle childhood in a Scottish city. Peer status and both the individual's own status position and the status distribution of the school class as a whole were considered as the respect of social relations. The number of children analysed was 13,932 and the number of school classes was 524. The results show a clear association at individual level: the higher the status position the more uncommon is malaise, which was supported by the teacher and by a parent report on malaise for both boys and girls. The association was generally present within school and existed regardless of grade, type of school and class size. Furthermore, a minority of the classes had a more compressed status distribution and here malaise was less common in all status positions. This was especially the case when the school class did not contain marginalized children. Consequently, that some children are marginalized in the group indicates problematic conditions for the persons in question but also for the other group members.

Aseltine and Gore (2005) examined how living situation, work school roles and experiences in those roles affect psychological functioning in high school. The sample consisted of 1325 students of seven communities and school districts in the Boston. The tools used were centre for epidemiological studies' depression (CES-D) scale (Radloff, 1977) to measure the depressed mood; Data was collected through both structured and open ended. Results showed that enrollment in college programmes and full-time are associated with lower levels of depressed moods and more positive quality of life. Disruptions in work were linked to higher levels of depressed mood, heavy episodic drinking and poorer quality of life; the negative effects of disruptions in post-secondary schooling are confined to high episodic drinking. The studies revealed that type of school management, medium of instruction influences the mental health of adolescents.

Studies Related to Transition and Mental Health

Transition of school calls for a lot of adjustment with the new environment. This in turn may affect the mental health of an individual.

Roeser *et al.* (1999) examined patterns of academic functioning and mental health in 184, middle school children and relation of such patterns to their prior and subsequent functioning. Data were collected from children during their 2nd, 3rd, 4th, 8th and 9th grade school years. Tools used were academic competence scale and academic value scale developed by Eccles (1983), general self-worth scale by Harter (1982). Cluster analysis was used to delineate patterns of academic functioning and mental health during 8th grade. These authors examined the relation of these patterns to academic functioning and mental health one year later the transition to high school, and then examined the long term development roots of the 8th grade patterns using data collected during elementary school years. There was no significant change in mental health among the full sample, in emotional functioning, the multiple problems youth mental health improved significantly across the transition.

Impact of Intervention on Mental Health

Kannappan and Bai (1994) assessed and compared the effect of different psychological training and tested the trend of different trainings over successive periods on 240 adolescent deviant boys (age range 14-16 years) identified by behavioural deviant checklist (Kannappan, 1992). The boys were assigned to seven experimental groups such as social skills training (SST), human relationship training (HRT), social skills with human relationship training (SS-HRT), yoga-cognitive training (YCT), cognitive skills training (CST), yoga with cognitive skills training (YCST), multiple training (MT) and control group randomly. Training was given for two months. The groups SST, HRT, YCT, CST and YCST had changes in few areas of mental health but group SS-HRT and MT had significant change in self-concept, perception of self among others, concept of life and perception of adjustment.

Gonzales *et al.* (2004) studied the efficacy of the bridges programme, an intervention designed to prevent school disengagement and negative mental health trajectories during transition to junior high school. The intervention included adolescent coping skills intervention, a parenting skills intervention and a family strengthening intervention. The programme was evaluated by examining pretest to posttest changes on targeted mediators and outcomes with a sample of 22 predominantly Mexican American families. Adolescents reported increased use of active and distraction coping strategies and decreased depressive symptoms for themselves from pretest to posttest. They also reported significant changes in their mothers' parenting skills, including increased monitoring and a decrease in inconsistent discipline. Maternal caregivers reported an increase in supportive parenting and a decrease in inconsistent discipline for themselves and fewer adolescent problem behaviours.

Hence the studies reveal that intervention programmes have positive impact on mental health, earlier the better.

Objectives

To understand and compare the extent of different types of problems faced by late adolescents boys and girls.

To compare the mental health status of students reporting higher *vs.* lower levels of problems among late adolescent boys and girls.

To study the relationship between different types of problems and mental health among late adolescent boys and girls.

Hypothesis

There will be no difference between the scores of late adolescent boys and girls on the problems in different areas.

Late adolescent boys and girls reporting higher levels of problems will be obtaining lower scores on mental health areas as compared to those reporting lower levels of problems.

Scores on problem areas will be negatively associated with mental health scores for both late adolescent boys and girls.

Sample

The sample consisted of 38 boys and 40 girls. The sample were taken from Kendriya Vidyalaya, B.H.U., Varanasi. All the samples were students of class 12th. The age range was 16-17 years.

Tools

Mental Health Inventory

Developed and standardized by Jagdish and Srivastava (1983) assess the various symptoms of sound mental health. There are 56 items in the inventory which are to be rated on four point scale. The items in the inventory cover the six dimensions of sound mental health—Positive self-evaluation, Integration of personality, Autonomy, Group oriented attitude and Environmental mastery.

Table 9.1: Self-Image Related Issues among Boys and Girls with High and Low Mental Health Status

		Boys			Girls		
		Mental Health Status		χ^2	Mental Health Status		χ^2
		Low	High		Low	High	
Nervousness While Conversing	Yes	8 (44.4%)	2 (10%)	5.80**	7 (33.3%)	1 (5.3%)	4.91*
	No	10 (55.6%)	18 (90.0%)		14 (66.7%)	18 (94.7%)	
Lonliness	Yes	8 (44.4%)	2 (10.0%)	5.80**	2 (9.5%)	1 (5.3%)	0.261
	No	10 (55.6%)	18 (90.0%)		19 (90.5%)	18 (94.7%)	
Superiority Complex	Yes	4 (22.2%)	2 (10.0%)	1.06	0 (0.0%)	3 (15.8%)	3.59*
	No	14 (77.8%)	18 (90.0%)		21 (100.0%)	16 (84.2%)	
No Self-Confidence	Yes	2 (11.1%)	2 (10.0%)	.012	5 (23.8%)	3 (15.8%)	0.401
	No	16 (88.9%)	18 (90.0%)		16 (76.2%)	16 (84.2%)	
No Enough Courage	Yes	4 (22.2%)	0 (0.0%)	4.97*	4 (19.0%)	1 (5.3%)	1.73
	No	14 (77.8%)	20 (100.0%)		17 (81.0%)	18 (94.7%)	
Unable to Understand Myself	Yes	3 (16.7%)	2 (10.0%)	0.39	8 (38.1%)	1 (5.3%)	6.17**
	No	15 (83.3%)	18 (90.0%)		13 (61.9%)	18 (94.7%)	
Unable to Control Self Behaviour	Yes	6 (33.3%)	1 (5.0%)	5.06*	6 (28.6%)	3 (15.8%)	0.94
	No	12 (66.7%)	19 (95.0%)		15 (71.4%)	16 (84.2%)	
Unable to Bear Even the Slightest Scolding	Yes	5 (27.8%)	1 (5.0%)	3.70*	13 (61.9%)	6 (31.6%)	3.70*
	No	13 (72.2%)	19 (95.0%)		8 (38.1%)	13 (68.4%)	
Don't Get Appreciation in Any Kind of Work	Yes	4 (22.2%)	0 (0.0%)	4.97*	3 (14.3%)	1 (5.3%)	0.902
	No	14 (77.8%)	20 (100.0%)		18 (85.7%)	18 (94.7%)	
Bad Complexion	Yes	7 (38.9%)		9.53**	1 (4.8%)	1 (5.3%)	0.005
	No	11 (61.1%)	20 (100.0%)		20 (95.2%)	18 (94.7%)	
Poor Appearance	Yes	5 (27.8%)	1 (5.0%)	3.70*	1 (4.8%)	1 (5.3%)	0.005
	No	13 (72.2%)	19 (95.0%)		20 (95.2%)	18 (94.7%)	
Get Tired Because of Many Activities	Yes	7 (38.9%)	2 (10.0%)	4.37*	3 (14.3%)	2 (10.5%)	0.13
	No	11 (61.1%)	18 (90.0%)		18 (85.7%)	17 (89.5%)	

(Contd.)

(*Contd.*)

		Boys			Girls		
		Mental Health Status		χ^2	Mental Health Status		χ^2
		Low	High		Low	High	
Afraid of failure in whatever I undertaken	Yes	8 (44.4%)	3 (15.0%)	3.99*	13 (61.9%)	3 (15.8%)	8.84**
	No	10 (55.6%)	17 (85.0%)		8 (38.1%)	16 (84.2%)	
Many problems at a time	Yes	8 (44.4%)	3 (15.0%)	3.99*	11 (52.4%)	4 (21.1%)	4.17*
	No	10 (55.6%)	17 (85.0%)		10 (47.6%)	15 (78.9%)	
Unable to do Good Work	Yes	5 (27.8%)	1 (5.0%)	3.70*	4 (19.0%)	1 (5.3%)	1.73
	No	13 (72.2%)	19 (95.0%)		17 (81.0%)	18 (94.7%)	
Unable to Solve Difficulties	Yes	5 (27.8%)	1 (5.0%)	3.70*	6 (28.6%)	1 (5.3%)	3.75*
	No	13 (72.2%)	19 (95.0%)		15 (71.4%)	18 (94.7%)	
Problems in Making Plans	Yes	4 (22.2%)	1 (5.0%)	2.46	4 (19.0%)		4.02*
	No	14 (77.8%)	19 (95.0%)		17 (81.0%)	19 (100.0%)	
Unable to do Many things Which Other Persons are Able to do	Yes	3 (16.7%)	3 (15.0%)	0.02	6 (28.6%)	1 (5.3%)	3.75*
	No	15 (83.3%)	17 (85.0%)		15 (71.4%)	18 (94.7%)	
Problems in Doing Things at Right Moment	Yes	3 (16.7%)	2 (10.0%)	0.37	8 (38.1%)	2 (10.5%)	4.04*
	No	15 (83.3%)	18 (90.0%)		13 (61.9%)	17 (89.5%)	
Cannot Decide Interests	Yes	5 (27.8%)	2 (10.0%)	1.99	10 (47.6%)	1 (5.3%)	8.97**
	No	13 (72.2%)	18 (90.0%)		11 (52.4%)	18 (94.7%)	
Unable to Change the Behaviour	Yes	4 (22.2%)	2 (10.0%)	1.06	6 (28.6%)	1 (5.3%)	375*
	No	14 (77.8%)	18 (90.0%)		15 (71.4%)	18 (94.7%)	
Waste time on Radio and Movies	Yes	5 (27.8%)		6.39**	9 (42.9%)	3 (15.8%)	3.48
	No	13 (72.2%)	20 (100.0%)		12 (57.1%)	16 (84.2%)	
Telling the Things Which Should Not Tell	Yes	8 (44.4%)	4 (20.0%)	2.62	8 (38.1%)	2 (10.5%)	4.04*
	No	10 (55.6%)	16 (80.0%)		13 (61.9%)	17 (89.5%)	
Doing the Things Which Should Not do	Yes	7 (38.9%)	3 (15.0%)	2.79	8 (38.1%)		9.05**
	No	11 (61.1%)	17 (85.0%)		13 (61.9%)	19 (100.0%)	
Nightmares	Yes	6 (33.3%)	1 (5.0%)	5.06*	3 (14.3%)	2 (10.5%)	0.13
	No	12 (66.7%)	19 (95.0%)		18 (85.7%)	17 (89.5%)	

Student's Problem Inventory

Developed by Dr. Badami (1977) was used to assess the extent of problems in various areas. It has 265 items which refer to problems experienced by adolescents, divided in 9 areas, viz. Physical problems, Self and Self-Image related problems, Economic problems, Friendship sex and marriage related problems, Problems related to Family, Social Problems, Educational problems, Vocational problems, Custom related problems.

On the area of nervousness while conversing the value of chi square among boys was significant ($\chi^2 = .86, p < 01$). 44.4 per cent students who scored low on the score of mental health had the problem in this area while 55.6 per cent who scored low in this area did not have the problem in this area. 10 per cent students who scored high on mental health had the problem in this area while 90.0 per cent students who scored high on mental health area did not have the problem in this area.

On the area of nervousness while conversing the value of chi square among girls was significant ($\chi^2 = 4.91, p < 05$). 33.3 per cent students who scored low on the score of mental health had the problem in this area while 66.7 per cent who scored low in this area did not have the problem in this area. 5.3 per cent students who scored high on mental health had the problem in this area while 94.7 per cent students who scored high on mental health did not have the problem in this area.

On the area of loneliness the value of chi square among boys was significant ($\chi^2 = 5.80, p < 01$). 44.4 per cent students who scored low on the score of mental health had the problem in this area while 55.6 per cent who scored low in this area did not have the problem in this area. 10 per cent students who scored high on mental health had the problem in this area while 90.0 per cent students who scored high on mental health area did not have the problem in this area.

On the area of loneliness the value of chi square among girls was not significant ($\chi^2 = 0.26$, NS). 9.5 per cent students who scored low on the score of mental health had the problem in this area while 90.0 per cent who scored low in this area did not have the problem in this area. 5.3 per cent students who scored high on mental health had the problem in this area while 94.7 students who scored high on mental health did not have the problem in this area.

On the area of superiority complex the value of chi square among boys was not significant ($\chi^2 = 5.80$, NS). 22.2 per cent students who scored low on the score of mental health had the problem in this area while 77.8 per cent who scored low on the score of mental health did not have the problem in this area. 10 per cent students who scored high on mental health had the problem in this area while 90.0 per cent students who scored high on mental health area did not have the problem in this area.

On the area of no self-confidence the value of chi square among boys was not significant (χ^2 = .012, NS). 11.1 per cent students who scored low on the score of mental health had the problem in this area while 88.9 per cent who scored low on the score of mental health did not have the problem in this area. 10 per cent students who scored high on mental health had the problem in this area while 90.0 per cent students who scored high on mental health area did not have the problem in this area.

On the area of no self-confidence the value of chi square among girls was not significant (χ^2 = 0.40, NS). 23.8 per cent students who scored low on the score of mental health had the problem in this area while 76.2 per cent who scored low on the score of mental health did not have the problem in this area. 15.8 per cent students who scored high on mental health had the problem in this area while 84.2 per cent students who scored high on mental health area did not have the problem in this area.

On the area of no enough courage the value of chi square among boys was significant (χ^2 = 4.97%, p < 05). 22.2 per cent students who scored low on the score of mental health had the problem in this area while 77.8 per cent who scored low on the score of mental health did not have the problem in this area. 0 per cent students who scored high on mental health had the problem in this area while 100 per cent students who scored high on mental health area did not have the problem in this area.

On the area of no enough courage the value of chi square among girls was not significant (χ^2 = 1.73, NS). 19 per cent students who scored low on the score of mental health had the problem in this area while 81 per cent who scored low on the score of mental health did not have the problem in this area. 5.3 per cent students who scored high on mental health had the problem in this area while 94.7 per cent students who scored high on mental health area did not have the problem in this area.

On the area of unable to understand myself the value of chi square among boys was not significant (χ^2 = 0.39, NS). 16.7 per cent students who scored low on the score of mental health had the problem in this area while 83.3 per cent who scored low on the score of mental health did not have the problem in this area. 2 per cent students who scored high on mental health had the problem in this area while 90 per cent students who scored high on mental health area did not have the problem in this area.

On the area of unable to understand myself the value of chi square among girls was significant ($\chi^2 = 6.17, p < .01$). 38.1 per cent students who scored low on the score of mental health had the problem in this area while 61.9 per cent who scored low on the score of mental health did not have the problem in this area. 1 per cent students who scored high on mental health had the problem in this area while 94.7 per cent students who scored high on mental health area did not have the problem in this area.

On the area of unable to control behaviour the value of chi square among boys was significant ($\chi^2 = 5.06, p < .05$). 33.3 per cent students who scored low on the score of mental health had the problem in this area while 66.7 per cent who scored low on the score of mental health did not have the problem in this area. 5.0 per cent students who scored high on mental health had the problem in this area while 95.0 per cent students who scored high on mental health area did not have the problem in this area.

On the area of unable to understand myself the value of chi square among girls was not significant ($\chi^2 = 0.94$, NS). 28.6 per cent students who scored low on the score of mental health had the problem in this area while 71.4 per cent who scored low on the score of mental health did not have the problem in this area. 15.8 per cent students who scored high on mental health had the problem in this area while 84.2 per cent students who scored high on mental health area did not have the problem in this area.

On the area of unable to bear even the slightest scolding the value of chi square among boys was significant ($\chi^2 = 3.70, p < .05$). 27.8 per cent students who scored low on the score of mental health had the problem in this area while 72.2 per cent who scored low on the score of mental health did not have the problem in this area. 5.0 per cent students who scored high on mental health had the problem in this area while 95.0 per cent students who scored high on mental health area did not have the problem in this area.

On the area of unable to bear even the slightest scolding the value of chi square among girls was significant ($\chi^2 = 3.70, p < .05$). 61.9 per cent students who scored low on the score of mental health had the problem in this area while 38.1 per cent who scored low on the score of mental health did not have the problem in this area. 31.6 per cent students who scored high on mental health had the problem in this area while 68.4 per cent students who scored high on mental health area did not have the problem in this area.

On the area of don't get appreciation in any kind of work the value of chi square among boys was significant ($\chi^2 = 4.97, p < .05$). 22.2 per cent students who scored low on the score of mental health had the problem in this area while 77.8 per cent who scored low on the score of mental health did not have the problem in this area. 0 per cent students who scored high on mental health had the problem in this area while 100 per cent students who scored high on mental health area did not have the problem in this area.

On the area of don't get appreciation in any kind of work the value of chi square among girls was not significant ($\chi^2 = 0.90$, NS). 14.3 per cent students who scored low on the score of mental health had the problem in this area while 85.7 per cent who scored low on the score of mental health did not have the problem in this area. 5.3 per cent students who scored high on mental health had the problem in this area while 94.7 per cent students who scored high on mental health area did not have the problem in this area.

On the area of bad complexion the value of chi square among boys was significant ($\chi^2 = 9.53, p < .01$). 38.9 per cent students who scored low on the score of mental health had the problem in this area while 61.1 per cent who scored low on the score of mental health did not have the problem in this area. 0 per cent students who scored high on mental health had the problem in this area while 100 per cent students who scored high on mental health area did not have the problem in this area.

On the area of bad complexion the value of chi square among girls was not significant ($\chi^2 = 0.01$, NS). 4.8 per cent students who scored low on the score of mental health had the problem in this area while 95.2 per cent who scored low on the score of mental health did not have the problem in this area. 5.3 per cent students who scored high on mental health had the problem in this area while 94.7 per cent students who scored high on mental health area did not have the problem in this area.

On the area of poor appearance the value of chi square among boys was significant ($\chi^2 = 3.70, p < .05$). 27.8 per cent students who scored low on the score of mental health had the problem in this area while 72.2 per cent who scored low on the score of mental health did not have the problem in this area. 5 per cent students who scored high on mental health had the problem in this area while 95.0 per cent students who scored high on mental health area did not have the problem in this area.

On the area of poor appearance the value of chi square among girls was not significant ($\chi^2 = .005$, NS). 4.8 per cent students who scored low on the score of mental health had the problem in this area while 95.2 per cent who scored low on the score of mental health did not have the problem in this area. 5.3 per cent students who scored high on mental health had the problem in this area while 94.7 per cent students who scored high on mental health area did not have the problem in this area.

On the area of get tired because of many activities the value of chi square among boys was significant ($\chi^2 = 4.37, p < .05$). 38.9 per cent students who scored low on the score of mental health had the problem in this area while 61.1 per cent who scored low on the score of mental health did not have the problem in this area. 10 per cent students who scored high on mental health had the problem in this area while 90.0 per cent students who scored high on mental health area did not have the problem in this area.

On the area of get tired because of many activities the value of chi square among girls was not significant ($\chi^2 = 0.13$, NS). 14.3 per cent students who scored low on the score of mental health had the problem in this area while 85.7 per cent who scored low on the score of mental health did not have the problem in this area. 10.5 per cent students who scored high on mental health had the problem in this area while 89.5 per cent students who scored high on mental health area did not have the problem in this area.

On the area of afraid of failure in whatever I undertaken the value of chi square among boys was significant ($\chi^2 = 3.99, p < .05$). 44.4 per cent students who scored low on the score of mental health had the problem in this area while 55.6 per cent who scored low on the score of mental health did not have the problem in this area. 15 per cent students who scored high on mental health had the problem in this area while 85 per cent students who scored high on mental health area did not have the problem in this area.

On the area of afraid of failure in whatever I undertaken the value of chi square among girls was significant ($\chi^2 = 8.84, p < .01$). 61.9 per cent students who scored low on the score of mental health had the problem in this area while 38.1 per cent who scored low on the score of mental health did not have the problem in this area. 15.8 per cent students who scored high on mental health had the problem in this area while 84.2 per cent students who scored high on mental health area did not have the problem in this area.

On the area of many problems at a time the value of chi square among boys was significant ($\chi^2 = 3.97, p < .05$). 44.4 per cent students who scored low on the score of mental health had the problem in this area while 55.6 per cent who scored low on the score of mental health did not have the problem in this area. 15 per cent students who scored high on mental health had the problem in this area while 85.0 per cent students who scored high on mental health area did not have the problem in this area.

On the area of many problems at a time the value of chi square among girls was significant ($\chi^2 = 4.17, p < .05$). 52.4 per cent students who scored low on the score of mental health had the problem in this area while 47.6 per cent who scored low on the score of mental health did not have the problem in this area. 21.1 per cent students who scored high on mental health had the problem in this area while 78.9 per cent students who scored high on mental health area did not have the problem in this area.

On the area of many problems at a time the value of chi square among boys was significant ($\chi^2 = 3.97, p < .05$). 44.4 per cent students who scored low on the score of mental health had the problem in this area while 55.6 per cent who scored low on the score of mental health did not have the problem in this area. 15 per cent students who scored high on mental health had the problem in this area while 85.0 per cent students who scored high on mental health area did not have the problem in this area.

On the area of unable to do good work the value of chi square among boys was significant ($\chi^2 = 3.70, p < .05$). 27.8 per cent students who scored low on the score of mental health had the problem in this area while 72.2 per cent who scored low on the score of mental health did not have the problem in this area. 5 per cent students who scored high on mental health had the problem in this area while 95 per cent students who scored high on mental health area did not have the problem in this area.

On the area of unable to do good work the value of chi square among girls was not significant ($\chi^2 = 1.73$, NS). 19 per cent students who scored low on the score of mental health had the problem in this area while 81 per cent who scored low on the score of mental health did not have the problem in this area. 5.3 per cent students who scored high on mental health had the problem in this area while 94.7 per cent students who scored high on mental health area did not have the problem in this area.

On the area of unable to solve difficulties the value of chi square among boys was significant ($\chi^2 = 3.70, p < .05$). 27.8 per cent students who scored low on the score of mental health had the problem in this area while 72.2 per cent who scored low on the score of mental health did not have the problem in this area. 5 per cent students who scored high on mental health had the problem in this area while 95 per cent students who scored high on mental health area did not have the problem in this area.

On the area of unable to solve difficulties the value of chi square among girls was significant ($\chi^2 = 3.75, p < .05$). 28.6 per cent students who scored low on the score of mental health had the problem in this area while 71.4 per cent who scored low on the score of mental health did not have the problem in this area. 5.3 per cent students who scored high on mental health had the problem in this area while 94.7 per cent students who scored high on mental health area did not have the problem in this area.

On the area of problems in making plan the value of chi square among boys was not significant ($\chi^2 = 2.46$, NS). 22.2 per cent students who scored low on the score of mental health had the problem in this area while 77.8 per cent who scored low on the score of mental health did not have the problem in this area. 1 per cent students who scored high on mental health had the problem in this area while 95 per cent students who scored high on mental health area did not have the problem in this area.

On the area of problems in making plan the value of chi square among girls was significant (χ^2= 3.75, p<.05). 19 per cent students who scored low on the score of mental health had the problem in this area while 81 per cent who scored low on the score of mental health did not have the problem in this area. 0 per cent students who scored high on mental health had the problem in this area while 100 per cent students who scored high on mental health area did not have the problem in this area.

On the area of problems in making plan the value of chi square among boys was not significant ($\chi^2 = 2.46$, NS). 22.2 per cent students who scored low on the score of mental health had the problem in this area while 77.8 per cent who scored low on the score of mental health did not have the problem in this area. 1 per cent students who scored high on mental health had the problem in this area while 95 per cent students who scored high on mental health area did not have the problem in this area.

On the area of problems in making plan the value of chi square among girls was significant ($\chi^2 = 4.02, p < .05$). 19 per cent students who scored low on the score of mental health had the problem in this area while 81 per cent who scored low on the score of mental health did not have the problem in this area. 0 per cent students who scored high on mental health had the problem in this area while 100 per cent students who scored high on mental health area did not have the problem in this area.

On the area of unable to do many things the value of chi square among boys was not significant ($\chi^2 = 0.02$, NS). 16.7 per cent students who scored low on the score of mental health had the problem in this area while 83.3 per cent who scored low on the score of mental health did not have the problem in this area. 15 per cent students who scored high on mental health had the problem in this area while 85 per cent students who scored high on mental health area did not have the problem in this area.

On the area of unable to do many things the value of chi square among girls was significant ($\chi^2 = 3.75, p < .05$). 28.6 per cent students who scored low on the score of mental health had the problem in this area while 71.4 per cent who scored low on the score of mental health did not have the problem in this area. 5.3 per cent students who scored high on mental health had the problem in this area while 94.7 per cent students who scored high on mental health area did not have the problem in this area.

On the area of problems in doing the things at right moment the value of chi square among boys was not significant ($\chi^2 = 0.37$, NS). 16.7 per cent students who scored low on the score of mental health had the problem in this area while 83.3 per cent who scored low on the score of mental health did not have the problem in this area. 10 per cent students who scored high on mental health had the problem in this area while 90 per cent students who scored high on mental health area did not have the problem in this area.

On the area of unable to do many things the value of chi square among girls was significant ($\chi^2 = 4.04, p < .05$). 38.1 per cent students who scored low on the score of mental health had the problem in this area while 61.9 per cent who scored low on the score of mental health did not have the problem in this area. 10.5 per cent students who scored high on mental health had the problem in this area while 89.5 per cent students who scored high on mental health area did not have the problem in this area.

On the area of problems in doing the things at right moment the value of chi square among boys was not significant ($\chi^2 = 0.37$, NS). 16.7 per cent students who scored low on the score of mental health had the problem in this area while 83.3 per cent who scored low on the score of mental health did not have the problem in this area. 10 per cent students who scored high on mental health had the problem in this area while 90 per cent students who scored high on mental health area did not have the problem in this area.

On the area of problems in doing the things at right moment the value of chi square among girls was not significant ($\chi^2 = 0.37$, NS). 16.7 per cent students who scored low on the score of mental health had the problem in this area while 61.9 per cent who scored low on the score of mental health did not have the problem in this area. 10.5 per cent students who scored high on mental health had the problem in this area while 89.5 per cent students who scored high on mental health area did not have the problem in this area.

On the area of cannot decide interests the value of chi square among boys was not significant ($\chi^2 = 1.99$, NS). 27.8 per cent students who scored low on the score of mental health had the problem in this area while 72.2 per cent who scored low on the score of mental health did not have the problem in this area. 10 per cent students who scored high on mental health had the problem in this area while 90 per cent students who scored high on mental health area did not have the problem in this area.

On the area of cannot decide interests the value of chi square among girls was significant ($\chi^2 = 8.97, p < .01$). 47.6 per cent students who scored low on the score of mental health had the problem in this area while 52.4 per cent who scored low on the score of mental health did not have the problem in this area. 5.3 per cent students who scored high on mental health had the problem in this area while 94.7 per cent students who scored high on mental health area did not have the problem in this area.

On the area of unable to change the behaviour the value of chi square among boys was not significant ($\chi^2 = 1.06$, NS). 28.6 per cent students who scored low on the score of mental health had the problem in this area while 71.4 per cent who scored low on the score of mental health did not have the problem in this area. 5.3 per cent students who scored high on mental health had the problem in this area while 94.7 per cent students who scored high on mental health area did not have the problem in this area.

On the area of unable to change the behaviour the value of chi square among girls was significant ($\chi^2 = 3.75, p < .05$). 28.6 per cent students who scored low on the score of mental health had the problem in this area while 71.4 per cent who scored low on the score of mental health did not have the problem in this area. 5.3 per cent students who scored high on mental health had the problem in this area while 94.7 per cent students who scored high on mental health area did not have the problem in this area.

On the area of unable to change the behaviour the value of chi square among boys was not significant ($\chi^2 = 1.06$, NS). 28.6 per cent students who scored low on the score of mental health had the problem in this area while 71.4 per cent who scored low on the score of mental health did not have the problem in this area. 5.3 per cent students who scored high on mental health had the problem in this area while 94.7 per cent students who scored high on mental health area did not have the problem in this area.

On the area of unable to change the behaviour the value of chi square among girls was significant ($\chi^2 = 3.75, p < .05$). 28.6 per cent students who scored low on the score of mental health had the problem in this area while 71.4 per cent who scored low on the score of mental health did not have the problem in this area. 5.3 per cent students who scored high on mental health had the problem in this area while 94.7 per cent students who scored high on mental health area did not have the problem in this area.

On the area of waste time on radio and movies the value of chi square among boys was significant ($\chi^2 = 6.39, p < .01$). 27.8 per cent students who scored low on the score of mental health had the problem in this area while 72.2 per cent who scored low on the score of mental health did not have the problem in this area. 0 per cent students who scored high on mental health had the problem in this area while 100 per cent students who scored high on mental health area did not have the problem in this area.

On the area of waste time on radio and movies the value of chi square among girls was not significant ($\chi^2 = 3.48$, NS). 42.9 per cent students who scored low on the score of mental health had the problem in this area while 7.1 per cent who scored low on the score of mental health did not have the problem in this area. 15.8 per cent students who scored high on mental health had the problem in this area while 84.2 per cent students who scored high on mental health area did not have the problem in this area.

On the area of telling the things which should not tell the value of chi square among boys was not significant ($\chi^2 = 2.62$, NS). 44.4 per cent students who scored low on the score of mental health had the problem in this area while 55.6 per cent who scored low on the score of mental health did not have the problem in this area. 20 per cent students who scored high on mental health had the problem in this area while 80 per cent students who scored high on mental health area did not have the problem in this area.

On the area of waste time on radio and movies the value of chi square among girls was not significant ($\chi^2 = 4.04, p < .05$). 38.1 per cent students who scored low on the score of mental health had the problem in this area while 61.9 per cent who scored low on the score of mental health did not have the problem in this area. 10.5 per cent students who scored high on mental health had the problem in this area while 89.5 per cent students who scored high on mental health area did not have the problem in this area.

On the area of doing the things which should not do the value of chi square among boys was not significant ($\chi^2 = 2.79$, NS). 44.4 per cent students who scored low on the score of mental health had the problem in this area while 55.6 per cent who scored low on the score of mental health did not have the problem in this area. 20 per cent students who scored high on mental health had the problem in this area while 80 per cent students who scored high on mental health area did not have the problem in this area.

On the area of doing the things which should not do the value of chi square among girls was significant ($\chi^2 = 9.05, p < .01$). 38.1 per cent students who scored low on the score of mental health had the problem in this area while 61.9 per cent who scored low on the score of mental health did not have the problem in this area. 0 per cent students who scored high on mental health had the problem in this area while 100 per cent students who scored high on mental health area did not have the problem in this area.

On the area of nightmares the value of chi square among boys was significant ($\chi^2 = 5.06, p < .05$). 33.3 per cent students who scored low on the score of mental health had the problem in this area while 66.7 per cent who scored low on the score of mental health did not have the problem in this area. 5 per cent students who scored high on mental health had the problem in this area while 95 per cent students who scored high on mental health area did not have the problem in this area.

On the area of nightmares the value of chi square among girls was not significant ($\chi^2 = 0.13$, NS). 14.3 per cent students who scored low on the score of mental health had the problem in this area while 85.7 per cent who scored low on the score of mental health did not have the problem in this area. 10.5 per cent students who scored high on mental health had the problem in this area while 89.5 per cent students who scored high on mental health area did not have the problem in this area.

Overall results indicate that within low subjects both boys and girls had the problems in conversing inability to bear even the slightest scolding, afraid of failure, facing many problems at a time, inability to solve difficulties.

Within boys mental health—low subjects suffered from problems of loneliness, not having enough courage, being unable to control their behaviour, not getting appreciation for any kind of work, felt that they had bad complexion, poor appearance, got tired of because of many activities. They get easily offended, unable to do good work, waste time on radios and movies and had nightmares.

Within girls mental health—low subjects, on the other hand more often felt that they suffered from inability to understand themselves, problems in making plans, thought that they were unable to do many things which other persons were able to do, had problems in doing right things at right moment, could not decide interests, were unable to change their behaviour. They felt that they were prone to telling the things which they should not tell and doing the things which they should not do.

Discussion

The overall result seem to convey that late adolescents irrespective and their sex appear to be facing a number of self-image related issues which are likely to influence their mental health (Anand, 1999).

However, there are also a number of issues that are paramount to the maintenance of mental health of boys and girls exclusively. The genetic make-up, time and rate of maturity differs between boys and girls especially during adolescents. In Indian society norms and perception are different for boys and girls. Hence the mental health of boys and girls will be different. At this stage boys are very conscious about their physical fitness and appearance because a larger body frame for boys defines and demarcates them as fully grown adults and being backward in this aspect may lead to being labelled as 'sissy' (Shephard, Lavallee & Lariviere, 1978). In this modern society they cannot control themselves so they generally waste there many times with radio, TV, computers, mobiles etc. Media is used as a third parent or servant. It is very important, as both parents are working, mother in kitchen and father busy in reading or out for his work and the child is having remote in his hand and does not know how to select the programmes and watches only movies or cartoons. Teenagers spend their lives immersed in electronic media. While doing homework on internet, they do instant messaging to their friends. They have television in background and listen to music on i-pod at the same time. Furthermore, time spent with media decreases the amount of time available for pursuing other more healthy activities such as sports, physical activity, community service, cultural pursuits, reading and family time (Dave & Dave, 2011). Boys generally do not share their problems easily with others because they are socialized in our society in such a way that they do not share their problems with other and generally they are more skilful controlling impulses. So they feel lonelier (Fernandz-Berrocal &

Extremera, 2006). In our society girls generally don't have independent right to take their own decisions, so they are unable to decide their interest. They generally don't have control on their thoughts and they seek generally more social support so they do and say the things which they think they should not (Redden, 2002).

Clinicians increasingly recognize that mental health and related problems are important and demanding parts of their practices, with pediatricians reporting that nearly one fifth of their patients have an emotional, behavioural, or school problem (Kelleher, McInerny & Gardner, 2000). Increasing to improve mental health, policy-makers and programme administrators need accurate information about the issue.

On the basis the result of this study it may be recommended that problems of adolescents should be identified and remedial measures should be taken at the inception itself. It should be recognized that crucial problem areas and mental health issues may differ for boys and girls and gender sensitive intervention should be instituted. Availability of counsellor in schools must be ensured by authorities as has already been recommended by NCERT.

The result show that within low mental health both boys and girls had the problems in conversing inability to bear even the slightest scolding, afraid of failure, facing many problems at a time, inability to solve difficulty. Within boys subjects with low mental health suffered from problems of lonliness, not having enough courage, being unable to control their behaviour, not getting appreciation for any kind of work, felt that they had bad complexion, poor appearance, got tired of because of many activities. They get easily offended, unable to do good work, waste time on radios and movies and had nightmares. Within girls subjects with low mental health, on the other hand more often felt that they suffered from inability to understand themselves, problems in making plans, thought that they were unable to do many things which other persons were able to do, had problems in doing right things at right moment, could not decide interests, were unable to change their behaviour. They felt that they were prone to telling the things which they should not tell and doing the things which they should not do.

References

Abraham, R.R., Zulkifli, E.M.B., Fan, E.S., Xin, G.N., & Lim, J. T. G. (2009). A report on stress among first year students in an Indian medical school. *South East Asian Journal of Medical Education,* 3(2), 78-81.

Abu-Rayya, H.M. (2006). Ethnic identity, ego identity and psychological well-being among mixed ethnic Arab-European adolescents in Israel. *British Journal of Developmental Psychology, 24,* 669-679.

Adalf, E.M., Demers, A., and Gliksman, L. (Eds.) (2005). *Canadian Campus Survey 2004.* Toronto, ON: Center for Addiction and Mental Health.

Andrews, G. & Jenkins, R. (eds) (1999). *Management of Mental Disorders* (1st edn). Sydney: WHO Collaborating Centre for Mental Health and Substance Misuse.

Aseltine, R.H. and Gore, S. (2005). Work, post-secondary education and psychological functioning following the transition from high school. *Journal of Adolescent Research,* 20(6), 615-639.

Badami, H.D. (1977). *Student Problem Inventory.* Varanasi: Rupa Psychological Centre.

Bhagi, S. and Sharma, P. (1992). *Encyclopedic Dictionary of Psychology.* New Delhi: Anmol Publisher.

Bhatia, B.D., (1982). *Mental Health in Education.* Advanced Educational Psychology, Sterlings.

Breier, A., Charney, D.S., and Heninger, G.R. (1986). Agoraphobia with panic attacks: development, diagnostic stability, and course of illness. *Archives of General Psychiatry, 43,* 1029-1036.

Brooks, T.L., Harris, S.K., and Thrall, J.S. (2002). Association of adolescent risk behaviour with mental health symptoms in high school students. *Journal of Adolescent Health, 31,* 240-246.

Brown, T.A., O'Leary, T.A., and Barlow, D.H. (2001). *Generalized Anxiety Disorder. In Clinical Handbook of Psychological Disorders: A Step-by-Step Treatment Manual* (3rd edn) (ed. D. H. Barlow), 154-208. New York: Guilford Press.

Busch, S.H., & Barry, C.L. (2007). Mental health disorders in childhood: Assessing the burden on families. *Health Affairs, 26(4),* 1088-109.

Cassano, P. and Fava, M. (2002). Depression and public health: An Overview. *Journal of Psychosomatic Research, 53,* 849-857.

Chauhan, S.S. (2008). *Advanced Educational Psychology.* New Delhi: Vani Educational Books, 415.

Dav., D. and Dave, A.C. (2011). Electronic Media and Child Behaviour. *National Journal of Medical Research, 1(2),* 87-89.

Dhoundiyal, (1984). Home environment and emotional disturbance among adolescents. *Indian Journal of Psychiatry, 59* (2), 17-22.

Dwairy, M. (2004). Parenting styles and mental health of Arab gifted adolescents. *Gifted Child Quarterly, 48* (4), 275-286.

Ensminger, M.E., Hanson, S.G., Riley, A.W. and Juon, H.S., (2003) Maternal psychological distress: Adult sons' and daughters' mental health and educational attainment. *Journal of American Academy of Child and Adolescent Psychiatry, 42* (9), 1108-15.

Fernandez, B.P., Alcaide, R., Extremera, N., and Pizarro, D. (2006). The role of emotional intelligence in anxiety and depression among adolescents. *Individual Differences Research, 4(1),* 16-27.

Foa, E.B., Keane, T.M., and Friedman, M.J. (2008). *Effective Treatments for PTSD: Practice Guidelines from the International Society for Traumatic Stress Studies.* New York: The Guilford Press.

Gerbcr, P.D., Barrett, J.E., Barrett, J.A., *et al.* (1992). The relationship of presenting physical complaints to depressive symptoms in primary care patient. *Journal of General Internal Medicine,* 7, 170-173.

Gonzales, N.A., Dumka, L. E., Deardorff, J., Carter, S. J. and McCray, A., (2004). Preventing poor mental health and school dropout of Mexican American adolescents following the transition to junior high school. *Journal of Adolescent Research 19* (1), 113-131.

Gulati, J.K. and Dutta, J. (2004). Mental health profile of rural adolescents living in persistent economic hardship. *Man in India, 84* (1&2), 113-121.

Jagdish & Srivastava, A.K. (1983). *Mental Health Inventory.* Varanasi: Manovaigyanik Parikshan Sansthan.

Jahoda, M., (1958). *Current Concepts of Positive Mental Health.* New York, Basic books, pp. 45-49.

Kannappan, R., and Bai, R.L. (1994). Positive change in mental health in adolescent deviant boys. *Indian Psychological Review, 42* (5-6), 28-36.

Kelleher, K.J., McInerny, T.K., and Gardner, W.P. (2000). Increasing identification of psychosocial problems: 1979-1996. *Pediatrics, 105(6),* 1313-1321.

Kessler, R.C.,. Chiu, W.T., Demler, O., *et al.* (2005b). Prevalence, severity and co-morbidity of 12-month DSM-IV disorders in the National Co-morbidity Survey Replication. *Archives of General Psychiatry, 62,* 617-627.

Lewinsohn, P.M., Solomon, A., Seeley, J.R., *et al.* (2000). Clinical implications of sub-threshold depressive symptoms. *Journal of Abnormal Psychology, 109,* 345-351.

Menninger, K.A., (1945). *Human kind.* New York.

Merikangas, K.R., Ames, M. Lihong, C, *et al.* (2007). The impact of co-morbidity of mental and physical conditions on role of disability in the US adult household population. *Archives of General Psychiatry, 64*(10), 1180-1188.

Ojha, S., (2002). A comparative study of social anxiety and mental health of handicapped and normal adolescents. *Indian Psychological Review, 59,* 114-120.

Ostberg, V. (2003). Children in classrooms: Peer status, status distribution and mental well-being. *Social Science and Medicine, 56*(1), 17-29.

Rahi, Manju, Kumavat, A.P., Garg, Suneela, and Singh, M.M., (2005). Socio-demographic correlates of psychiatric disorders. *Indian Journal of Pediatrics, 72*(5), 395-398.

Rask, K., Astedt-kurki, P. and Laippala, P., (2002). Adolescent subjective well-being and realized values. *Journal of Advanced Nursing, 38* (3), 254-263.

Ray, V.K. and Yadav, V. C. (1993). A study of mental health of higher secondary students in relation to socio-economic status. *Journal of Psychological Researches,* 37(182), 39-46.

Redden, C.E. (2002). *Social alienation of African American College Students: Implications for Social Support Systems*. Paper presented at the National Convention of the Association for Counsellor Education and Supervision, Park City, UT, USA.

Reddy, S. Rao, G.B., and Nagarathnamma, B., (2002). Mental health status of students of co-educational and non-co-educational schools. *Indian Psychological Review, 58*(1), 31-36.

Resnick, M.D. (2000). Protection, resiliency, and youth development. *Adolescent Medicine: State of the Art Reviews, 11*(1), 157-164.

Roeser, W. Robert, Eccles, S. Jacquelynne, Doan, F., and Carol, (1999). Academic functioning and mental health in adolescence: Patterns, progressions and routes from childhood. *Journal of Adolescent Research, 14*(2), 135-17.

Shek, D.T., (2002). Family functioning and psychological well-being, school adjustment, and problem behaviour in Chinese adolescents with and without economic disadvantage. *Journal of General Psychiatry, 163*(4), 497-502.

Shephard, R.J., Lavallee, H., and Lairview, G. (1978). Competitive Selection among age-class ice-hockey players. *British Journal of Sports Medicine, 12*, 11-13.

Srivastava, S. K., Prasad, Deepesh, C., and Kumar, V. (1999). A study of mental health of Hindi and English medium students. *Journal of Educational Research and Extension, 36(3)*, 23-28.

United States Department of Health and Human Services (1999). *Mental Health: A Report of the Surgeon General.* Rockville, MD: Office of the Surgeon General, U.S. Public Health. Service. [Available at: http://www.surgeongeneral.gov/library/mentalhealth/home.html].

Wittchen, H.U., Kessler, R.C, Beesdo, K., *et al.* (2002). Generalized anxiety and depression in primary care: prevalence, recognition, and management. *Journal of Clinical Psychiatry, 63*, 24-34.

World Health Organization (2004). *Promoting Mental Health: Concepts, Emerging Evidence, Practice (Summary Report).* Geneva, Switzerland: Department of Mental Health and Substance Abuse.

10

Family Climate and Happiness

Towards Cultural Perspective

Aradhana Shukla

Happiness is a state of mind which comprised (*i*) physical support, (ii) being socially acceptable and easily getting along with others, (iii) free of worries and hardships, and (iv) possessing a healthy and normal mind. According to Wilson (1967) the healthy person is "young, healthy, well-educated, well paid extroverted, optimistic, worry free, religious, and full of high self-esteem, job morale, modest aspiration and of a wider range of intelligence. In addition, it conveys several different meanings including momentary satisfaction with life and long term enjoyment. (Diener & Diener, 1995). This term is also used as a popular and short hand description of well-being.

In everyday parlance happiness refers to most generic and unqualified state of feeling good, term such relaxed, elated, and calm are used for the (Watson, J.B., 1930). However, the speotic circumstances of happiness and the meanings attached to it, depend crucially on the contrual of the self as independent or as interdependent. Evidence suggests that people experience this unqualified good feeling when they have successfully accomplished the cultural task of either independence or interdependence.

Until recently, the orientation of Psychology has been negative. As reported by *Myers and Diener* (1995) that psychological articles researching negative states outnumber those examining positive states by a ratio of 17 to 1. Also, in past research on emotion revealed that 83 per cent of researches in psychology dealt with negative feelings (Cejka, 1986). However, psychologists like Maslow and Rogers focused attention to more positive side of human existence.

There have been two popular definitions of happiness:

1. **Happiness as a warm puppy definition**: According to this group of definition happiness is just about anything person could imagine. Happiness is a "good job", "good health", "being loved" etc. Happiness, according to this popular definition, is just about anything, anyone, anywhere might think of as making themselves happy. But the flow in this definition lies in cause *versus* effects. Many people claim, happiness is/are actually are things that cause happiness. These are not what happiness actually is. Things as money, health, success can make people happy but those things are not "happiness" itself.
2. **The second popular definition:** It states that "happiness is satisfaction, contentment, fulfilment, etc. However, this definition falls victim to a fallacy of circular logic. It does not define "happiness" but merely describes it using other words that mean essentially the same.

   Words like contentment, well-being, bliss, harmony, etc. are nowhere closer to the definition of happiness, since these words are simply synonymous of happiness.

   In fact, happiness is part of special category of mental experiences that includes such positive things as joy, pleasure, satisfaction, etc. Some researchers have attempted to measure the emotional side of happiness, including being in good mood while the other have attempted to measure cognitive reflective side associated with quality of life. Happiness occurs in various ways and it is often seen as a reflection of satisfaction with life.

Thus, it can be claimed that happiness is an inner state and it appears in many forms of behaviour; In addition, it is a consequent variable which is stated with many aspects and goals of life directly and indirectly. Moreover, it is a positive and sustainable condition which enables a person to live in and interact properly with society. Truly speaking, it is a culturally relative phenomenon.

Happiness is also related with motivational and personality variable. It has been noted that those who feel happy, think and do good for self/ others (Shukla, 2006) and their other forms of behaviour seems better than others. It is caused by mental strength, personality trait, personal advantage achievement and freedom of life, self-acceptance, personal growth, and purpose of life, autonomy and relationship with others. In addition, Malhorta (2007) has described certain aspects of happiness which need to be mentioned. They are—stability, definiteness, time emphasis, conscientiousness and appropriateness.

Argyle, Martin and Lee (1995) believed that happiness is comprised three related components, namely positive affect (pleasant mood and emotion), absence of negative effect (unpleasant mood and emotion), and satisfaction with life as a whole (Bhandari, 2005; Dwivedi, 2001; Joshi, 2006).

As it has been mentioned happiness is revealed in the deeds of people and it is based on satisfaction with oneself and the surrounding. That is to say that the causes of happiness are deeply rooted in the family and occupational surroundings. It has been found that people living in supportive family and occupational climate evidence positive state of mind and high level of satisfaction with their life. Moreover, it has also been observed that the children reared in authoritative parenting show higher level of happiness and better scholastic performance.

Keeping these views in consideration this study was planned in factorial perspective and it was aimed to find out the impact of cultural variation, sex, age and family climate on happiness. The hypotheses were as follows:

- Cultural variation would cause variation in the magnitude of happiness.
- Boys and girls would differ in the degree of happiness.
- Variation in chronological age would provide variation the experience of happiness.
- Supportive family climate would evince higher level of happiness.

Method

Sample: One hundred sixty children in the age-range of 10 to 14 years served as participants and they were arranged according to the requirements of 2 × 2 × 2 × 2 factorial design with 2 levels of cultural variation (*non-tribal/tribal*), two sex (*boy/girls*), two levels of age (*10-11 yrs/13-14 yrs*) and two levels of family climate (***highly supportive/ less supportive***).

Measures: In this study two measures were used and they were as follows:

Measure of family climate: In order to assess the pattern of family climate the Home Environment Scale (may be abbreviated as HES later on) (Dhaundiyal, 1993) was used. It is comprised 74 statements and deals with ten dimensions of home climate, namely attention and care, facilities, impartiality, parental approval of child's and adolescent's activities, sharing of ideas, trust, confidence, decision-making, parental support and encouragement and harmony among family members. It is a questionnaire of true-false items. Two scores are given for true answer and one for false answer. Thus, the score ranges between 74-148. Low score indicates supportive family climate and high score and *vice versa*. Split half reliability is .79 and test/retest reliability is .70. This is successfully used in other studies (Bhandari, 2006; Dwivedi, 2001; Joshi, 2006).

Measure of happiness: In order to get the profile of happiness, the happiness scale (Shukla, 2006) was taken in consideration. It is consisted of 40 five-point items dealing with general well-being, expectation, achievement, congruence, and confidence in coping, transcendence, family group support, social support, primary group concern, independence mental mastery, perceived ill health, deficiency in social contacts and general well-being. Scores range between 40-200. Low scores indicate higher level of happiness and well-being and high score *vice versa*. Split half reliability of the measure is .64 and test-retest reliability is .71.

Procedure: At first the investigator contacted 400 families, i.e. 200 from Sitarganj measure is .61 and test-retest reliability is .66. The tribal area and 200 from Almora, the non-tribal area, i.e. 50 in each cell and administered the HES on them. This administration was aimed to find out the pattern of perceived family climate of the participants, i.e. how they experience their family. Since, we had to take only the children of high supportive and low supportive families so 10 highest and 10 lowest participants of each cell were taken and thus, the sample was constructed of 160 participants. On these participants the measure of happiness was administered. Data collection was done individually and but attempts were made to avoid external distractions.

Results

Obtained data were analysed by 4 ways ANOVA and interpreted in terms of happiness as affected by cultural variation, sex, age and family climate. Data analysis was done in three phases. In first phase sample section will be presented and in second phase impact of cultural variation, sex, age family climate on happiness will be discussed. The third phase will deal with area-wise analysis of happiness scale. Findings are presented below:

(i) *Classification of the participants as highly or less supportive about their family climate:* The aim of this analysis was to select the participants on the basis of their scores on HES and entitle them as the members of high/less supported families. The means of the sample is given below.

Table 10.1: Classification of the participants on the basis of their scores on Home environment scale

	A			
	A1		*A2*	
	B1	*B2*	*B1*	*B2*
C1	109.5	98.47	101.19	108.05
C2	115.76	126.68	106.57	141.00

Legends

A	*Cultural Variation*		*Sex*		*Age*
A1	Non-tribal	B1	Boys	C1	10-11 yrs
A2	Tribal	B2	Girls	C2	13-14 yrs

Table 10.1 shows that all groups were different in relation to their experience about their families. Non-tribal experienced more supportive family climate as compared to tribal group. Moreover, higher supportive climate was experienced by boys and young ones.

(ii) *Impact of cultural variation, sex, age and family climate on happiness:* In addition to the analysis given is phase one 4-way ANOVA was also computed and it is reported in Table 10.2.

Table 10.2 reveals that the main effect of cultural variation was insignificant ($F1$, 144 = 1.17 $P > .05$) and it revealed that non-tribal and tribal were more or less equally happy. The next main effect of sex was significant ($F1$, 144 = 4.26 $P < .05$). It revealed that boys did significantly less magnitude of happiness than girls. The third main effect of age was significant ($F1$, 144 = 4.96 $P < .05$) and it revealed that older participants revealed less magnitude of happiness as compared to young participants. The fourth main effect of family climate was significant ($F1$, 144 = 4.48 $P < .05$) and it was found that the participants of highly supportive and less supportive families were highly different in the experience of happiness. It was noticed that highly supportive family climate did provide higher level of happiness.

Table 10.2: Summary table showing the impact of cultural variation, age, sex and family climate on happiness

Sources of variation	*SS*	*df*	*MS*	*F*
A	0.28	1	0.28	1.17
B	3.24	1	3.24	4.26
C	3.77	1	3.77	4.96
D	3.41	1	3.41	4.48
AB	4.88	1	4.88	6.42
AC	7.35	1	7.35	6.59
AD	3.80	1	3.80	5.01
BC	0.82	1	0.82	1.19
BD	3.05	1	3.05	4.01
CD	3.18	1	3.18	4.19
ABC	3.41	1	3.41	4.48
ABD	4.70	1	4.70	6.18
ACD	4.25	11	4.25	5.59
BCD	7.92	1	7.92	6.02
ABCD	4.42	1	4.92	6.48
Errpe	189.46	144	189.46	
Within		159		

The cultural variation × sex interaction was highly significant (F1, 144 = 6.42 $P < .01$). It was found that both variables yielded their impact on happiness. The cultural variation × age interaction was also significant (F1, 144 = 6.42 $P < .01$) and it was noticed that the magnitude of happiness was influenced by cultural variation and age although the magnitude of discrepancy was not uniform. The cultural variation × family climate interaction was also significant (F 1, 144 = 5.01 $P < .01$) and it was found that both variables yielded their impact on the magnitude of happiness.

The sex × age interaction was in significant (F 1, 144 =1.19 P > .05) and it was noted that both variables were not able to yield their impact on happiness. The sex × family climate interaction was significant (F 1, 144 = 4.01 $P < .01$). The age × family climate interaction (F 1, 144 = 4.1 $P < .01$) revealed that the pattern of happiness was influenced by both variables.

The three-way interaction of cultural variation × sex × age was significant (F, 1, 144, 4.48 $P < .05$) and it is appeared in Fig 10.1.

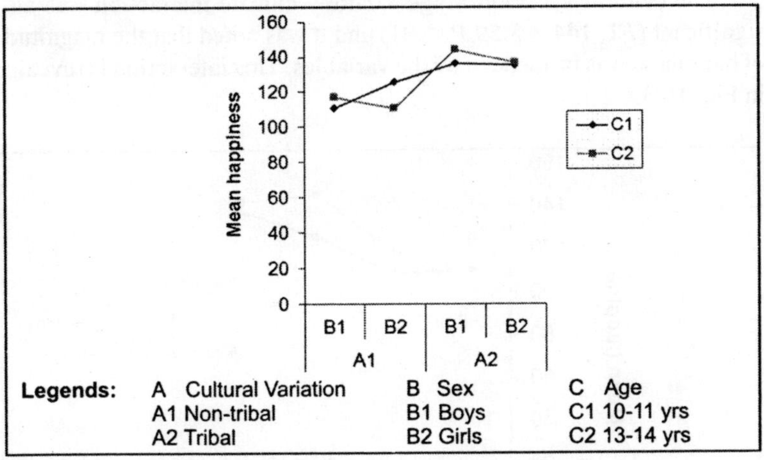

Fig. 10.1: Impact of cultural variation, sex and age on happiness

The cultural variation × sex × family climate interaction was also significant (F 1, 14 = 6.18 $P < .01$) and it was found that these variable evinced their impact on happiness. This interaction is presented in Figure 10.2.

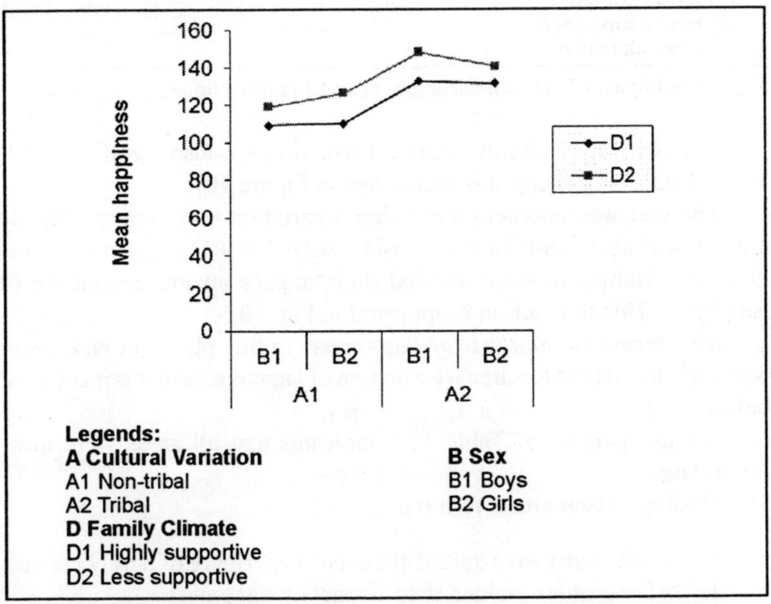

Fig. 10.2: Impact of cultural variation, sex and family climate on happiness

The cultural variation × age × family climate interaction was also significant ($F1, 144 = 5.59$ $P < .01$) and it was noted that the magnitude of happiness was influenced by the variables. This interaction is revealed in Fig. 10.3.

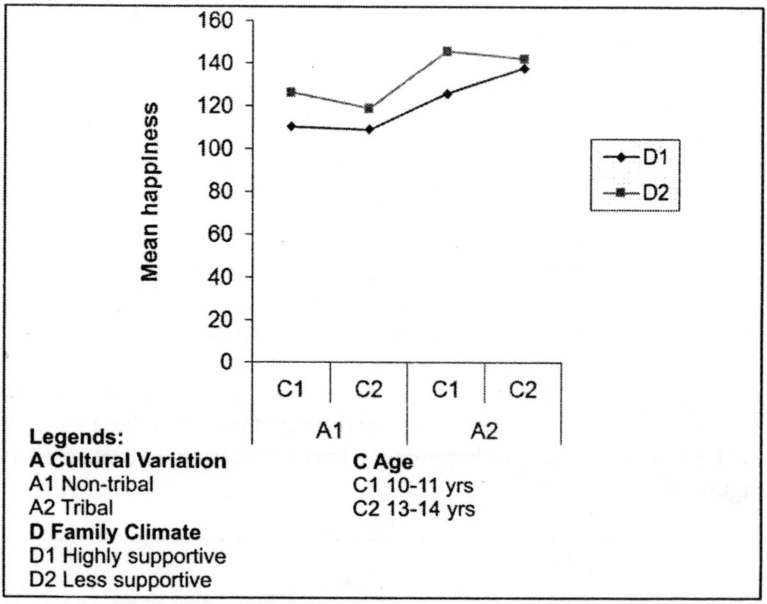

Fig. 10.3: Impact of cultural variation, age and family climate on happiness

The sex × age × family climate interaction was also significant ($F1, 144 = 6.02$ $P < .01$) and it is mentioned in Figure 10.4.

The four way interaction of cultural variation × sex × age × family climate was also significant ($F1, 144 = 6.19$ $P < .01$) and it was found that all variables in sum, yielded their impact on the magnitude of happiness. This interaction is appeared in Fig. 10.5.

(iii) Area-wise analysis of happiness: In this phase an endeavour was made to find out the area wise pattern of happiness and it is mentioned below:

A close perusal of Table 10.3 indicates that all areas were quite interrelated.

Finding in sum are as follows:

1. Participants were quite different on experience of family climate.
2. All variables yielded their impact on happiness.

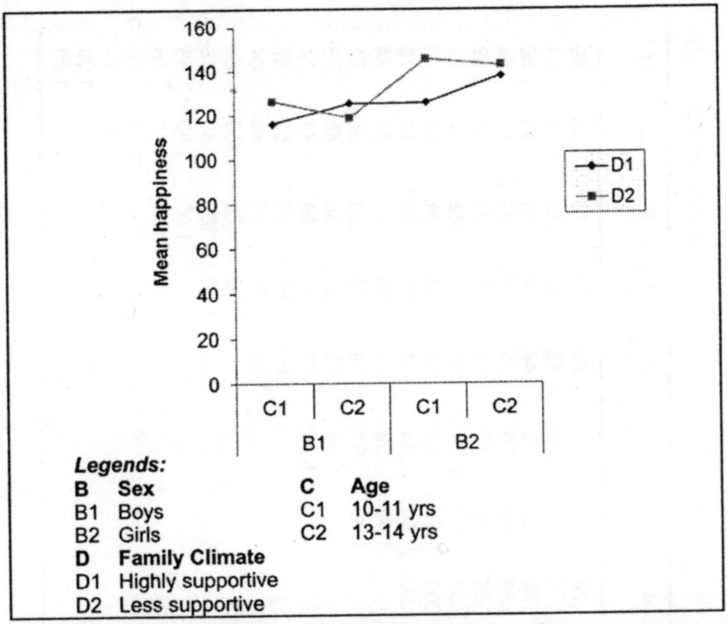

Fig. 10.4: Impact of sex, age and family climate on happiness

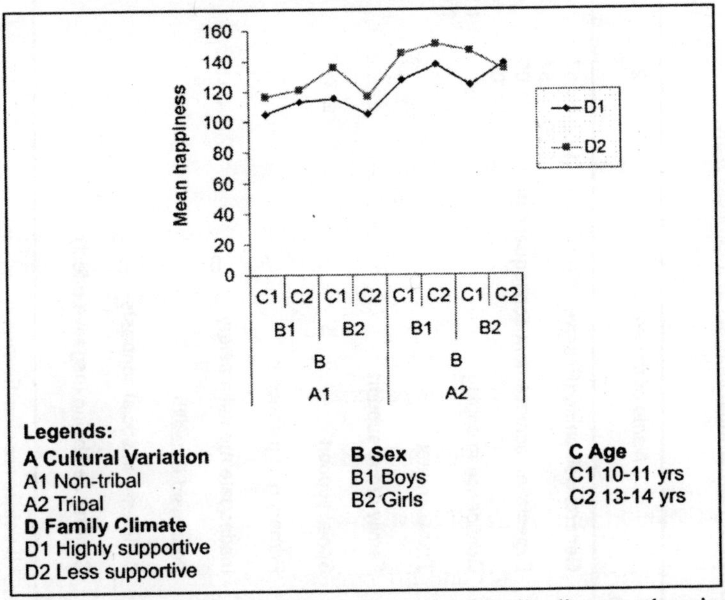

Fig. 10.5: Impact of cultural variation, sex, age and family climate on happiness

Table 10.3: Corelational analysis of happiness scale

(Co-relational values)

Sl. No.	*Name of the areas*	*1*	*2*	*3*	*4*	*5*	*6*	*7*	*8*	*9*	*10*	*11*
1.	General well-being (Positive effect)	1.00	.57	.49	.73	.49	.56	.46	.75	.78	.58	.69
		1.00	.57	.50	.74	.51	.49	.48	.81	.89	.59	.61
2.	Expectation achievement consequences		1.00	.46	.59	.56	.76	.46	.74	.81	.49	.56
			1.00	.41	.56	.50	.79	.51	.76	.79	.51	.54
3.	Confidence in coping			1.00	.56	.64	.72	.49	.76	.79	.51	.59
				1.00	.54	.62	.74	.54	.74	.68	.52	.60
4.	Transcendent				1.00	.79	.64	.54	.74	.71	.50	.76
					1.00	.64	.68	.51	.72	.69	.58	.79
5.	Family group support					1.00	.58	.78	.69	.72	.52	.74
						1.00	.61	.74	.64	.68	.56	.71
6.	Social support						1.00	.79	.61	.56	.46	.79
							1.00	.71	.62	.64	.44	.74
7.	Primary group concern							1.00	.68	.59	.51	.67
								1.00	.64	.56	.46	.64
8.	Inadequate mental mastery								1.00	.60	.53	.64
									1.00	.69	.59	.68
9.	Perceived ill health									1.00	.56	.68
										1.00	.46	.56
10.	Deficiency in social contrasts										1.00	.70
											1.00	.71
11.	General well-being (negative effect)											1.00
												1.00

Note: All values are significant.

3. The areas of happiness were related with each other.

Discussion

Obtained data were analysed by analysis of variance and interpreted in terms of cultural variation, sex, age and family climate as affectors of happiness. Prior to the study some hypotheses were formulated and the findings will be discussed on the lines of these hypotheses.

(i) *Cultural variation would cause variation in the magnitude of happiness*: Our first and foremost concern was related with the impact of cultural variation on happiness. It was contended that variation in cultural setup would cause variation in the magnitude of happiness. It was found that a nominal difference between tribal and non-tribal group was noticed and tribals found more happier than the non-tribals. Although it was a hairline difference yet it established the fact that the tribals experience more happiness (in spite of their cultural impoverishment) as compared to their non-tribal counterparts.

During recent years considerable attempts have been made to trace the demographical determinants of happiness (Andrews & Withy, 1976; Gurin, Veroft and Feld, 1960). It was decided that many socio-cultural variables play important role in this regards. It was known as social indicate. Movements in well-being researches (Ryff, 1989) highly hold that same socio-demographically defined groups were happier because of differential availability of Psychological, Physical and Material recourse. But more recent work has raised doubt in this regard. The studies carried out by Bradburned and Caplovitz (1965), Diener (1989, 1994) Myers and Diner (1995) and Ryff (1989) have shown that the influence of socio-demographics is modest, explaining only a mark portion of the individual difference in happiness.

Another issue related to this view is that whether material enjoyment cans really to be relative source of happiness/well-being. Numerous studies conducted on subjective well-being (Diener & Diener, 1995) show that economically poor and rich nations do not differ significantly on the index of life satisfaction. A number of cross-national evidences (Diener & Lucas; Myers, 2000) revealed that national wealth as well as economic growth has no positive correlation with indices of life satisfaction and happiness and they follow the low of diminishing return beyond a certain point. Diener (1989, 1994) elicited that some orientation is needed to ascertain the impact of materialism on enjoy'ng the life and thus, its contribution to the society.

4. *Vigyanamaya Kosh* refers tointellect involving ideas, concepts which are use to know the world.
5. *Anandmaya Kosh* reflects bliss, the characteristics of true self.

Vedanta accepts only the self—as subject to be true self, dismissing the identification of the self with any object as ultimately deceptive. Self as subject is a consciousness based construct. Self as an object is a manifestation of ego and is an aspect of mind. Since *Atman* is similar to *parmatman*, it becomes the duty of human beings to cultivate in themselves divine like qualities which would subsequently bring well-being not only at personal level but at transpersonal level. What one needs to do for it? He is required to remind himself all the time that I am divine like and I should act divine like. This will enable him to approach divinity. The more are does it, greater will be well-being.

Human beings fail to understand true self and its limitlessness because of three misbeliefs about themselves. These three limitations are sorrow, mortality and ignorance. If we are limited by nature, we should not shive against limitations which we generally do. And these limitations should have been acceptable to us (Dayanand, 1991).

According to *Gita* knower and known cannot be the same. We know we are hurt, we feel jealous, we experience pain. Since we know our sorrow we cannot be sorrow. Similarly, only when we confuse body with self we associate mortality with the self. Lord Krishna says,

> देहिनोऽस्मिन् यथा देहे कौमारं यौवनं जरा।
> तथा देहान्तरप्राप्तिर्धीरस्तत्र न मुह्यति।।

Just as the self embodied in this body must pass through childhood, youth and old age, so it will assume another body (at death) with reference to that the wise do not come to grief. All agents of destruction are incapable of destroying *I-awareness* which is explicitely described in the following *shloka*:

> नैनं छिन्दन्ति शस्त्राणि, नैनं दहति पावकः।
> न चैनं क्लेदयन्त्यापो न शोषयति मारुतः।।
> (Weapon cannot cut it, fire cannot burn it, water cannot wet it, even wind cannot dry it).

We are aware of our ignorance too. So we cannot be ignorant. In all our pursuits we seek freedom from these limitations as these are not our true nature. We are aware of these limitations (known) there the knower the self is different from the known. When these limitations are overcome, we tend not to explore happiness in outside world. No particular object can provide happiness. It is the self which is the source of happiness. It is manifested only in a satisfied mind, a mind that desires nothing. According to Swami Dayanand, "A person who understands that the self is the source of all happiness will be free from all desires".

Thus the main thrust of development of personality according to *Vedanta* is towards realization of the true self (i.e. the devine) which is all pervading, indescribable and impersonal. The course of development of personality is charted along a successive transcendence from the empirical to spiritual pot in other words from phenominal to nominal.

Aids for Self Realization: Four Methods of *Advait Vedanta* are suggested as the aids of self-realization.

These are as follows:

1. Making a wise discrimination between the permanent and the impermanent with regard to the self.
2. Detatchment from the gains of either this or the other worldly life.
3. Development of the following:
   (i) *Sama*: It refers to control of mind so that mind may rest firmly on a single object.
   (ii) *Dama*: Which means withdrawal of senses from the objects of pleasure.
   (iii) *Uparati*: It cannot prevent the mind from being controlled by external objects.
   (iv) *Titiksha*: It is endurance of hardships without lamenting or becoming anxious.
   (v) *Shraddha*: It refers to faith in the reality of teachings of the scriptures and the advice of a capable teacher.
   (vi) *Samadhan*: Fully resting the mind as the formless *Brahman* without being enticed by desires.
4. Desire for liberating oneself from egoism and the perpetual chain of actions and their consequences.
5. With the vast and varied experiences of life and maturity of adulthood, elderly persons may assure themselves of the worth and salience of acquiring these six values which would assist them to attain well-being in their life. The above method may be considered as a form of applied psychology as it helps in changing the human condition from a less desirable to a more desirable state.

and Adelison (1966), defined a democratic family as one "in which the child is allowed a fair degree of autonomy, is included in important discussion massing and is controlled primarily by reasoning and verbal discipline." On the other hand an authoritarian family is that in which rules are set without consulting the children autonomy is limited and discipline is predominant by physical.

According to Cronbach (1977), "home differ in many respects warmth encouragement of independence, pressure for achievement and so on. Warm parents express their own love and encourage the child to express his feeling. Family members react to each other on emotional level. Other extreme is hostile rejection. The parents dislike children and are continuously critical and punitive. In some homes the child has little influence and freedom while other homes are often caused by democratic practices. Here, policies are worked out between parent and child or explained carefully." Danesh (1978) pointed out "authoritarian families are power oriented, tend to have dichotomous conceptions, have emotional and intellectual rigidity. In contrast democratic homes and permissive home bows to the whims of the child."

Slee (1996) investigated mothers' perception of family climate of normal and disordered children. Mothers completed the moss family environment scale. In addition, 9 mothers and their conduct disordered children and their matched comparisons were video-taped interacting in their homes. Mothers with a conduct-disordered child perceived the family climate as less cohesive, less encouraging of the expression of feeling and more conflict than their counterparts. The same mothers also perceived families to be more control oriented and less organized then their matched controls. Mothers of conduct disordered children were more controlling during interactions. Mothers of conduct disordered children reported that the family in which they were raised was less cohesive and less encouraging of independence than their counterparts.

Kardek and Fine (1993), investigated the relationship between parenting transitions due to changes in family structure and perceived family climate and parenting style. 1,017, 5th-7th graders who lived with both biological parents, a single divorced mother a single divorced father, a mother and a step father, a father and a step mother or a multiply divorced parent-appraised supervision with warmth, conflict, and order in family climate and indicated that different family structures varied on different dimensions of family process. Adolescents who did not experience parenting transitions rated their family climates more positively than these who had experienced transitions.

Aurora and Singh (1994) investigated the dependence of the quality of mothering behaviour upon the nature of the family-climate, with emphasis on high class families of mothering behaviour. The study includes of mothering behaviour. The study includes 2 factorial experiments. Ss were 160 adult high caste Hindu mothers with at least 2 children. Analysis showed that the demographic climate constituted by 3 variables, cultural determination, work involvement, and education, determines. Quality of mothering and mothers' education denotes mothering of conservative behaviour univariately.

Keeping these views in consideration it is surly fair to say that happiness is a psychological state that is caused by personal and demographic variables.

References

Andrew, F.M. and Withy, S. (1976). Social indicators of well-being. *Americans perception of life quality.* New York, Plenum.

Argyle, M., Martin M. and Lu, L. (1995). Testing for stress and happiness: the role of social and cognitive factors in C.D. Spielberger and I.G. Sarason (eds.). *Stress and Emotion*, Washington, DC: Taylor and Francis, 15, 173-187.

Aurora, S. and Singh, A. (1994). Demographic background of high earth mothering. The progressivistic conserve atavistic dimension. *Indian Journal of Psychology and Education*, 25(12), 47-52.

Bhandari, V. (2005). A Study of disruptive Behaviour in Children of Rural and Urban Setting. *Unpublished Ph.D. thesis.* Department of Psychology Kumaun University, Nainital.

Bradburn, N.M. and Coplovitz, D. (1965). *Reports on happiness.* Chicago, Aldine.

Brandtstadlter, J. and Greve, W. (1994). The aging self: Stabilizing and protective processes. *Development Review*. 14, 52-80.

Cejka, E. (1986). Inter-correlation data between happiness measure, *Psycap Inventory and other mood test.* (Unpublished data, reported in Fordyce, 1987).

Cronbach, L.J. (1977). *Educational Psychology.* IIIrd Has Const Brace Jovanovich, New York.

Danish, H.B. (1978). The authoritative family and its adolescents. *Canadian Psychiatric Association Journal* 23, 7. pp. 479-485.

Dhaundiyal, V.R. (1993). *Emotionally Disturbed Adolescents of the Himalaya*, Almora, Shyam.

Diener, E. (1989). Subjective well-being. *Psychological Bulletin.* 1995, 542-575.

Diener, E. (1994). Assessing subjective well-being: progress and opportunities. *Social Indicator Research.* 31, 103-157.

Diener, E. and Diener, M. (1995). Cross cultural correlates of life satisfaction and self esteem. *Journal of Personality and Social Psychology.* 68, 653-663.

Do van, E. and Adelson, J. (1966). *The adolescents experience*, Wiley, New York.

Dwivedi, V. (2001). Impact of family climate and school climate an academic stress and stress management in adolescents: A study of open and closed culture, *Unpublished Ph.D. Thesis.* Department of Psychology, Kumaun University, Nainital.

Filipp, S.H. (1996). Motivation and emotion in J.E. Birren and K.W. Schale (eds). *Handbook of the psychology of aging.* (pp. 218-235). San Diego, C.A.: Academic Press.

Gurian, G. Veroff, J. and Felds, S. (1964). *Americans view their mental health.* New York: Basic Books.

Joshi, U. (2006). Climate variation, disruptive behaviour and Attributional style among children as a function of age, sex and residential local. *Unpublished Ph.D. thesis*, Department of Psychology, Kumaun University, Nainital.

Kakkar, R. (2006). Development of Emotional disturbance and well-being as affected by Gender and Level of Employment. *Unpublished Ph.D. thesis.* Department of Psychology.

Kurdek, L.A. and Fine, M.A. (1993). The relation believe family strictness and younger adolescents appraisal of family climate and parenting behaviour. *Journal of Family* Issues, 14, 2, 279, 290.

Lawton, M.P. (1996). Quality of life and effect in later life in C. Magai and S.H. Mcfadden (Eds.), *Handbook of emotion, adult development and aging* (pp. 327-348). San Diego, CA: Academic Press.

Malhotra, S. (2007). Happiness its sociodemographic correlates in R. Singh and R. Shyam (Eds.) *Psychology of well-being.* Delhi: Global.

Maslow, A.H. (1941). The dynamics of Psychological Security and Insecurity. *Character and Personality,* 10, 331-334.

Myer, D.G. and Diener, E. (1995). Who is happy *Psychologies Science*, 6, 10-19.

Ryff, C.S. (1989). Happiness is everything or is its. Explanations on PW meanings psychological Well-being. *Journal of Personality and Social Psychology.* 5-7, 1069-1081.

Shukla, A. (2006). The happiness scale. *Unpublished Scale,* Departmental of Psychology. Kumaun University, Nainital.

Shukla, A. (2008). Resilience: being-well in difficulty. *Paper presented in the National Seminar on Learned Behaviour and Happiness in Life* held at Newing Christian College. Allahabad on 13-14 September.

Shukla, A. and Kamalak, S. (1998). Academic Motivation Scale. *Unpublished Scale*, Department of Psychology, Kumaun University, Nainital.

Slee, P.T. (1996). Family climate and behaviour in families with conduct disordered children. *Child Psychiatry and Humans Development*. 26, 4, 255-265.

Staudinger, V.M., Marsiske, M., and Baltes, P.B. (1995). Resilience and reserve capacity in later adulthood: Potentials and limits of development across the life span. In D. Ciccetli and D.J. Cohen (Eds.) *Developmental of Psychology* (Vol. 2, pp. 801-847). New York: Wiley.

Watson, J.B. (1930). Psychology from the stand point of a behaviourist. *Phyladelpia*, Lippincott.

Wilson, W. (1967). Correlates of avowed happiness. *Psychological Bulletin*, 67, 291-306.

11

Poverty, Social Position and Mental Health of Women

Anubhuti Dubey

An array of mental disorders and associated disabilities are common to women. In contemporary times there has been a change from a spotlight on "women" to a focus on "gender" as a critical determinant of health. Ottawa Charter for Health Promotion (1986) observes health as multidimensional and espouses a social model of health and defines health as *'a positive concept emphasising social and personal resources, as well as, physical capacities.'*

The social dimensions of mental health is previously emphasized by World Health Organization (WHO) in its definition of mental health used in 1981 as *'Mental health is the capacity of the individual, the group and the environment to interact with one another in ways that promote subjective well-being, the optimal development and use of mental abilities (cognitive, affective and relational), the achievement of individual and collective goals consistent with justice and the attainment and preservation of conditions of fundamental equality.'*

By the year 2020, it is estimated that depression will become the second most important cause of disease burden in the world (Global Burden of Disease). In many countries women are approximately twice as likely as men to experience depression. Depression is the most prevalent psychiatric disorder in women.

Women's mental health is a significant public health issue. Gradually, it has become a concern that any substantial decline in the over representation of women who are depressed would make a crucial contribution in reduction of the global burden of disease. Furthermore, two of the fifteen leading causes of disease burden, particularly significant for women who are estimated for year 2020 are—violence against women at number twelve and self-inflicted injuries at number fourteen. Depression, violence and self-injuries have particular relevance to women's mental health (Stark and Flitcraft, 1995, 1996).

A gender approach has been used when taking into account the differences between women and men. When talking about health both physical and mental health, this does not exclude biological or sex differences, however, it bear in mind the vital roles that social and cultural factors may play. Additionally, researches had accounted so for that unequal power relations between men and women are pertinent in promoting or impeding mental health. Inequalities in social position of men and women promote or retard gender development and empowerment (UNDP, 1997). Through the means of education and economic independence women can be equipped with the competence and capacity to deal with different problems (Kumar and Dubey, 2012).

Social factors can and do amend within and between countries in ways that detection and alteration of the social factors that affect women's mental health put forward the prospect of primary prevention of certain mental disorders by reducing their incidence. The social factors generate, maintain and aggravate the risk factors that imperil women's mental as well as physical health (Dubey, 2013).

Social Position and Mental Health

Considering the 10 major risk factors for the global burden of disease the social position determines that women will be disproportionately exposed to several of the health risk factors. The ten risk factors, in order of importance, are malnutrition, poor water supply, sanitation and personal/ domestic hygiene, unsafe sex, tobacco use, alcohol use, occupation, hypertension, physical inactivity, illicit drug use and air pollution. It is crucial, therefore, that women's health in general and women's mental health in particular should mull over social determinants like women lack autonomy, decision making power and access to independent income, many other aspects of their lives and health necessarily be outside of their control (Okojie, 1994) including their susceptibility to communicable diseases (Hartigan, 1999). Speedy social changes in many areas already beleaguered by poverty, negatively distress the health of the population. The utilization of health services was related with their affordability. People from the poorest strata, despite having more health problems are six times less likely to get access to hospitalization than people from the richer sections. This implies that women, especially from *dalit*, *advasi* and other marginalized communities are less likely to meet the expense of and get access to hospitalization when requisite (National Coordination Committee, Jan Swasthaya Abhiyan, 2006). The low social status of women prevents them from voicing their concerns about health related needs. Dubey (2013) reported that only 40 per cent of rural females said that significant males of their family have knowledge about the health problems of females, however, nearly 60 per cent of the males had said so. Hence, it is clear that in spite of the fact that females are primary care giver in the family; they are deprived of basic health information, treatment and holistic health (Rani and Banu, 2003). In rural north India during pregnancy only 30-40 per cent husbands' escorted their wives to hospital and this was mainly for a visit to bigger hospitals in cities/towns and they decided regarding the treatment agency in the majority of cases (Singh and Arora, 2008). Women have to seek permission to men folk to go to avail available health facilities. They cannot move alone, any man or elderly woman of the family escort them as they are socially and economically dependent on them (Hunte and Sultan, 1992; Dubey, 2013).

SES and Mental Health

The link between mental health and low income amongst urban women has also been recognized in Bombay, Olinda and Santiago (Blue, Ducci, Jaswal *et al.*, 1995) and reported that compared with people in high socio-economic groups, those in low socio-economic groups are far more likely to have lower levels of resources, education, poorer living and working environments and lower levels of social support. Health inequalities also originate from other sources including differences related to age, marital status, genetic factors, ethnic background and access to health care and health related information. As well as there are disparities in access and the qualities of the health care women receive.

Women's socio-economic status or class are not well established or calculated. Cross-sectional population-based studies time and again demonstrated that the poor and marginalised are at greater risk of having common mental disorders (Patel and Kleinman, 2003). Women are at greater risk, including in low and middle income countries. Review of the probable explanations for this set-up is no evidence to maintain a hormonal or biological mechanism (Piccinelli and Wilkinson, 2000). Problems in measurement of SES include whether a woman's own or her partner's occupation, if she has one, should be used as a pointer of her social class. Unemployment, if defined as not being in paid work, may have quite different connotations for women than for men. These may arise from disagreeing conceptions of role and identity which affect whether or not unemployment is perceived as the deprivation of a primary role and the primary source of income. Many a women are not in paid employment, however, are taking care for small children or other adults, undertaking productive but unpaid work in the home and possibly accomplishing training or study, may or may not feel unemployed or underemployed.

The highest rates of ill health and morbidity occur amongst women living in the most socio-economically disadvantaged circumstances (Blaxter, 1990; Arber, 1991, 1997; Arber and Cooper, 2000; Popay, Bartley and Owen, 1993). The baseline socio-economic factors most strongly associated with the risk for common mental disorders were related to deprivation and poverty, i.e. low level of education, low household income, lack of access to running water in the home, having experienced hunger and difficulties in making both ends meet. Compared with single woman, married and divorced/widowed woman were at significantly elevated risk (Patel *et al.*, 2006). In many countries, poverty is disproportionately experienced by women, and our study demonstrates the double burden of gender disadvantage and poverty on the risk of common mental disorders in women. National surveys in India and twelve other developing countries clearly demonstrate that the strong link ages between gender disadvantage and poverty with women's health and global health policy are increasingly influenced by this evidence (Patel, *et al.*, 2006). Lack of social security and economic polarization further aggravates the situation and makes the poor more vulnerable because of the lack of affordability and limited choice of health care provider (Sheikh and Hatcher, 2005; Chuma, Gilson and Molynex, 2007).

Stress at both paid and unpaid can negatively affect levels of self-care. Large numbers of women turn to smoking and alcohol in an attempt to relieve stress (Kolander, Ballard and Chandler, 1999; Frone, 1999). Stress can also cause headaches, muscular pain, insomnia, anxiety attacks, ulcers, colitis, asthma, amenorrhea, diabetes and cancer (Kolander, Ballard and Chandler, 1999; Thoits, 2010 Rogers and Pilgrim, 2010). Researchers had recognized that overwork is a health hazard both for physical health as well as for mental health. When men are overworked in their paid jobs it is difficult for wives to negotiate sharing unpaid work. Furthermore, women world-wide work longer total hours (in paid and unpaid work) than men (Briar, 2000). Major sources of stress to women in paid works are 'Role spillover', where demand from paid work spill over into family time. In some occupations particularly where the work is boundless create frequent conflicts in home and family life. Low-control jobs with high demands are known to be a major source of stress, exhaustion, depression, burnout and physical illness (Tausig and Fenwick, 2012) and mental fatigue (Carter Danford, Howcroft, Richardson, Smith and Taylor, 2013). Men are far more likely than women to have high control over their work process, which compensates for high demands and so can be a source of positive stress (Karasek and Theorell, 1993). Longer paid maternity leave was also generally associated with better mental health and longer duration of breastfeeding (Borrell, Palència, Muntaner, Urquía, Malmusi and O'Campo, 2014).

Unpaid Work and Mental Health

Women who are at home full time also have different kinds of stress (Kolander, Ballard and Chandler, 1999). Some researchers find that women who go out to work and women who stay at home have similar levels of depressive illness (Lennon, 1994). However, the representation is multifarious, and the condition of both employed and non-employed mothers depends a great deal on social circumstances, particularly levels of support (Lee, 1998). High total work load—including reduced time for rest, recovery, and sleep—is a risk factor for women's mental health and symptoms 12 months after childbirth. Women's postpartum health was positively associated with social support, which may help to decrease the negative effects of excess work (McGovern *et al.*, 2011). Working in isolation from other adults, as mothers at home do can combine with low income and status produces poor physical and mental health. Whether they also have unpaid work or not, mothers report worse health than fathers. In particular women with very young children are almost twice as likely as men with children the same age to report being constantly tired (Graham, 1993: 170; Popay, 1991:106).

Gender division of labour within the family, undoubtedly, differ significantly within and across countries. Such as, a woman living in a very traditional household—she being the one bearing the bulk of household activities, including child rearing—might report a very different level of happiness if this household is located in Sweden, where generally gender inequality is less pronounced, compared with a country such as Greece, where strict gender roles prevail (Mencarini and Sironi, 2012).

Regardless of women's greater than before partaking in paid work, many of women's unpaid work responsibilities have mounted in recent decades. Men have only slightly increased their involvement in family tasks, not acquiring a full share of family responsibility in childcare and housework (Blossfeld and Drobnic, 2001; Bernhardt, 2004; Neuwirth and Wernhart, 2008). Hence, gender relations within the family have changed very little. The observed increase in women's employment, not followed by men increasing their responsibility for domestic chores and care, characterizes the 'stalled revolution' (Hochschild, 1990). The increase of women's work participation without a consequent redistribution of housework and childcare has often generated a real 'dual-burden' for them, other than a 'dual-presence'. However, men's participation in the routine repetitive chores of cooking, cleaning and washing relieves women's burden, contributes to their sense of fairness, and hence lowers their chances of being depressed (Coltrane, 2000). In Indian organizations the biggest challenge faced by women managers today is managing their dual role of organizational managers and housewives. Women experience tremendous stress caused by either work overload or underload. Women's overload comes from the pressure to work harder to prove them. While Indian men do not mind having women as subordinates, they do not like them as bosses. Dissatisfaction from subordinates is a source of stress for women managers, which they see as a challenge to be confronted (Rao *et al.*, 2013).

Depression in Women

Depression in women is the leading cause of disease related disability among women (Noble, 2005). Epidemiological studies have shown that the life time prevalence of a major depressive disorder in women (21.3%) is almost twice that in men (12.7%) (Kessler, *et al.*, 1994). Mothers of young children constitute a group at particularly high risk for depressive symptoms (Kahn *et al.,* 1999; Heneghan *et al.,* 1998). Depression is not only the most frequently encountered women's mental health problem, but ranks as the most important women's health problem overall. The search for biological causes of women's higher rates of depression continues unabated (Crow, 1986; Rubinow, 1992; Halbreich and Lumley, 1993; Nolen-Hoeksma and Girgus, 1994; Blehar and Oren, 1995; Nolen-Hoeksema, 2002; Dumit, 2003). It has long been known that the social environment is of critical importance for health. Variations in both mortality and morbidity rates by social class are consistent findings of epidemiology (Dohrenwend, 1990; Dohrenwend, *et al.*, 1992; Najman, 1993; Bartley and Owen, 1996; MacIntyre and Hunt, 1997; Stansfield,

Head and Marmot, 2000; Kessler *et al.*, 2003). The evidences suggest that environmental stressors such as life events and chronic difficulties contribute significantly to the lower social class predominance for non-psychotic disorders like depression and anxiety. These non-psychotic or neurotic mental disorders are also referred to as Common Mental Disorders (CMD) in reference to their high prevalence in the community. CMD are the third most frequent causes of morbidity in adults and represent a significant public health problem (Ormel *et al.*, 1994). Psychiatric co-morbidity, with depression as a common factor, is a characteristic finding of many studies on women's mental health (Brown and Anderson, 1991; Ustin and Sartorius, 1995; Kessler *et al.*, 1994; Spataro *et al.*, 2004; Husky, Mazure, Paliwal, and McKee, 2008). The first in depth study of the role of social factors in the development of depression in working class British women was carried out by Brown and Harris in their book 'Social Origins of Depression: A Study of Psychiatric Disorder in Women', published in 1978, represented a significant departure at the time from the theorising about depression in women that dwelt on intrinsic biological, hormonal and reproductive factors in its model of mental health (Brown, Harris and Eales, 1996).

Social model of depression continues to contain three interconnecting main components. These are provoking elements or severe life events such as important losses and disappointments or major difficulties lasting for two or more years, vulnerability factors, such as a non-entrusting marriage which intensify the risk in the company of a provoking agent and symptom formation factors.

Social Rank Theory (Gilbert, 1992; Price, Sloman, Gardner, Gilbert, and Rohde, 1994; Price, 2000) underlines several key variables in the development of depression. These include perception of the self as inferior or in an unwanted subordinate position, low self-confidence and behaving in submissive or non-assertive ways, having a sense of defeat in relation to important battles, and at the same time, wanting. Stansfield, Head and Marmot (1998) found that the rank or grade of employment was significantly related to well-being to escape but being trapped. Women traditionally receive less pay and have lower status jobs than men. Even when men and women report similar workload demands, Karasek (1979) found that women often had to cope with such demands while exercising less control over the pace of the demands than men and for this reason he concluded that women's jobs can be more stressful. Psychosocial conditions have been examined in terms of their effects on women's mental health, and a number of risk factors identified. For instance, high mental demands and time pressure have been found to result in the highest levels of distress and reduced psychological well-being of women (Karasek and Theorell, 1993). Moreover, low status itself is a source of stress. Although 'executive stress' is real, however, the subordinates who experience most of the stress and women occupy most of the subordinate positions (Rodriguez, 2012).

Other psychosocial issues that have been identified in the literature having implications for the mental health of both men and women include: low levels of social support, poor job satisfaction, fear of making mistakes and disjuncture between personal values and those of the organisations—add sources. In addition women may suffer as a result of sex discrimination and/or sexual harassment at work (Thorbjornsson, 2000).

In women social capital the gender specific nature of the humiliation and defeat related to the beginning of depression. Psychosocial resources and the means to exercise choice and have a sense of control over one's life appears crucial safeguard against depression regardless of a woman's age. The bio-psychiatric model of depression, a disease model which emphasizes the roots of the disorder in anatomy, heredity, and disease processes, is more common in Western societies than elsewhere (Keyes, 1985). Conversely, a "situational" model that describes psychological distress in the context of social and interpersonal situations may be a more common explanatory strategy in traditional societies and minority communities in the West (Patel, 1995).

Conclusion

If programmes to promote women's mental health focus on the reduction of individual 'lifestyle' risk factors, they may neglect the very factors that bring that lifestyle into being. Utilization of gender analysis in the development of mental health policies and programmes social factors and women's social position affect their mental and emotional well-being is crucial to the development of a workable model of women's mental health promotion. At the present time, an accurate needs assessment of women's mental health, an essential element in effective health promotion, remains hampered by inadequate sources of data, an overly biological, individual focus in research and theoretical models which often neglect to consider how women's low social status and material circumstances intersect with their family roles and their participation in paid employment in determining mental health outcomes.

References

Arber, S. (1991). Comparing inequalities in women's and men's mental health: Britain in 1990s. *Social Science Medicine*, Vol. 44(6), 773-787.

Arber, S. (1991). Class, paid employment and family roles: Making sense of structural disadvantage, gender and health status. *Social Science and Medicine*, Vol. 32, 425-436.

Aeber, S. and Cooper, H. (2000), "Gender and inequalities in health across the life course", in E. Annandale and K. Hunt, eds., *Gender Inequalities in Health* (pp. 123-149). Open University Press, Buckingham.

Bartley, M., and Owen, C. (1996). Relation between socio-economic status, employment, and health during economic change, 1973-93. *British Medical Journal*, 313(7055), 445-449.

Bernhardt, E.M. (2004). Is the Second Demographic Transition a useful concept for demography? *Vienna Yearbook of Population Research*, 25-28.

Bildt Thorbjornsson, C. (2000) 'Working conditions and mental health amongst women' in Sherr, L. and St. Lawrence, J.S. (Eds) *Women, Health and the Mind* Chichester, John Wiley and Sons Ltd.

Blaxter, M. (1990). *Health and Lifestyles. London: Routledge.*

Blehar, M.C. and Oren, D.A. (1995). *Mood, Anxiety, and Personality Disorders Research Branch,* National Institute of Mental Health, Rockville, *Medscape Women's Health*, 2(2): 3.

Blossfeld, H.P. and Drobnic, S. (2001). A cross-national comparative approach to couples' career. In Blossfeld, H.P. and Drobnic, S. (Eds.), *Careers of Couples in Contemporary Society* (pp. 3-15). New York: Oxford University Press.

Blue, I., Ducci, M.E., Jaswal, S., Ludermir, A., and Harpham, T. (1995). The mental health of low-income urban women: Case studies from Bombay, India; Olinda, Brazil; and Santiago, Chile. In T. Harpham, and T. Blue (Eds.), *Urbanization and mental health in developing countries*, (pp. 75-101). Aldershot: Avebury.

Borrell, C., Palència, L., Muntaner, C., Urquía, M., Malmusi, D., and O'Campo, P. (2014). Influence of macrosocial policies on women's health and gender inequalities in health. *Epidemiologic reviews*, 36(1), 31-48.

Briar, C. (2000). 'In search of gender-sensitive concepts and measures of poverty, inequality and well-being', *Social Policy Journal of New Zealand,* 14, 17-29.

Brown, G.R. and Anderson, B. (1991). Psychiatric morbidity in adult inpatients with childhood histories of sexual and physical abuse. *American Journal of Psychiatry*, 148(1), 55-61.

Brown, G.W., Harris, T.O., and Eales, M.J. (1996). Social factors and co-morbidity of depressive and anxiety disorders. *British Journal of Psychiatry*, 168, 50-57.

Carter, B., Danford, A., Howcroft, D., Richardson, H., Smith, A., and Taylor, P. (2013). 'Stressed out of my box': employee experience of lean working and occupational ill-health in clerical work in the UK public sector. *Work, Employment and Society*, 27(5), 747-767.

Chuma, J., Gilson, L., and Molynex, C. (2007). Treatment-seeking behaviour, cost burdens and coping strategies among rural and urban households in Coastal Kenya: an equity analysis. *Tropical Medical Internal Health*, 12: 673-86.

Coltrane, S. (2000). Research on household labour: modeling and measuring the social embeddedness of routine family work. *Journal of Marriage and Family*, 620, 1208-1233.

Crow, T.J. (1986). The continuum of psychosis and its implication for the structure of the gene. *British Journal of Psychiatry*, 149, 419-429.

Dohrenwend, B.P. (1990). Socioeconomic Status and Psychiatric Disorders: Are the Issues Still Compelling? *Social Psychiatry and Psychiatric Epidemiology*, 25, 41-47.

Dohrenwend, B.P., Levav, I., Shrout, P.E., Schwartz, S., Naveh, G., Link, B.G., Skodol, A.E., and Stueve, A. (1992). Socioeconomic status and psychiatric disorders: The causation-selection issue. *Science, 255*, 946-952.

Dubey, A. (2013). *Psychosocial Dynamics of Health in Women of Rural Eastern Uttar Pradesh.* Research Project Report submitted to ICSSR, New Delhi.

Dumit, J. (2003). Is it me or my brain? Depression and neuro scientific facts. *Journal of Medical Humanities*, Vol. 24(1/2), 35-47.

Frone, M.R. (1999). Work stress and alcohol use. *Alcohol Research and Health*, 23(4), 284-291.

Gilbert, P. (1992). *Depression: The evolution of powerlessness.* New York: Guilford Press.

Graham, H. (1993) *Hardship and Health in Women's Lives Hemel* Hempstead, Harvester Wheatsheaf.

Gwatkin, D.R. (1997). Global Burden of Disease. The Lancet, Vol. 350, 9071-141.

Hartigan, P. 1999. *Communicable Diseases, Gender, and Equity in Health.* Working paper 99.08. Cambridge: Harvard Center for Population and Development Studies.

Halbreich, U. and Lumley, L.A. (1993) the multiple interactional biological processes that might lead to depression and gender differences in its appearance. *Journal of Affective Disorders*, 29, 159-173.

Heneghan, A.M.; Silver E.J. Bauman, L.J., Westbrook, L.E., Stein, R.E.K. (1998). Depressive symptoms in inner-city mothers of young children: who is at risk? *Paediatrics*, 102: 1394-1400.

Hochschild, A. (1990). The Second Shift. New York: Avon Books.

Hunte, P. and Sultan, F. (1992). Health seeking behaviour and meaning of medication in Balochistan, Pakistan. *Social Science Medicine*, 34, 1385-1397.

Husky, M.M., Mazure, C.M., Paliwal, P., and McKee, S.A. (2008). Gender differences in the co morbidity of smoking behaviour and major depression. *Drug and alcohol dependence*, 93(1), 176-179.

Karasek, R.A. (1979). Job demands, job decision latitude, and mental strain: Implications for job redesign. *Administrative science quarterly*, 24(2).

Karasek, R.A. and Theorell, T. (1990) *Healthy work, stress. productivity and the reconstruction of working life*, New York, Basic Books.

Kessler, R.C., McGonagle, K.A., Zjao, S., Nelson, C.B., Hughes, M., Eshleman, S., Wittchen, H., Kendler, K.S. (1994). Lifetime as 12-month prevalence of DSM-III-R psychiatric disorders in the United States. *Archives of General Psychiatry*, 51, 8-19.

Kessler, R.C., Berglund, P., Demler, O., Jin, R., Koretz, D., Merikangas, Rush, A.J., Walters, E.E., and Wang, P.S. (2003). The epidemiology of major depressive disorder: Results from the national co-morbidity survey replication. *Journal of the American Medical Association*, 289(23), 3095-3105.

Keyes, C. (1985). The interpretive basis of depression. In A. Kleinman, and B.J. Good (Eds.), *Culture and depression*. Berkeley: University of California Press.

Kahn, R.S, Wise, P.H., Finkelstein, J.A., Bernstein, H.H., Lowe, J.A., and Homer, C.J. (1999). The scope of unmet maternal health needs in paediatric settings. *Paediatrics*, 103, 576-581.

Kumar, D. and Dubey, A. (2012). Empowerment and Sources of Power as perceived by women of Eastern Uttar Pradesh. *International Journal of Social Science Tomorrow*, Vol. 1, No. 4, 1-5, ISSN 2277-6168.

Lee, C. (1998). *Women's Health: Psychological and Social Perspectives*. London, Sage.

MacIntyre, S. and Hunt, K. (1997). Socio-economic position, gender and health: How do they interact. *Journal of Health Psychiatry*, Vol. 2 (3), 315-334.

McGovern, P., Dagher, R.K., Rice, H.R., Gjerdingen, D., Dowd, B., Ukestad, L.K., and Lundberg, U. (2011). A longitudinal analysis of total workload and women's health after childbirth. *Journal of Occupational and Environmental Medicine*, 53(5), 497-505.

Mencarini, L., and Sironi, M. (2012). Happiness, housework and gender inequality in Europe. *European Sociological Review*, 28(2), 203-219.

Mullen, P.E., Martin, J.L., Anderson, J.L. *et al*. (1993). Childhood sexual abuse and mental health in adult life. *British Journal of Psychology*, 168, 721-732.

National Coordination Committee, *Jan Swasthaya Abhiyan* (2006). *Women's Health.*

Najman, J.M. (1993). Health and poverty: past, present and prospects for the future. *Social Science Medicine*, 36(2), 157-166.

Nolen-Hoeksema, S. (2002). Gender differences in depression. In I.H. Gotlib and C.L. Hammen (Eds.), *Handbook of Depression* (pp. 492-509). New York: The Guilford Press.

Nolen-Hoeksema, S. and Girgus, J.S. (1994). The emergence of gender differences in depression during adolescence. *Psychological Bulletin*, 115(3), 424-443.

Noble, R.E. (2005). Depression in women. *Metabolism*, 54, 49-52.

Neuwirth, N. and Wernhart, G. (2008). *Work-life balance reconsidered. Time allocation within partnerships: Germany, UK and Austria*. OIFS working paper 67. Vienna: Austrian Institute for Family Studies, University of Vienna.

Okjie, C.E.E. (1994). Gender inequalities of health in the third world. *Social Science Medicine*, Vol. 39(9), 1237-1247.

Ormel, J., VonKorff, M., Ustun, T.B., Pini, S., Korten, A., and Oldehinkel, T. (1994). Common mental disorders and disability across cultures: results from the WHO Collaborative Study on Psychological Problems in General Health Care. *JAMA*, 272(22), 1741-1748.

Ottawa Charter for health promotion (1986). World Health Organization, Geneva.

Patel, V. (1995). Explanatory models of mental illness in sub-Saharan Africa. *Social Science Medicine,* 40, 1291-1298.

Patel, V., and Kleinman, A. (2003). Poverty and common mental disorders in developing countries. *Bulletin of the World Health Organization*, 81, 609-615.

Patel, V., Kirkwood, B.R., Pedneker, S., Weiss, H. and Mabey, D. (2006). Risk factors for common mental disorders in women: Population based longitudinal study. *British Journal of Psychiatry*, 189, 547-555.

Piccinelli, M., and Wilkinson, G. (2000). Gender differences in depression. Critical review. *British Journal of Psychiatry*, 177, 486-492.

Popay, J. (1991). "My health is all right, but I'm just tired all the time". Women's experiences of ill health, in Helen Roberts (Ed) *Women's Health Matters* London, Routledge.

Popay, J., Bartley, M., and Owen, C. (1993). Gender inequalities in health: Social position, affective disorders and minor physical morbidity. *Social Science and Medicine,* Vol. 36, 21-32.

Price, J. (2000). Subordination, self-esteem, and depression. In L. Sloman & P. Gilbert (Eds.), *Subordination and defeat: An evolutionary approach to mood disorders and their therapy* (pp. 165-177). Mahwah, NJ: Erlbaum.

Price, J., Sloman, L., Gardner, R., Gilbert, P., and Rohde, P. (1994). The social competition hypothesis of depression. *British Journal of Psychiatry, 164,* 309-315.

Rabinow, P. (1992). Artificiality and enlightenment: From sociobiology to biosociality. In J.C.S. Kwinter (Ed.), *Incorporations* (pp. 190-201). New York: Zone (distrib: MIT Press).

Rani, M. and Banu, S. (2003). Rural Indian women's care seeking behaviour and choice of provider for gynecological symptoms. *Study of Family Planning,* 34, 173-185.

Rao, D.K.L., Yadav, S. and Chellayya, B. (2013). Income and marital factors influence on women leadership (with reference to public and private sectors in Andhra Pradesh), *Spectrum*, 2(1).

Rodriguez, L.L. (2012). Patriarchy and Women's Subordination in the Philippines. *Review of Women's Studies*, 1(1).

Rogers, A., and Pilgrim, D. (2010). *A sociology of mental health and illness.* McGraw-Hill International.

Shaikh, B.T., and Hatcher, J. (2005). Health seeking behaviour and health service utilization in Pakistan: Challenging the policy makers. *Journal of Public Health*, 27, 49-54.

Singh, A. and Arora, A.K. (2008). How much do rural Indian husbands care for the health of their wives'? *Indian Journal Community Medicine*, 33(1): 19-25.

Spataro, J., Mullen, P.E., Burgess, P.M., Wells, D.L., and Moss, S.A. (2004). Impact of child sexual abuse on mental health prospective study in males and females. *The British Journal of Psychiatry*, 184(5), 416-421.

Stansfeld, S.A., Head, J., and Marmot, M.G. (2000). *Work-related factors and ill health: The Whitehall II Study.* Norwich, UK: HSE Books.

Stark, E., and Flitcraft, A. (1995). Killing the beast within: Women battering and female suicidality. *International Journal of Health Services,* Vol. 25 (1), 43-64.

Stark, E., and Flitcraft, A. (1996). *Women at risk: Domestic violence and women's health.* Thousand Oaks: Sage.

Tausig, M., and Fenwick, R. (2012). Job Structures, Job Stress, and Mental Health. In *Work and Mental Health in Social Context* (pp. 25-49). Springer New York.

Thoits, P.A. (2010). Stress and health major findings and policy implications. *Journal of Health and Social Behaviour*, 51(1 suppl), S41-S53.

UNDP, (1997). *Human Development Report 1997.* Oxford University Press, New York.

Ustin, T.B. and Sartorius, N. (1995). *Mental illness in General Health Care: An international study*: John Wiley on behalf of the World Health Organization.

Vaananen, A., Buunk, A.P., Kivimaki, M., Vahtera, J. and Kiskenvo, M. (2008). Change in reciprocity as predictor of depressive symptoms: A prospective cohort study of Finnish women and men. *Social Science Medicine,* Vol. 67 (11), 1907-1916.

12

Scholastic Culture and Quality of Life

Shraddha J. Kapoor and *Aradhana Shukla*

Orthopedic disabilities are also known as locomotors disabilities or physical disabilities and health impairments. The term Orthopedic is related to a physical deformity or disability of the skeletal system and associated with motor function (Dutch, Smith and Luckasson 1992). A child with a physical disability has a problem with the structure or functioning of the body. A child with health impairment has a limitation on the body's physical well-being that requires on going medical attention. Berdine and Blackhurst (1985) defined orthopedic children as those who are physical or health problem results in an impairment of normal interaction with society to the extent that specialized services and programmers are required. Hallahan and Kauffman (1991) defined such children with disabilities as those whose non-sensory physical limitations or health problem interfere school attendance or learning to such an extent that special services, training, equipment, materials, or facilities are required.

The individuals with Disabilities Act (Idea-1977) USA, provides a definition of orthopedic disabilities as an impairment, which adversely affects a child's educational performance. This term includes impairments caused by congenital anomaly (e.g. clubfoot, absence of a limb etc., impairments caused by disease (e.g. poliomyelitis, bone tuberculosis, etc.) and impairments from other causes (e.g. cerebral palsy, amputations, and burns which causes contracture).

The PWA Act, 1996 refers to orthopedic disability as locomotors disability and defines it as disability of bones, joints or muscles leading to substantial restriction of the movement of the limbs or any form of cerebral palsy.

Orthopedic disabilities can broadly be categorized into four sets each including a number of impairments. They are:

1. Neurological Impairment
   (i) Cerebral Palsy
   (ii) Epilepsy
   (iii) Spina Bifidra
2. Masculoskeletal Condition
   (i) Osteogenesis Imperfeeta
   (ii) Tuberclosis of Bones and Joints
3. Cogenital Malinformations
   (i) Common Malinformations
   (ii) Malinformation due to Teralogens

Causes of orthopedic disability are as follows:

- Poor nutrition during pregnancy. Babies born prematurely or severely under weight may often have cerebral palsy and other disabilities.
- Genetic factors.
- Infectious disease such as diarrhoea can lead to dehydration, high fever and sometimes brain damage resulting in fits or cerebral palsy.
- Poor sanitation and eroded living conditions together with poor food make disease such as tuberculosis and the other severe disabilities.
- Lack of immunization against diseases such as polio, rubella etc.
- Birth defects and mental retardation on account of inappropriate medicines during pregnancy.
- Accidents resulting in loss of limbs, blindness and other disabilities.
- Leprosy infection.
- Disability caused by poisons in food, water, air or work place. Pesticides particularly can cause serious damage, e.g. fluoride poisoning mainly from drinking water can cause bone damage.
- Ageing.

Concept of Family Environment

Three terms have been used in respect to the type and quality of environment prevailing in home. These are authoritarian, democratic and permissive; these terms have been used in relation to both home and school environments and defined in behavioural terms by different authors.

Platt *et. al.* (1962) state that authoritarian control is employed by parents. This continuum stems from parents who are restrictive and coercive, permitting the child little freedom or limit the range of activity, to the parents who are lax and ineffectual and unable to control the child. Between those two extremes are the parents who allow the child freedom but who is capable of asserting when and where desired. According to Shah (1982), Authoritarian parents rely too heavily on one's means to enforce obedience. For this purpose they use many repressive restraints. They hold a strong concentration that child must obey and that it is the responsibility of parents to mark children to obey their parents. Authoritarian parents take advantage of child's weakness to secure complaints even subservience.

Maslow (1941) in contrast stated that "A good home is said to be one in which the child is given fullest opportunity for self-expression within the limits of parental affection and supervision". Malm (1952) characterized, "A home with affection; democracy, lack of conflict; comradeship; good personal adjustment, security and appropriateness of attitude: Douvan and Adelison (1966), defined a democratic family as one, "in which the child is allowed a fair degree of autonomy; is included in important discussion massing and is controlled primarily by reasoning and verbal discipline." One the other hand an authoritarian family is that in which rules are made and implemented without consulting the children, autonomy is limited and discipline is predominant by physical punishment.

According to Cronbach (1977), "home differs in many respects warmth encouragement of independence, pressure for achievement and so on. Warm parents express their own love and encourage the child to express his feeling and family members reacts to each other on emotional level. Other extreme is hostile rejection. The parents dislike children and are continuously critical and punitive. In some homes the child has little influence and freedom while other homes are often caused by democratic practices. Here, policies are worked out between parent and child or explained carefully." Danesh (1978) pointed out, "authoritarian families are power oriented, tend to have dichotomous conceptions, have emotional and intellectual rigidity. In contrast democratic homes bow to the whims of the child."

Keeping these views in consideration this study was planned in four-way factorial design and aimed to ascertain the pattern of familial culture of Orthopedically disabled and non-disabled young participants as affected by their age, types of physical condition, types of residential setting and family. The hypotheses were as follows:

- Variation in age would cause variation in familial culture.
- Variation in physical condition would cause variation in familial culture.
- Variation in residential type would cause variation in familial culture.
- Variation in family type would cause variation in familial culture.

Method

Sample

One hundred and sixty participants ranging between 10-16 years served as participants and they were arranged according to the requirements of 2×2×2×2 factorial design with 2 levels of age (10-12 and 13-15 yrs), 2 levels of physical condition (Orthopedically disabled and non-disabled), 2 residential settings (urban and rural) and types of family (joint and nuclear) i.e.; 10 participants were placed in each cell.

Table 12.1: Experimental Design used in the Study

		A							
		A1				A2			
		B				B			
		B1		B2		B1		B2	
		C		C		C		C	
		C1	C2	C1	C2	C1	C2	C1	C2
D	D1	10	10	10	10	10	10	10	10
	D2	10	10	10	10	10	10	10	10

Legends

A = Levels of chronological Age
A1 = 10-12 years
A2 = 13-15 years
B = Levels of Physical Condition
B1 = Orthopedically Disabled
B2 = Non-Disabled

C = Types of Residential Setting
C1 = Urban
C2 = Rural
D = Types of Family
D1 = Joint
D2 = Nuclear

Measure

In this measure only one tool was employed and it is mentioned below:

Family Environment Scale (FES). It was constructed and standardized by Vohra. It is a scale having 98 items which can be answered in Yes/No form. It consists of seven areas which are considered as most important dimension in order to access the environment of any family. The dimensions are Competitive Framework, Cohesion, Expression, Independence, Moral Orientation, Organization, and Recreational Orientation.

Data collection was done individually and best attempts were made to avoid the external distractions.

Result

Obtained results were analysed by four-way analysis of variance and interpreted in terms of chronological age, physical condition, residential settings and family type as the effectors of familial culture. Findings are given in Table 12.2.

Table 12.2: Summary table of ANOVA showing the impact of chronological age, level of physical conditions, residential setting and types family type on familial culture

Source of variations	*SS*	*Df*	*MS*	*F*
A	1.26	1	1.26	1.17
B	5.85	1	5.85	5.42
C	5.81	1	5.89	5.46
D	6.68	1	6.68	6.19
AB	6.37	1	6.37	5.90
AC	7.03	1	7.03	6.51
AD	8.08	1	8.08	7.48
BC	5.60	1	5.60	5.19
BD	6.63	1	6.63	6.14
CD	6.24	1	6.24	5.78
ABC	7.76	1	7.76	7.19
ABD	7.28	1	7.28	6.74
ACD	7.81	1	7.81	8.44
ABCD	8.81	1	8.81	8.16
ABCD	7.73	1	7.73	7.16
Error (within)	155.52	144	1.08	
		159		

A close perusal of Table 12.2(i) reveals that the main effects of chronological age was insignificant (F, 1,144 = 1.17, P > .05). Mean values of older (X = 124.89) and younger (X = 133.48) children revealed nominal difference. The next main effect of physical condition was significant (F 1, 144 = 5.42 P < 0.01) and it revealed that the disabled children felt more distortion (X = 120.01) as compared to their non-disabled (X = 131.01) counterparts. The third main effect of residential settings revealed its significance (F, 1,144 = 5.46 P < 0.01). It was that urban participants felt less distractions (X =) rather than rural participants (X = 131.43). The last main effect of family type was also significant (F, 1,144 = 6.19 P < 0.01) and it was noticed that children of joint family (X = 117.03) experienced more familial distortion than nuclear family (X = 133.98).

The two way interaction of chronological age * physical condition was also significant (F, 1,144 = 5.90 P < 0.01). Similarly, chronological age * residential setting interaction was also significant (F, 1,144 = 6.51 P < 0.01). Likewise, chronological age * family type interaction was significant (F, 1,144 = 7.48 P < 0.01). All these interactions showed significant influence on familial culture. The physical condition * residential setting interaction was also significant (F, 1,144 = 5.19 P < 0.01). The physical condition * family type interaction was also significant (F, 1,144 = 6.14 P < 0.01) and revealed its influence of familial condition. The residential setting * family type interaction was significant (F, 1,144 = 5.78 P < 0.01) and it was found that both the variables yielded their significant impact on familial culture.

The chronological age* physical condition * residential setting interaction was significant (F, 1,144 = 7.19 P < 0.01) and it was shown in Fig. 12.1.

Figure reveals that all the variables displayed their influence on familial culture. The chronological age * physical condition * family type interaction was significant (F, 1,144 = 6.79 P < 0.01) and it is appeared in Fig. 12.2.

In this way context chronological age * residential setting * family type interaction was also significant (F, 1,144 = 8.44 P < 0.01) and it is appeared in Fig. 12.3.

The physical condition * residential setting * family type interaction showed its impact in significant manner (F, 1,144 = 8.16 P> 0.01) and it is appeared in Fig. 12.4.

The four-way interaction of chronological age * physical condition * residential setting * family type was significant (F, 1,144 = 7:16 P > 0.01) and it is appeared in Fig. 12.5.

A close perusal of figure 12.5 reveals that all variables exhibited their impact on familial culture.

In order to ascertain the pattern of relationship among the areas of Family Environment Scale a correlational analysis was made and the findings are given in Table 12.3.

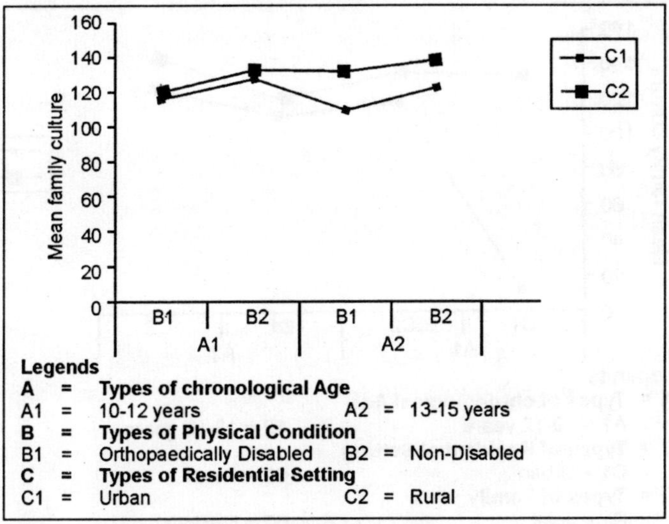

Fig. 12.1: Mean values showing the impact of types of chronological age, types of physical condition and types of residential setting on familial culture

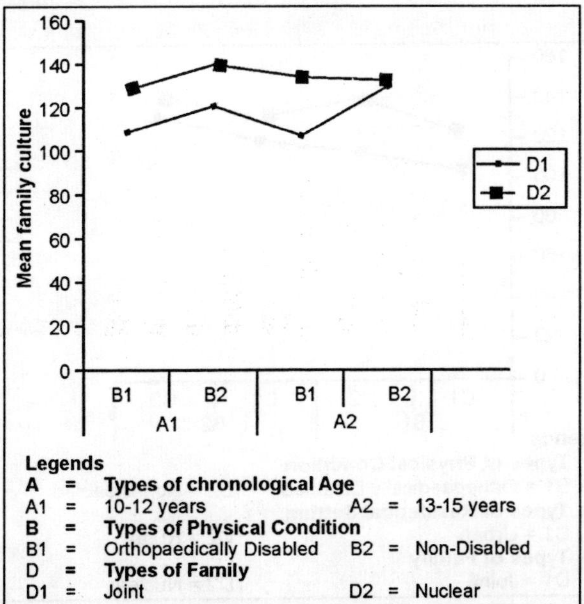

Fig. 12.2: Mean values showing the impact of types of chronological age, types of physical condition and types of family on familial culture

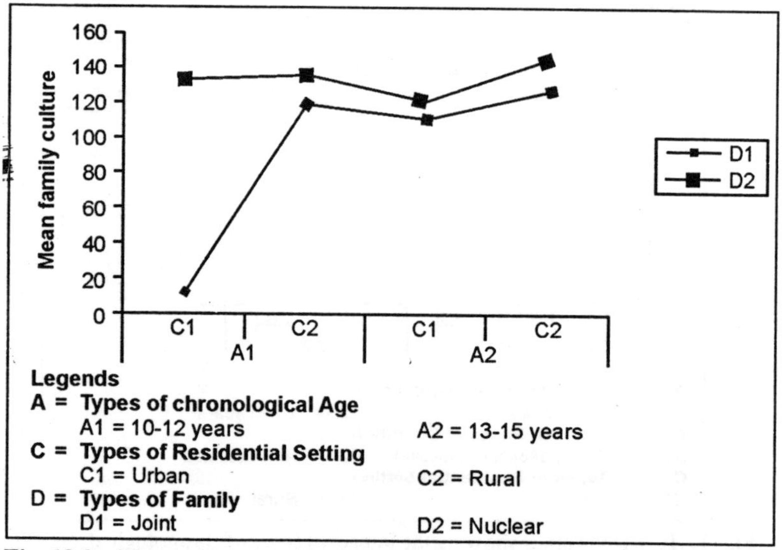

Fig. 12.3: Mean values showing the impact of types of chronological age, types of residential setting and types of family on familial culture

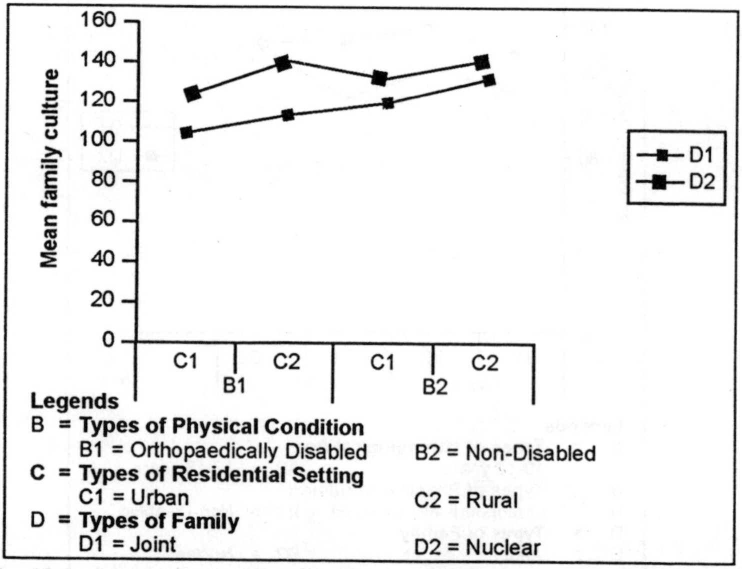

Fig. 12.4: Mean values showing the impact of types of physical condition types of residential setting and types of family on familial culture

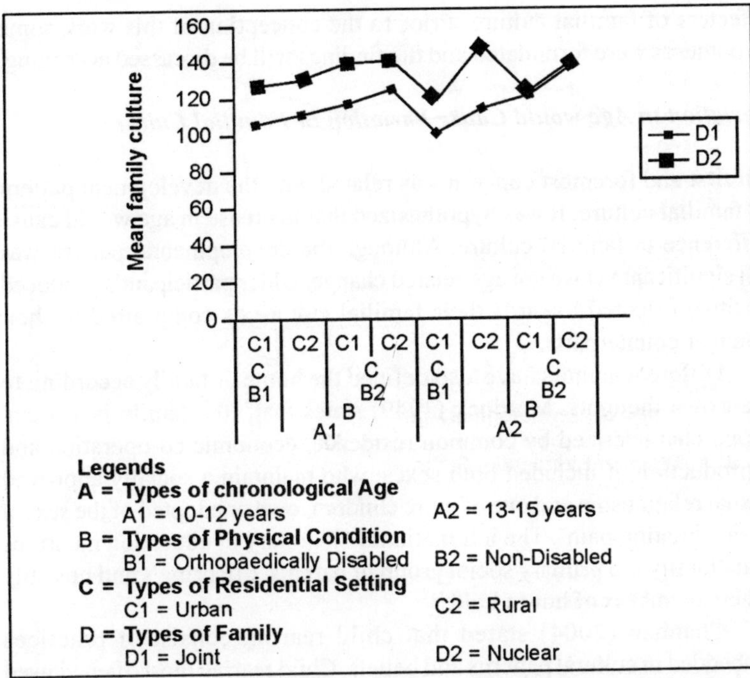

Fig. 12.5: Mean values showing the impact of types of chronological age types of physical condition, types of residential setting and types of family on familial culture

Table 12.3: Correlational analysis of data

Sl. No.	*Name of the areas*	*Correlation coefficients*						
		1	*2*	*3*	*4*	*5*	*6*	*7*
1	Competitive framework	—	.56	.48	.76	.49	.59	.61
2	Cohesion		—	.59	.49	.61	.74	.59
3	Expression			—	.51	.58	.46	.61
4	Independence				—	.59	.61	.68
5	Moral orientation					—	.64	.71
6	Organization						—	.76
7	Residential orientation							—

A close perusal of Table 12.3 indicates that all the dimensions are closely related to each other and it was shared by all variables.

Discussion

Obtained data were analysed by analysis of variances and interpreted in terms of age, disability, residential setting and family types of age, as affecters of familial culture. Prior to the conception of this work some hypotheses were formulated and the findings will be discussed according.

Variation in Age would Cause Variation in Familial Culture

On first and foremost concern was related with the development pattern of familial culture. It was hypothesized that in crease in age would cause difference in familial culture. Although the developmental pattern was not significant yet we got age related change. Older participant's produced positive oriented towards their familial culture as comp aired to their younger counterparts.

Different authors have also defined the home or family according to their own thoughts. Murdock (1949) states that, 'the family is a social group characterized by common residence, economic co-operation and reproduction, it included both sexes, who maintain a socially approved sexual relationship and one of more children, own or adopted of the sexual co-habituating pain'. The international dictionary of education mentions that "family is a primary social group of parents, offspring's and possibly others members of house hold."

Chauhan (2004) stated that child rearing consist of practices embedded in cultural patterns and beliefs. Child rearing most often viewed in the context of the personality development of an individual. To a large extent these practices determine the behaviour and the expectations surrounding a child's birth and infancy. They also influence childhood, adolescence and also the way these children parents in future. Theorists like Bronfenbrenner and Super and Harkness have forwarded their thought regarding personality development in a cultural context.

Tripathi (2004) investigated the self-perception of physically disabled girls and their mother's perception of their disabled daughters. Fifty four disabled girls and their mothers were interviewed. The age range of disabled girls was 14 to 19 years and their mother age range was 35 to 56 years. The data was quantitatively and qualitatively themselves negatively and their mothers also did not perceive them positively.

Mendiratta (2004) stated that culture provides context wherein child's development takes place. The beliefs, values, practices that parents have for child's development are rooted within this context. Socialization of child thus cannot be viewed in isolation. There are various factors like, parenting style, personality traits, family type, socialization situation provide to they child, parents understanding about socially context that influence adults perspective regarding self and the child which in turn influences the adult child interaction. This adult child interaction influences the adult child development. The present paper attempts to understand the linkages between the parental beliefs and child development within the cultural context.

On the basis of this discussion it is surely fair to say that variation in age causes variation in financial experiences.

Variation in Residential Type would cause Variation in Familial Culture

Villages are heterogeneous in terms of location, life style and their relationship with urban centers (Muthayya, 1988). When we talk about rural development it represents a process of change from existing level to a planned new level where quality of life is better. In this way rural development seems to be a continuous process which remains positive and purposive (Reddy, 1982; Singh and Ray, 1980). The main objective of rural development is to improve the psycho-social conditions and lifestyle of the people of villages. However, this fact seems to have been over looked in the process of developmental planning (Sinha, 1984). On this context it is also important to note that the way people interpret the developmental programme determines their acceptance and adoption. The interpretation of programmes depends on peoples past experiences, their general attitudes towards life and the values of the social system. (Muthayya, 1980) the existing level of socio-economic development also plays an important role. Socially disadvantaged, for instance, perceive their problems in a different framework. According to them the village problems include poverty, unemployment, and lack of roads. They perceive lesser accessibility to the facilities and lesser degree of satisfaction (Annesudin and Naidu, 1984; Muthayya, 1980).

Variation in Family Type would cause Variation in Familial Culture

Last but not least was the hypothesis in which impact of family on familial culture was measured. Here, it was assumed that perception of family set would vary with variation in family type, i.e. joint and nuclear families. Our hypothesis was confirmed and we found that the participants residing in joint or nuclear families did produce variation in the experience of familial set-up.

In affirmation of the salience of family as a context of development, numerous studies have investigated the role of family variables on various aspects of development in early years. Misra and Tewari (1984) determine the influence of digital variables and proximal variables on the cognitive development of school. Using regression analysis the researchers observed higher contribution of proximal have variables compared to that of distal variables. Studies with older children have explored the links between their perceptions and recollections of child rearing practices and some aspects of social and moral development (Sethi and Gupta, 1984; Sahoo and Nanda, 1990).

Studies on familial influences on children with special needs cover a wide range of topics from parent's and sibling's knowledge about familial set-up and circumstances prevailing there variables pertaining to familial influences assume greater significances for the care and development of the children with special needs, since parental knowledge and understanding about the disability affects their behaviour in terms of acceptance, help seeking, future aspirations, and support given to the child. Several of these links have been empirically substantiated (Kapur, 1992).

The review of studies pertaining to the relation between familial variables and developmental outcomes shows that rarely here the family been treated as a unit and the intra familial interaction pattern studied properly. The family unit as a whole is likely to change its modes and areas of functioning as consequences of social change, as indicated by Kumar's conception of the changed manifestations in modern's families of the traditional norms of continuity between the adults and child's world (Kumar, 1993). Any change in the family structure needs to be understand in terms of what caused the change and for how long the change has persisted, for example a family may follow a joint structure other due to emotional cohesiveness or due to emotional compulsion on the other hand a family may be rendered nuclear by one individual's derive to achieve independent success leaving the other members in another nuclear structure. The two units, however, will not be isomorphic as context for child's socialization. There is a need to articulate and contextualize the transitions that a primary group such as family experiences (Anand Lakshmy, 1993) in order to understand their salience in child development.

References

Anand Lakshmy, S. (1993). Psychosocial experiences of childhood in india; implications for mental health. In M. Kapur, S. Kelaur, R. Tarter and R. Wilson (Eds.), *Child mental health: Proceedings of the Indo-US Symposium*. Bangalore: NIMHANS.

Bajaj, B. and Raut. P. (2004). Trait-Anger and Anger Expression Among Parent and Child, *14th Annual Conference of National Academy of Psychology on Psychology and Development in Department of Humanities and Social Sciences,* Indian Institute of Technology, Kharagpur.

Biswas, A. and Aggrawal, J.C. (1971). *Encyclopedic Dictionary and Directory of Education,* Vol. I, New Delhi: Academic Pub.

Bloom, M. (1968). *Stability and change in human characteristics*, New York: John-Willy & Sons.

Chapman, J.W. (1988). Learning disabled children self's concept. *Review of Educational Research,* 58, 3, 347-371.

Chauhan, G.S. (2004). A Cross Cultural view of child Rearing practices and construction of personality and behaviour, *14th Annual Conference of National Academy of Psychology on Psychology and Development in Department of Humanities and Social Sciences,* Indian Institute of Technology, Kharagpur.

Cooley, E.J. and Ayers, R.R. (1988). Self-Concept and Success failure attributions of non-handicapped students with learning and disabilities. *Journal of Learning Disabilities*, 21, 3, 174-178.

Cronbachl, I. (1977). *Educational Psychology*, IIIrd Ed, Harcourt Brace Jovanovich, New York.

Danesh, H.B. (1978). The Authoritarian family and its Adolescence. *Canadian Psychiatric. Association Journal*., 23, 7, pp. 479-485.

Douvan, E. and Adelison, J. (1966). The *Adolscence experience,* New York: Willey, pp. 95-98.

Good, C.V. (1973). *Dictionary of Education*, IIIrd Ed., New York: McGraw Hills.

Grolniek, W.S. and Ryan, R.M. (1990). Self Perception motiratm and adjustment in children with learning disabilities: A multiple group comparison study. *Journrl of Learning Disabilities,* 23, 3, 177-184.

Harter, S. (1985). Competence as a Dimension of Self-Evaluation: Towards a Comprehensive Model of Self Worth in Leahy, R.L. (ed). *The Development of Self.* Orlando: Academic Press, Inc.

Hussain, A. (2006). Self concept of Physically challenged adolescents, *Journal of the Indian Academy of Applied Psychology,* Vol. 32, No.1, pp. 43-46.

Kapur, M. (1992). Siblings relationship in families with mentally handicapped children. *Unpublished masters dissertation*, Lady Lrwin College, University of Delhi, Delhi.

King, G.A., I.Z. Sted, K. Gilpin, M. and Cathers, T. (1993). Self Evaluation and Self Concept of adolescents with physical disabilities, *American Journal of Occupational Therapy*, 47, 2, 132, 140.

Kumar, K. (1993). Study of childhood and family. In T.S. Saraswathi and B. Kaur (Eds). *Human development and studies in India: An agenda for research and policy, Sage.*

Mahapatra, P. Rani, C. Moltra, J. and Alam, P. (2004). Impact of disability on social adjustment: An Empirical study on Orthopendically challenged, *14th*

Annual Conference of National Academy of Psychology on Psychology and Development in Department of Humanities and Social Sciences, Indian Institute of Technology, Kharagpur.

Malm, M. and Jamison O.G. (1952). *Adolescence,* New York: McGraw Hill, pp. 282-283.

Maslow, A.H. (1941). The Dynamic of Psychological security and Insecurity, *Character and Personality,* 10, pp. 331-334.

Mendiratta, A. (2004). Parental beliefs, Child Development within cultural context, *14th Annual Conference of National Academy of Psychology on Psychology and Development in Department of Humanities and Social Sciences,* Indian Institute of Technology, Kharagpur.

Misra, G. and Tiwari, B.K. (1984). Environmental correlates of cognitive development. *Indian Journal of Applied Psychology*, 24, 1, 41-52.

Mishra, U. (2001). The Experience of Social change in Rural India: A Qualitative Analysis of Panchayati Raj in selected villaged. *Unpublished Ph.D. Works,* C.C.S. Meerut University, Meerut.

Murdock, G.P. (1949). *Social Structure*, New York: McMillan Co.

Muthayya, B.C., Aneesddin, M. and Naidu, K.K. (1984). The rural disadvantaged: a psychosocial study in Bihar and Orissa. *Journal of Rural Development,* 3(3) 175-248.

Muthayya, B.C. (1988). Dynamics of Rural Development in J. Pandey (Ed). *Psychology in India: The state-of-the-art*, Vol. 2 (pp. 225-278). New Delhi: Sage.

Platt *et al.* (1962). Comparison of Child Rearing Attitude of Mothers and Fathers of Emotionally Disturbed Adolescents, *Child development*, 33, 117-122.

Reddy, G.R. (1982). Panchayati Raj and rural development in Andhra Pradesh, India. In Norman T. Uphaff (Ed), *Rural Development and Social Organization in Asia*, (vol. 1), New Delhi: MacMillan.

Sahoo, F.M. and Nanda, U. (1990). Socialization parameters of learned helplessness. *Psychological Studies*, 35, 1, 52-61.

Sethi, A.S. and Gupta (1984). Moral judgment level and perceived maternal child rearing attitudes of boys and girls. *Journal of Psychological Researches*. 28, 2, 102-106.

Singh, S. and Ray, J.J. (1980). Modernization and Development among Indian Farmers. A modern proof of some old theories, *Economic Development and Cultural Change*, 28(2), 509-522.

Shah (1982), *Personality Development in Children*, Multi-Tech. Pub. Co., Bombay.

Stott (1974). *The Psychology of Human Development*, New York: Holt, Rinehart and Winston, p. 208.

Tripathi, N. (2004). Perception of disability: Disabled girls and their mothers, *14th Annual Conference of National Academy of Psychology on Psychology and Development in Department of Humanities and Social Sciences,* Indian Institute of Technology, Kharagpur.

Wolman, B.B. (1977). *International Encyclopedia Psycholonalysis and Neurology*, Van Nostrand Reinholt Co., New York.

13

Dynamic Constructs and Static Gender

Constructing Higher Education by Deconstructing Well-being

Tanu Shukla and *Kalyan Kumar*

Introduction

In the contemporary age, analyzing changes in working conditions requires an understanding of gender relations at work place. The nature of the work is undergoing transformation to a greater extent and demand understanding of the various intricacies involved in it. Freedom is intrinsically trapped and restrained in the matters of normative frameworks in relation to gender. There is an inertia associated with the socio-cultural constructs; its views any change or push in any of the social structure as a path to instability by inducing anarchic elements. Any anarchic introduction undermines complete domination or oppressive impositions; this is always viewed as a negative and destructive ailment, which is not necessarily true in every given faculty. Therefore, these norms and constructs breed on interpreting gender as a fundamental necessity which needs to be nurtured adequately to avoid any dislocation. This phenomenon completely disguises the desire to view gendered practices as a matter of choice or associate it with freedom. It has become institutional than instinctual.

Human pride is frequently violated on grounds of sex which by the meaning refers to the biological difference between men and women that is determined by birth. Gender connotes the socially constructed and culturally determined characteristics associated with social roles. At every sphere, women are experiencing inequalities and claiming their rights to be respected. Development of women is one of the crucial agendas of the state from the very first plan (1951-56), the successive plans reflected in the similar welfare approach, but the major shift was seen in the approach of 'welfare' to 'development' in the current plan lay emphasis on a multidisciplinary approach with a special thrust on the core sectors of health, education and employment. The current plan highlights the notion of human development as it focuses on the development of women that ensures benefits to women in different sectors including gender equality as the major concern. The current scenario indicates new challenges for the gender equality which involves rights that deserves respect from laws and social institutions and the idea of functional capabilities.

In a patriarchal society like India, the authority of men is considered as the primary causal factor for the oppression of women. It survives by stereotyping the role of gender (women). These roles that are adopted or rather enforced after unjust exercise of power, maintaining and nurturing it in disguise to frame the identity of a particular. These identities always implicate in itself a subordinate nature of the being. Mill refutes, criticizes and expresses this outlook in *The Subjugation of Women* as—

> There are no means of finding what either one person or many can do, but by trying—and no means by which anyone else can discover for them what it is for their happiness to do or leave undone (Mill, 1869).

The boundaries of socio-cultural roles of gender remain undisturbed even with vast shifts and progress in various events of life, but the advancement and changes in a society recommend a deviation from the structural impositions. The confinement of gender to a role, limitations within a social norm account of repression of human instincts instilling fear and an element of extra caution and self-surveillance on one hand and are simultaneously exposed to different scenarios in the changing times. There is a constant sense of anxiety for any given stimulus. These alterations, shifts, repression and impositions unsettle and invoke frustration, leading to mental disturbances in an individual. It is often said that women supposedly need to work twice as hard as men with double social restrictions by men in a discriminating organizational ambience driven by psychological subordination to men just to achieve an equal status to men. This study identifies itself with the gender discrimination and inequality and its relation to the women's mental health (exclusively the well-being) in the context of Indian higher education.

Gender discrimination is rampant in every sphere of activity in India. Trend analyses of professional segregation based on gender connotes the transparent glass-ceiling effect that also depicts double marginalization, discrimination and inequality experienced by women especially belonging to minority ethnic backgrounds. The motive subjugates the consciousness and women's social and economic status over the past few years. There is a strong interaction of psychological characteristics, experiential factors, processes of socialization and social expectations which leads to differences in the input and output of women. Stereotyping the role of women has led to repression at an individual level and marginalization at a group level, which inevitably influences the mental well-being of women.

Objectives

- To identify the factors and the invisible barriers that prevent or curb women's professional growth.
- To analyze the impact of social and psychological constructs that impact the well-being of women in the context of higher education.

Gender in Higher Education

Education is by large viewed as a potential tool to avoid, solve or reform these imbalances (Chanana, 1993). With achievement of relatively genuine enrollment rates of girls at primary and secondary educational levels in India and yet the persisting challenges for women, it is fair to hope that higher education would turn out to be more effective (Pascarella and Terenzini, 1991; Klein, 1984; Freeman, 1975). It is only at the level of higher education, people tend to attain necessary employable skills, and in case of girls it is very essential as it guarantees economic independence and social respect (Nussbaum, 2000). Benavot's (1989) research claims that educating girls ensures more economic development than in comparison to educating boys. But the model or organization of higher education is itself turning out to be non-inclusive and hostile in regard to women (Chanana, 1993). A sustainable model is essential for its better functioning and in achieving gender empowerment through equality. Gender inequality is heavily imbalanced in the higher education arena than in primary and secondary (according to the Statistics of Higher and Technical Education 2009-10, Provisional). Higher education is not seen merely as a process of academic growth, but also as self-development. The process in here is depriving the purpose itself. Reducing the gender gap below 10 per cent is included in the twelfth five year plan and UGC has taken up several schemes for the benefit of women (Annual Report 2012-13, MHRD).

There are a decent proportion of female teachers at primary level, but this could not be maintained as we reach a top of the higher education (NIEPA). Ironically, higher education in India, which is believed to empower the marginalized and oppressed is itself suffering from the lack of women professional representatives. Lack of women professionals and persistence of growth barriers, in regard to gender equality (Sen, 1984), in the organizations of academia is firstly an injustice and then hindrance to reforming the social system at large. There must be apriority and, as much emphasis on removing the barriers within higher education institutes as much on removing barriers through higher education.

As an effect of globalization and goals to internationalize higher education, the social circle and cross-cultural interaction is expanded and encouraged. There is also an expansion of the marginalization of women (Chatterjee, 1992). This invariably distorts the gendered role prevailing in developing countries with rural backgrounds and social stigmas. The burden of any small shift biasedly affects women and a further gender disparity is observed (Sen, 1999; Banerjee, 1989).

Higher education of women is not a fundamentally essential component like in the case of men. In the case of women, higher education is viewed as an end in itself, but in the case of men it is a means to achieve further ends; to move up the ladder. This has a very resonating effect as every social-culture construct has similar implications in the domain of gender reinforcing the subordinate or the unequal status of women.

Conceptualizing Well-being and Its Link to Women's Mental Health

Mental health is often conceptualized in two directions. One being the absence of any disorder or, with the emergence of positive psychology, it can be seen as a positive attribute that is evaluating psychologically how well a being is, what are her opportunities and functioning's as an individual in a social realm and how one maintains a balance with self and the changing contexts of the surrounding world. The emphases are more about the lifestyle than on the individual and furthermore on the factors that contribute to the persistence of these lifestyles, which affect the well-being. The empowerment for a quality life has occupied precedence over eradication of illness. For effective treatment of illness is a means, but not an end in itself. The idea of mental health has gained a multi-dimensional approach. The constitution of WHO views Health as "*a state of complete physical, mental and social well-being and not merely the absence of disease or infirmity*". In regard to social factors of mental health, the WHO reports 1986 states—

> "Mental health is the capacity of the individual, the group and the environment to interact with one another in ways that promote subjective well-being, the optimal development and use of mental abilities (cognitive, affective and relational), the achievement of individual and collective goals consistent with justice and the attainment and preservation of conditions of fundamental equality."

Many studies have enabled in constructing suitable models for better contemplation and further application of the conceptual framework of well-being. In the present study of various constructs (limited to gender) in the domain of higher education (in India) follows the similar conceptual framework of well-being and mental health of women. Studies that have been consistently conducted on the parameters that would affect or contribute in determining and evaluating the well-being of individuals would help in justifying this study. For instance, Sweeney and Witmer (1991), Witmer and Sweeney (1992), in the wheel of wellness have identified work-leisure as one among the five important determinants of well-being that possess a significant role in affecting the quality of life. Further down, Myers, Sweeney, and Witmer (2000) have sub-categorized the tasks in relation to well-being; gender and cultural identity being two among them.

The focus of this study is also to expose the factors that contribute to the barriers which hinder the growth of women and cause discrimination and marginalization. In addition, it is equally important to note the visible effects of these invisible barriers in the chosen domain. As mentioned above, it is evident that the note should point towards the well-being of women. The succeeding questions in the process would be how these social, cultural and psychological phenomena are addressed? How does it impact the well-being of an individual and the over all mental health of people in the community? What are the fundamental causes behind these ill effects?

Liberal Feminist theories argue that the subordination and oppression of women are unjust and appeals for an effective reform in the context of the socio-economic and political structures. They emphasize on the equality of opportunity and right to protection and social dignity in an evolved and civilized world.

Likewise in other feminist discourses, scholars are constantly challenging the discrimination and the prevailing status of women. Marxist Feminists criticize the subordinate and unequal status of women in society and attribute these defects to the nature of profit seeking and the struggle for superiority amongst the individuals or groups in an institution. The subjugation of women is observed right from the birth, in the institution of marriage, in domestic work, at work place, at wages and in distribution. The abnormalities in the functioning of any domain of the society are linked to the means that have been chosen to meet the necessary ends. Harstsock, a Marxist-feminist scholar, mentions that a class society is a resultant of the oppression (women) and not oppression being a product of existence of class. This feminist discourse also describes how domination and exploitation have been an essential part of the social structure in forms of capitalism and patriarchy.

Psychoanalytic feminist discourse argues on the process of how a biological woman is made into a cultural feminine individual. The arguments are based on Freud's and Lacan's theory of psychosexual development. It refers to how the self is gendered and the role of subconscious structures in constructing gender identity and inducing the personality traits of asymmetry, inferiority and lack in girls. The focus of the discourse if on the oppression of a female individual self within the structures of culture and in the process of socialization. Radical Feminism views the oppression of women as the primary causal factor for various cultural imbalances, social inequalities and economic differences in a society. Women as a whole is suggested to form into a single class to fight against the oppression. Radical feminists hold that the authority of one class and the inferiority of the other is maintained by strategies such as intimidation, fear, violence and terror by one class towards other.

The whole nemesis of the study is the gender inequality in the domain of higher education. This inequality persists because of the lack of the opportunity for women to become equal, the lack of opportunity (Sen, 1993) to choose, to refrain, to disagree, to have their agency (Sen, 1985c, 203) and to be well. Women in higher education are found not to be deficient in abilities but in opportunities. These barriers, at group or individual level, impair primarily not growth, but the freedom and opportunity to grow and be well.

Methodology

There have been a plethora of empirical studies on women in higher education and also on gender and mental health. Moving away for the quantitative works over period and in comprehending the dynamics of the socio-cultural and psychological constructs, it is important to note that these abstractions and its implications are non-uniform, ever varying and subjective. Therefore, the more suitable, inclusive and chosen method is a qualitative study. Higher education in India is considered to be post-secondary education. The population is the entire female teachers from the two universities from Hyderabad selected by incidental sampling technique. Likewise, for the purpose of the interview, the sample size included female teaching staff of various faculties of two different universities where factors like academic, administrative and experience were also considered.

The interview encompassed questions regarding working environment, social circle, flexibility of rules, time spent at work, family relationships, opportunities, prejudices and preferences, satisfaction levels, tolerance, attitude and mood shifts, derogatory incidents, ambitions and hopes.

Findings and Discussions

Reviewing literature included the theoretical frameworks of gender and feminism, studies conducted on gender, mental health and well-being etc. Analyzing the semi-structured interview conducted on how stereotyping gender in the domain of higher education and its implications on the their well-being have led to the following discussions.

Broadly, the constructs which act as barriers to achieve well-being of women can be delineated into social and psychological form. One can conceptualize social as the explicit influence of external parameters, invisible structures of gender (the social norms having a direct impact on females). Psychological barriers being the implicit influence exerted on an individual personality. Psychological barriers are conceptualized keeping individual as the base, whereas social barriers are organizational and effect on community/frames of society as the base.

Social Constructs as Barriers

Social barriers in higher education in regard to gender that affect the well-being of women as a whole is largely due the whole organizational culture persisting in India. The hierarchic nature with rigidity is adopted and justified by organizations citing efficiency and greater productivity. But this is achieved only at the cost of well-being of women, inciting oppression and marginalization in a system. There has been a consistent discrimination of gender right from recruitment process (Tolbert and Oberfield, 1991; Konrad and Pfeffer, 1991) stretching to the promotions (Hulbert and Rosenfeld, 1992; Long and Fox, 1995). The notion of equality is disturbed right from the inception; the basic prerogative of an equal opportunity is subjugated and effectively disguised. The universities opt for men over women; as a result, they perceived heavily discriminated while the rules and norms are framed to avoid even the least discrimination. Most of the women unanimously agree that men are more favoured for promotion in spite of seeking extra advantage in the recruitment process. The most common reason meted out is to tackle immense pressure and heavy workload. One of the excerpts of the interview exhibit the discrimination that lies in organizational structure—

> "... Unequal means cannot produce equal ends. Several reasons in organizational framework like faster output, tight competence and undisturbed dedication are mentioned as reasons for preferring men over women. Men have the means and preference over women to work and grow in an institute. They hold most of decision making posts and all of the key posts.... This obviously leads to relatively low output, and most of the times, this is taken as an alibi to substantiate the decisions that have been taken or would be taken. Women have inevitably ended up in a loop of subjugation; it has evolved as a systemic flaw..."

One of the toughest challenges that are observed and also unique to higher education is a balance between the administrative positions *versus* academic research. Most women are overlooked for handling two tasks. This trend has had its influences from viewing women in other walks of life too. This has matured into pure insensitivity towards the gender undermining their ability. They are sometimes shown unjust sympathy and unwanted protectiveness under the assumption of an imaginative burden. Proposing this reason, women are narrowed down only to academic affairs. There is a male dominance in administrative affairs. All administrative positions are hierarchic and attach to themselves the notions of power, order, restrictions and making decisions behalf of all and for all. It is observed that there is a complete lack of control of women in decision-making due to the need of adequate representation.

The power dynamics between any two sects or groups are said to fair and productive if it is not oppressive and unjust. Women do not get to choose but are assigned the role in which they are forced to adhere to. Many men are found to be stereotypical in matters of gender and professional work, in case they are not; the rigid culture of the organization restricts their approach to a stereotypical one. The discrimination of women is not always mandatory by negative oppressive forces. A few professors, relatively young, have mentioned that over politeness, undue care and extra attention shown to women are also features contributing to discrimination.

Many social scientists over a period have elaborated on the dual shift, work-home responsibilities, enforced on women. One of the excerpt includes:

> "Women need to work hard to equal men in their professions and have to deal with similar burdens at home. Work at home is not relaxing or free from stress esp. In the context of joint families or with only a single, young or middle aged woman. It certainly affects the focus and energy needed for other things we desire to work on. Work at home is disguised and is not accounted as strained labour.... Home happens to be the only place on earth, which is gendered with a preference for women over men, this preference of women over men is again without the consent of women..."

To enjoy a similar social status of men, women have to score in two parallel endeavours. This invariably decelerates the professional progress. Women in an organization are judged not only as an employee (teacher/researcher/student) but also in a traditional sense of being feminine (family member, wife, mother etc.). Women in research programmes are very low in number (Ransom, 1990). Though equally passionate, find it difficult to study further to specialize or gain expertise in a chosen field by moving into doctoral programmes, post doc or advanced research programmes. The invisible barriers which stop women from these are the restrictions that are imposed by the family. In a patriarchal sense, the family finds it difficult to accept, or perceive it to be demeaning for the husband of the respective lady, for a woman to have superior educational qualifications or additional degree. Even as per the institution, they place more trust on men to rejoin the same job after a doctoral or a post-doctoral research than on women. They discern that, the decision of women is dependent on several factors and is mostly influenced by the male support in her family. They are often engaged in the sphere of teaching and very less in research.

Women in academics also experience a severe lack of exposure to conferences and workshops. Safety, extra burden and other consequences are the most cited reasons causing this lack. The majority of them agree to the fact that they are avoidable and can be reformed. The inhuman part is some of them blame opportunity and prejudice for the lack. However, most of them agree that the above factors indirectly lead again to the same deprival of opportunity. They could not avail the funding opportunities for seminars, workshops and field research due to the lack of security and company. The excerpts of a senior faculty who has volunteered to participate in the interview assert:

> "... In a globalized world, the flow of information and the availability to equip oneself with changing technology and methods is abundant. But the opportunities and social norms in India in regard to women have failed to change sufficiently... The training opportunities and level of training attained by women in academic research is meagre, this is not because of the ability but taboo, lack of freedom and stereotyping the gender roles...
> ... Even in the process of socialization and association, men are at a vastly advantageous level over women. Women are yet restrained by social force or diverting responsibilities... and this has a resonating effect on their careers."

The approach and reach of women to larger audience, academic associations and external networks are restricted and discouraged due to the stereotypical view on socialization and informal interactions with women. Few women have complained that informal interactions in making new acquaintance are often met with discouraging gestures and character remarks from the prior collegues. This phenomenon is commonly observed in state universities with a rural back drop. It has wider repercussions in shaping the psychological well-being of an individual associated with academia.

Psychological Constructs and Barriers

Hitherto the above discussion deals with the effects of social structures on females as a whole. The constructs of gender in higher education are far reaching effect, notwithstanding at the level of a group, they have precise implications at the individual level. These barriers cease to fully retain their invisibility in the psychological categorization.

Intrinsically, with discrimination and subjugation, women have lower levels of self-confidence and self-respect. This is immensely because of the limited pool of opportunities available or rather 'made available' to women and the inconsistency between changing times/goals and existing expectations. Women have to outstretch in order to compete with men with these barriers, they have to undergo quite a few sacrifices with little hope of desired outcome. All these amounts to decent compromises individual's mental health.

As the effects of the above mentioned causes, there is a lack of authoritativeness and the locus of control for women is observed to be low. Due to the socio-economic factors and the patriarchal culture, from generations, women are found to have a dependent role. Though things have progressed, it has not been adequately proportionate with rapid advancements in various genres of life. Most of the faculty members spell out that a centre of women's studies, workshops and seminars in a university would accelerate the gender sensitivity amongst people. Universities in India still lack behind having or implementing these approaches. One of the faculties asserts—

> "... At family level and even in the professional arena, the achievements of women are often attributed chance, low competition, whereas in the case of men it is looked as a constructive step to move forward. Inequality is observed at the stage of low expectations for women and the indifference towards their passions and dislikes; their voice is unheard and they assume a role of subaltern... The levels of motivation are shaped out to be absolutely low; self-respect and identity exist only in crisis. These phenomena are very depressing, things seem only as a matter of chance with women it is never a matter of choice..."

The chances of depression are found more in the case of women in comparison to men (Patel *et al.*, 1999). Most of them can be corrected by a change in the attitudes rendered in regard to or against them. At a personal level, women feel there is an immense lack of mentorship and companionship. Solitude and egoistic attitudes in a professional race make them more prone to depression and other mental disturbances. Ironically,

Orpen (1995) and Scandura and Lankau (1997), state their findings that females possess more commitment and flexibility with respect to the work, which is positively correlated with job satisfaction.

This is rampantly observed in every section of the society in almost every walk of life. Women need to be extra conscious and vigilant in classrooms to staff meets and fieldwork. Many women hold the impression that a strong anti-sexual harassment policy in the university and more importantly, an effective implementation of the policy could largely help (Williams, 1992; Paludi and Barickman, 1991) in curbing incidents like voyeurism, stalking and teasing of female employees from the students and administrative sections. The committee that deals with the causes of discrimination and sexual harassment ought to work with rigour and under the oath of secrecy and not disturbing privacy. This would help secure women and reduce the gradient of mental disturbances to an extent.

An inadequate representation of women has its repercussions extended from the section of social constructs to the psychological ones. Low numbers of women faculty do not attract or support women enrollments. The lack of role models is seen as a critical issue. This adds to the prevalence of the under-representation for a length of time, for decades in India. Women faculty if found to be directly proportional to the number of achievers and enrollments in the succeeding generation (Tidball, 1980). Under-representation also discourages women to pursue further (Rothstein, 1995; Ehrenberg *et al.*, 1995; Erkut and Mokros, 1984). The levels of satisfaction for both female students and faculty are higher with a balanced representation.

Diet control and limited food intake are no a longer a matter of availability and economic affordability, but striving to fit into the social and normative definitions and limits of beauty. In management, Human Resources and administrative sectors in the professional stream consider face value, shapes and gestures of the body as an added asset. The cults of thinness, healthy diet restrain, the aggressive weight reduction has entered into the mainstream education and play a conveniently significant role in the university ambiences. Mental well-being is never more endangered for women than it is in the case of sexual harassment, voyeurism and improper advancements.

Psychologically, the normative frameworks, these burdens and stereotyping impair creativity in research. Impairing creativity and professional freedom affect the quality and output of academics and growth, fueling discrimination on an individual basis and the marginalization of gender in the socio-organizational structure.

Conclusion

Gender equality and empowerment lean to occupy the centre of the web of many social issues. It has intervened and played a significant role in every strata of the community we dwell. One of the significant means chosen to address gender inequality is education. Ironically, the system of education is itself harbouring discrimination, social and cultural barriers, domination and marginalization. These are the very traits that nurture and help in sustainment of inequality in society. This study sheds light on the consequences of the discriminating elements of the deprived gender in a system. It destabilizes and disturbs the whole well-being of individuals and consequently that of the society.

The qualitative nature of the study helped to capture the subtle ailments which are largely invisible and ignored. The semi-structured interview did not deal with the frequency and extent of discrimination, but on the nature, forms, causes and effects of this discrimination and inequality. The nature of the questions included on how different individuals perceived the causes of discrimination, how have they conceptualized the reasons of gender inequality (only in higher education), the role of family relations, the nature of work that they subscribe and that which is imposed, their personal goals and ambitions and the targets expected by the institute. In continuation, as another section, the effects of the above have been requested for a brief discussion. These include the satisfaction levels, the reasons for continuing or changing the jobs, levels of self-confidence and self-respect, the extent of choice and the availability of opportunities in the job and between life and job.

The influence of stereotyping the role of gender and the image of women has penetrated even into the academic and the intellectual circles of the society. Large proportions of women still believe that their entitlements and endeavours are vastly a matter of chance or limitations and less a matter of choice or interest. Independence and freedom for women remain distant, even with education and also in the system of education. As a consequence, the mental well-being and the social well-being are severely affected by psychological and social barriers. The idea of gender has remained static over time; or rather it has been maintained static with the influence of social and psychological constructs. The dynamics of these constructs in higher education, exercise, force which is responsible for pushing the conceptions of gender into a state of inertia. These barriers in the higher education have been disguised within the structural and organizational frameworks, they have a significant impact on hindering the growth of working women.

Gender equality, higher education and mental health, occupy a very pivotal role in determining the state of the society we inhabit today. It has been receiving an increasing focus currently, in the Millennium Development Goals chalked out by the United Nations. India seems to lag behind in addressing issues involving the above three parameters. Though efforts have begun to address the concerned issues, that which needs to be done largely out beat that which has been done.

References

Acker, J. (1990). Hierarchies, jobs, bodies: a theory of gendered organizations. *Gender Soc.,* 4, 139-58.

Ahmad, K. (1979). Equity and women's higher education. *Journal of Higher Education*, 5(1).

Ahmad, K.C. (1985). The social context of women's education in India 1921-81. *New Frontiers in Education*, 15(3), 1-36.

Alexander, K.L., and Eckland, B.E. (1974). Sex differences in the educational attainment process. *Am. Social. Rev*., 39, 668-82.

Anderson, M.S., and Hearn, J.C. (1992). Equity issues in higher education outcomes. In the *Economics of American higher education*, ed. W.E. Becker, D.R. Lewis, 301-34. Boston: Kluwer Acad.

Baatjes, I. (2003). The new knowledge-rich society: perpetuating marginalisation and exclusion. *Journal of Education* 2, 7, 179-204.

Banerjee, N. (1989). Trends in women's employment, 1971-81: Some macro-level observations. *Economic and Political Weekly*, 24(17) (April 29), 10-22.

Baugh, S.G. (1997). On the persistence of sexual harassment in the workplace. *Journal of Business Ethics*, 16(9), Women in Corporate Management, 899-908.

Benavot, A. (1989). Education, gender, and economic development: A cross-national study. *Sociol. Educ*., 62, 14-32.

Blackmore, J. (2002). Globalisation and the restructuring of higher education for new knowledge economies: New dangers or old habits troubling gender equity work in universities. *Higher Education Quarterly* 5, 6(4), 419-441.

Borgida, E., and Fiske, E.T. (1995). Gender stereotyping, sexual harassment and the law. Special issue. *J. Soc. Issues,* 51(1), 1-195.

Butler, J. (1985). Variations on sex and gender: Behaviour Wittig and Foucault, PRAXIS International (PRAXIS International), 505-516.

Buvinic, Mayra. (1997). *Women in poverty: A new global underclass*. Foreign Policy (Fall), 38-53.

Chanana, K. (1993). Accessing higher education: The dilemma of schooling women, minorities, scheduled castes and scheduled tribes in contemporary India. *Higher Education*, 26(1), 69-92.

Chanana, K. (1993). Partition and family strategies: Gender-education linkages among Punjabi women in Delhi. *Economic and Political Weekly*, 28(17), 25-34.

Chanana, Karuna. (ed.) (1988). *Socialisation, education and women: Explorations in gender identity.* New Delhi: Orient Longman.

Chitnis, Suma. (n.d.). *Education for the integration of the Indian polity*, mimeographed.

Constitution of World Health Organization, Basic Documents, Forty-fifth edition, Supplement, October 2006.

Costera Meijer, Irene. (1991). Which difference makes the difference? On the conceptualization of sexual difference. In *Sharing the Difference: Feminist Debates in Holland*, ed. Joke J. Hermsen and Alkaline van Lenning, 32-46. New York and London: Routledge.

Diener, E. (2000). Subjective well-being. *American Psychologist*, 55, 34-43.

Ehrenberg, R.G., Goldhaber, D.D., and Brewer, D.J. (1995). Do teachers' race, gender and ethnicity matter? Evidence from NELS. *Indust. Labor Related. Rev.*, 48(3), 547-61.

Erkut, S., and Mokros, J.R. (1984). Professors and models and mentors for college students. *Am. Educ. Res.* J., 21(2), 399-417.

Feingold, A. (1994). Gender differences in personality: A meta-analysis. *Psychological Bulletin*, 116, 429-456.

Freeman, J. (1975). *The politics of women's liberation.* New York: Longman

Gruber, J. (1989). How women handle sexual harassment: A literature review. *Sociol. Soc. Res.*, 74, 3-9.

Gruber, J. (1992). A typology of personal and environmental sexual harassment: Research and policy implications for the 1990s. *Sex Roles*, 26, 447-64.

Henry, M. (2001). Globalisation and the politics of accountability: issues and dilemmas for gender equity in education. *Gender and Education*, 13(l), 87-100.

Hochschild, Arlie. (1997). *The time bind: When work becomes home and home becomes work.* New York: Metropolitan Books.

Hulbert, J.S., and Rosenfeld, R.A. (1992). Getting a good job: Rank and institutional prestige in academic psychologists' careers. *Sociol. Educ.*, 65(3), 188-207.

King, J. (1971). Unequal access in education—sex and social class. *Social and Economic Administration*, 5, 167-175.

Klein, E. (1984). *Gender politics*. Cambridge: Harvard University Press.

Konrad, A.M., and Pfeffer, J. (1991). Understanding the hiring of women in minorities in educational institutions. *Sociol. Educ.* 64, 141-57.

Long, J.S., and Fox, M.F. (1995). Scientific careers: Universalism and particularism. *Annu. Rev. Sociol.*, 21, 45-71.

Marsh, H.W. (1990). A multidimensional, hierarchical model of self-concept:

Theoretical and empirical justification. *Educational Psychology Review,* 2(2), 77-172.

Mill, J.S. (2007). *On liberty and the subjection of women.* Revised edition, London: Penguin Classics.

Myers, J.E., Sweeney, T.J., and Witmer, J.M. (2000). The wheel of wellness counselling for wellness: A holistic model for treatment planning. *Journal of Counselling and Development*, 78, 251-266.

Nancy, F. (1989). *Unruly practices: Power, discourse and gender in contemporary social theory.* Minneapolis: University of Minnesota Press.

Nussbaum, M. (2000). *Women and human development: The capabilities approach.* Cambridge: Cambridge University Press.

Paludi M., (ed.) (1990). *Ivory power: Sexual harassment on campus.* Albany, NY: Suny Press.

Paludi, M.A., and Barickman, R.B. (1991). *Academic and workplace sexual harassment: Aesource manual.* Albany, NY: State University Press.

Patel, V., and Oomman, N. (1999). Mental health matters too: Gynaecological symptoms and depression in South Asia. *Reproductive Health Matters*, 7(14), Access to Reproductive Health: A Question of Distributive Justice, 30-38.

Ransom, M.R. (1990). Gender segregation by field in higher education. *Res. Higher Educ.*, 31(5), 477-94.

Roiphe, K. (1993). *The Morning after: Sex, Fear and Feminism on campus.* Boston, MA: Little, Brown and Co.

Rosenfeld, R.A. (1987). Patterns and effect of geographic mobility for academic women and men. *J. Higher Educ.*, 58(5), 493-515.

Rothstein, D. S. (1995). Do female faculty influence female students' educational and labour market attainments? *Indust. Labor Relat. Rev.*, 48(3), 515-30.

Scandura, T.A., and Lankau, M.J. (1997). Relationships of gender, family responsibility and flexible work hours to organizational commitment and job satisfaction. *Journal of Organizational Behaviour*, 18(4), 377-391.

Sen, A. (1985c). *The Standard of Living (The Tanner Lectures in Human Values).* Cambridge, Englnad: Cambridge University Press.

Sen, A. (1993). Markets and Freedoms: Achievements and limitations of the market mechanism in promoting individual freedoms. *Oxford Economic Papers*, New Series, 45(4), 519-541.

Sen, A. (1999). The Possibility of social choice. *The American Economic Review*, 89(3), 349-378.

Sen, A.K. (1984). *The Living standard.* Oxford: Oxford Economic Papers.

Sen, A.K. (1984). *Resources values and development*, Blackwell II, Oxford.

Subrahmanian, R. (2003). *Gender equality and the millennium development goals: Is the Glass Half-empty or Half-full?* R. Black and H. White (eds.), Targeting Development, London: Routledge.

Sweeney, T.J., and Witmer, J.M. (1991). Beyond ocial interest: Striving toward optimal health and wellness. *Individual Psychology*, 47, 527-540.

Terenzini, P.T., and Pascarella, E.T. (1991). Twenty years of research on college students: Lessons for future research. *Research in Higher Education*, 32(1), AIR Forum Issue, 83-92.

Tidball, M.E. (1980). Women's colleges and women achievers revisited. *Signs*, 5(3), 504-17.

Tinsley, H.E.A., and Stockdale, M.S. (1993). Special issue on sexual harassment in the workplace. *J. Vocat. Behav*., 42(1), 1-153.

Tolbert, P.S., and Oberfield, A.A. (1991). Sources of organizational demography: Faculty sex ratios in colleges and universities. *Sociol. Educ*, 64, 305-15.

Williams, E.A., Lam, J.A., and Shively, M. (1992). The impact of a university policy on the sexual harassment of female students. *J. Higher Educ.*, 63(1), 50-64.

Witmer, J.M., and Sweeney, T.J. (1992). A holistic model for wellness and prevention over the life span. *Journal of Counseling and Development*, 71, 140-148.

14

Positive Mental Health

Vijendra Nath Pathak, Priyanka Singh and *Santosh Kumar Singh*

Mental health problems are among the most important contributors to the burden of disease and disability worldwide. There is growing evidence of the global impact of mental illness. Five of the 10 leading causes of disability worldwide are mental health problems. They are as related to low-income countries as they are to rich ones, cutting across age, gender and social strata. Furthermore, all predictions indicate that the future will see a dramatic increase in mental health problems.

The WHO definition of mental health is as: *state of well-being in which the individual realizes his or her own abilities, copes with the normal stresses of life, works productively and fruitfully, and makes a contribution to his or her community* (WHO, 2001: 1).

In 1981, WHO adopted primary health care as the way to achieve the goal of health for all. As a strategy, primary health care seeks reorientation of health systems to enable the whole population to have effective and essential care and to promote individual and community involvement in health, as well as inter-sectoral collaboration. Appropriate treatment of common diseases and injuries and mental health care are integral components of primary health care. Much of the attention of WHO's Department of Mental Health and Substance Abuse is focused on the most effective ways to ensure the highest quality of life for persons with serious mental health problems.

There is increasing recognition throughout the world of the need to address mental health as an integral part of improving overall health and well-being (WHO, 2001, 2002, 2005a). Mental health is fundamental to good health and quality of life, it is a resource for everyday life and it contributes to the functioning of individuals, families, communities and society. The WHO phrase '*there is no health without mental health*' conveys clearly this emphasis on positive sense of mental health.

Positive Mental Health

In the mid-19th century, William Sweetzer was the first to clearly define the term "mental hygiene", which can be seen as the precursor to contemporary approaches to work on promoting positive mental health (Johns Hopkins University, 2010). Positive Mental Attitude has been touched upon since the concept of free will, but the concept was first developed and introduced in 1937 by Napoleon Hill in the book *Think and Grow Rich.* The book never actually uses the term, but develops the importance of positive thinking as a principle to success (Hill, 1960). He, along with W. Clement Stone, later wrote *Success Through a Positive Mental Attitude* which defines positive mental attitude as "The right mental attitude comprised of the 'plus' characteristics symbolized by such words as faith, integrity, hope, optimism, courage, initiative, generosity, tolerance, tact, kindliness and good common sense (Hill and Stone, 1987). Positive mental attitude is the philosophy that having an optimistic disposition in every situation in one's life attracts positive changes and increases achievement. It employs a state of mind that continues to seek, find and execute ways to win, or find a desirable outcome, regardless of the circumstances. It opposes negativity, defeatism and hopelessness.

A positive mental attitude is developed by constant reinforcement of one's goals, positive values and beliefs. Optimism and hope are vital to the development of positive mental attitude (Chang and Edward, 2001). One technique for positive reinforcement is with the use of "self-talk" such as the quote, "I feel happy. I feel healthy. I feel terrific." A variety of other techniques have been created over the years such as motivational posters, daily devotionals, accountability partners, and cause wristbands. Learning to control one's emotions is a key part to developing and maintaining positive mental attitude so as to expel the negative thoughts and feelings that could influence your actions and behaviour.

Positive mental health has been conceptualized as a positive emotion or affect such as subjective sense of well-being and feelings of happiness, a personality trait encompassing concepts of self-esteem and sense of control, and resilience in the face of adversity and the capacity to cope with life stressors (WHO, 2004a).

Marie Jahoda in her 1958 book *Current Concepts of Positive Mental Health*—one of the few publications addressing this topic—sought to define positive mental health in terms of a list of attributes such as an efficient perception of reality, self-knowledge, exercise of voluntary control over behaviour, self-esteem and self-acceptance, the ability to form affectionate relationships and productivity. Kovess-Masfety and associates (2005) pointed out that the definition of mental health is clearly influenced by the culture that defines it, and may have different meanings depending on socio-economic and political influences. From a cross-cultural perspective it is important to realize that our understanding of what constitutes positive functioning is likely to be very influenced by cultural beliefs about health and illness, societal values, norms and social influences. As mental health is embedded in the social and cultural framework of societies, the development of culturally sensitive and reliable indicators of mental health poses an important, though difficult, methodological challenge (Barry *et al.*, 2007).

The concept of positive mental health, therefore, encompasses the abilities to develop psychologically, emotionally, intellectually, socially and spiritually. Empirical work by (Keyes, 2002, 2005; Huppert and Whittington, 2003) reported the points to the independence of positive and negative well-being and shows that mental health and mental disorders are not opposite ends of a single continuum, but rather constitute distinct, though correlated, axes. Thus the absence of mental disorder does not equal the presence of mental health, and individuals without a mental disorder may experience varying degrees of positive mental health.

The emergence of positive psychology also brings a greater focus on the study of optimal human functioning (Seligman and Csikszentmihalyi, 2000; Seligman *et al.*, 2005), which includes studying positive psychological constructs such as optimism, love, emotional intelligence, creativity, hope, humour and a focus on positive subjective experiences, positive individual characteristics (strengths and virtues) and positive institutions and communities. To date, much of the scientific endeavour has focused on individual-level interventions to increase happiness and enhance positive emotions and characteristics. While the focus on positive emotions, such as happiness, has indeed captured the public imagination, as (Gable and Haidt, 2005) point out, there has been a lack of progress in studying the positive institutions and social conditions necessary for flourishing and optimal functioning.

Positive mental health should be sought in the attitudes of an individual towards his own-self. Various distinctions in the manner of perceiving oneself are regarded as demonstrating higher or lower degrees of health. Another group of criteria designates the individual's style and degree of growth, development, or self-actualization as expressions of mental health. This group of criteria, in contrast to the first, is concerned not with self-perception but with what a person does with his self over a period of time. Autonomy singles out the individual's degree of independence from social influences as most revealing of the state of his mental health. A number of proposals suggest that mental health is manifested in the adequacy of an individual's perception of reality. Finally, there are suggestions that environmental mastery be regarded as a criterion for mental health.

Model of Positive Mental Health

Humanistic psychologists—such as Abraham Maslow, Carl Rogers, and Ishizuka—developed theories and practices that involved human happiness and positivity. Recently, the theories of human flourishing have found empirical support from studies by positive psychologists.

Maslow Model: Maslow model is defined that the model of positive mental health provides a means to understand the same individual at different points in their cycle of life, whether in dire distress or optimal health. This differs with Maslow's studies of self-actualization, which focus on historical figures such as Lincoln, Jefferson, Thoreau, Einstein, and others as ideal candidates.

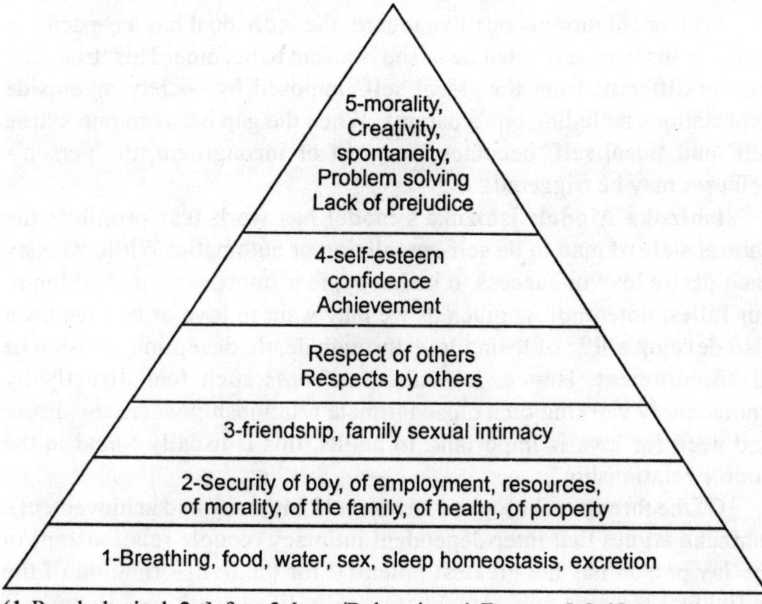

(1-Psychological, 2-Safety, 3-Love/Belonging, 4-Esteem, 5-Self-Actualization)

Although Maslow contributed much to the field by balancing the darker side of the human psyche with an understanding of love, well-being, and exuberance, some say he fell short of integrating the two halves; the positive and the negative. In this sense, the Lifetrack positive mental health approach may represent a middle ground, integrating the mind (or personality) both in distress and in well-being.

Carl Rogers Model: Rogers model has developed a theory based on self-actualization, in which the individual strives to develop optimal health in three spheres of psychological existence: self, intimacy and achievement. Like Rogers, growth is unlimited. Growth in the Life track model is frustrated by fear and can be experienced in the form of stress symptoms such as anxiety, anger, physical symptoms, depression or psychosis.

Carl Rogers is renowned for his work on Self-Actualization, which he viewed as an internal biological force to develop one's capacity to the fullest. Human beings, according to Rogers, strive for optimal health and require resilience in the face of adversity. Such resilience is fostered or nurtured by unconditional positive regard (a form of unconditional love) which can be experienced as a child from the relationship with one's parents.

With unconditional positive regard, the individual has a capacity to discover his 'true self' what he or she is meant to become. This 'true self' can be different from the 'ideal self' imposed by society or outside expectations including one's parents. When the gap between one's 'true self' and 'ideal self' becomes too great or incongruent, the person's defenses may be triggered.

Ishizuka Model: Ishizuka's model has work fear prohibits the natural state of man to be self-actualizing or automatic. While we may each desire love or success to be happy, fear impedes us to develop to our fullest potential. As much as we may want to love or be loved, we also develop a fear of losing love through death, deception, illusion or disappointment. Hence, Ishizuka confronts such fear directly by immediately working on a close intimate relationship where the desire and need for love is important. In adults, this is usually found in the couple relationship.

Of the three psychological needs (self, intimacy and achievement), Ishizuka argues that inter-dependent intimacy (couple relationship) in the lay person has the greatest potential for the transformation of the individual towards self-actualization. His life's work and therapy is based on the process of using breakthrough intimacy to trigger fundamental human change in all spheres of life: self, intimacy and achievement.

Sphere of Positive Mental Health: Yukio Ishizuka (1975) hypothesized that these three basic psychological needs or spheres that determined psychological health were: the search for self, the need for intimacy, and the quest for achievement. These three spheres—Self, Intimacy, and Achievement.

Self: Traditionally, the integrity of the Self refers to the entire personality of the individual. The Life track model defines Self more narrowly as the ability and willingness to be "in touch," "at peace," and "in control," of one's own thoughts, feelings and actions. Such self-awareness distinguishes human beings from their achievements and from their close relationships. To be "in touch," "at peace," and "in control" of self requires the capacity to recognize and accept both positives and negatives in life, integrating them into a balanced perspective. It also includes the flexibility to initiate, modify, and control thoughts, feelings, and actions. We can do this by observing our Self and remaining present in the given moment.

Intimacy: Intimacy requires us to extend our thoughts, feelings, and actions beyond the self and become close to another human being. Many different types of intimate relationships such as those with a parent, spouse, significant other, children, and friends, God or the universe bolster the psyche. A couple relationships, however, enables human beings to experience fullest union of personality, in all three dimensions of human intimacy—Intellectual/Social, Emotional, and Physical/Sexual. It is for this reason, that in Life Track Therapy, the therapist will focus on marriage intimacy or the development of an equivalent close couple relationship.

Achievement: Achievement is the capacity to reach beyond the Self through the productive, creative, and the constructive expression of one's capacities. It is an indirect way of finding an intimate union or relationship with the world in which one lives. Behind one's work, career, athletics, hobbies or other intellectual and productive activities is the desire not only to subsist, but also to find meaning and achieve value, acceptance, respect, admiration and deep down love by doing something difficult or meaningful. A person who is either unable or unwilling to build a relationship with the world through his or her constructive capacities may turn in desperation to destruction—an attempt to be noticed and counted and freed from total insignificance by a forced relationship of dominance.

The Scope of Positive Mental Health

These dimensions give a general sense of positive mental health. It will be helpful to give a partial list of topics that may be studied by a positive psychologist (a complete or comprehensive list would be quite exhaustive). Evidently, people are quite good at doing things well. In fact, the ways in which a person can excel is much more extensive than has been recognized in psychology.

Here is an A to Z list of possible topics: altruism and empathy, building enriching communities, creativity, forgiveness and compassion, the role of positive emotions in job satisfaction, the enhancement of immune system functioning, lifespan models of positive personality development, styles of psychotherapy that emphasize accomplishments and positive traits, savoring each fleeting moment of life, strengthening the virtues as way to increase authentic happiness, and the psychological benefits of Zen meditation (Lopez, 2002 and Snyder; Aspinwall and Straudinger, 2003; www.positivepsychology.org). One of positive psychology's early accomplishments was to help psychologists pay attention *to what people do right.* Once psychologists began to notice the many ways that human beings succeed in life, these neglected aspects of behaviour became the focus of theory, research, and intervention strategies.

Dimension of Positive Mental Health

Positive Mental Health is a broad concept, and there are a range of constructs and theories relevant to its understanding and assessment. As outlined above, positive mental health is usually conceptualized as encompassing aspects of emotional (affect/feeling), psychological (positive functioning), social (relations with others and society), physical (physical health) and spiritual (sense of meaning and purpose in life) well-being. The emerging literature on positive mental health and well-being considers the necessary or sufficient elements of positive functioning (Keyes, 2002; Huppert, 2005; Kovess-Masfety *et al.*, 2005; Zubrick and Kovess-Masfety, 2005; Ryff *et al.*, 2006). At least two dimensions of positive mental health have been identified:

- The hedonic component, which refers to subjective well-being and life satisfaction.
- The eudaimonic component, which includes positive functioning, engagement, fulfilment and social well-being.

Positive Mental Health: Balance the Cycle of Life

Regardless of one's willingness or natural ability, experiencing well-being in any one sphere of life requires presence, dedication and perseverance. There are trade-offs. There are moments when one sphere becomes dominant. However, when a person continuously chooses one sphere over the others, efforts become counter-productive. At the end of one's life one may regret having leaned too much towards the self, having thrown oneself into a love relationship at any cost, or having been consumed by achievement.

Positive Mental Health: Studies in India

The positive psychology movement has such an impact worldwide that it has become an integrated fabric of psychology all over. Jitendra Mohan and Meena Sehgal have so far supervised theses on various topics in Positive Psychology of Interpersonal Forgiveness, Happiness, Gratitude, Successful Aging and Work Engagement.

Mohan *et al.* (2007) studied dispositional forgiveness in relation to personality and spiritual well-being among Indian adolescents and reported positive correlations between dispositional forgiveness, spiritual well-being and personality dimensions of extroversion and social desirability and a negative correlation between dispositional forgiveness and personality dimensions of neuroticism as well as psychoticism. Similarly, Mohan *et al.* (2008a) studied Spiritual Well-being among adolescents in relation to their emotions and the results indicated significant relationships emerged between spiritual well-being along with its components and positive emotions, viz. optimism, hope, happiness and negative emotions, state and trait anger, anger-in, anger-out and anger control.

Mohan *et al.* (2008b) investigated relationship of psychological well-being with spiritual well-being and personality among adolescents and the results clearly revealed positive correlations between various dimensions of psychological well-being and spiritual well-being. Results also revealed negative correlations between various dimensions of psychological well-being and personality dimensions of neuroticism and psychoticism. Positive correlations were found between some dimensions of psychological well-being and personality dimensions of extraversion and social desirability.

Mohan *et al.* (2009) studied the structure of dispositional forgiveness in relation to happiness and well-being among Indian adolescents and the results revealed positive correlations between the dimensions of forgiveness, happiness and well-being. Two factors emerged significantly with Factor-I as a unipolar factor with significant loadings on forgiveness of self, happiness, life satisfaction, positive relations with others, self-acceptance, environmental mastery and positive affect. This implies that who are high on forgiving oneself are happier, experience more positive feelings, more accepting of one, share positive relations with others, seek environmental mastery, perceive their life to be purposeful and are satisfied with their life. Another factor emerged as a bipolar factor with significant loadings on all the three dimensions of forgiveness, i.e. forgiveness of self, others and situations, the dimension of autonomy and negative effect which implies that people who are overall forgiving (oneself, others and situations) experience less negative feelings in day-to-day life.

Mohan *et al.* (2010) have compared males and females on the dimensions of interpersonal forgiveness and results clearly revealed that males are higher on the various dimensions of forgiveness. Sehgal and associates (in 2010) have worked in the field of spiritual well-being and positive healthy aging and psychological well-being, parental bonding and gratitude among adolescents. The keynote addresses by Jitendra Mohan on Spiritual Psychology and well-being in Malaysia (2007), Eastern Viewpoints in Well-being in U.K. (2009) and Challenges in Positive Psychology in India (2010, 2011 and 2012) highlighted the questions and the answers merging in this field.

Banth *et al.* (2011) compared the 24 character strengths in leaders in the Indian Army and Civilian Sector. Results revealed that both army officers and civilian managers scored high in all the character strengths, and there were significant differences among army officers and bank managers on 14 out of 24 character strengths that can be attributed to their disparate work environment and organizational expectations.

Banth *et al.* (2010) examined the relationship of *Anasakti* with well-being and the three distinct happiness orientations. *Anasakti*, a Sanskrit term for traits like non-attachment, equipoise, selfless duty orientation, and effort in the absence of concern for the outcome, can be regarded as a Hindu-ideal cluster of personality traits. It was explored through a study of 676 college students and a sample of 65 yogic practitioners in India. The findings revealed that the yogic practitioners were markedly higher in *Anasakti* than the secular population. For the yogic population, there was a large correlation between *Anasakti* and the Orientation to Meaningful Life, and it accounted for more than 20 per cent of the variance in the regression of *Anasakti* against all the measures of well-being. The yogic population's scores also correlated with several other measures of well-being. The scores of the secular population were less strongly related to the well-being scores; though, several correlation coefficients were statistically significant.

Positive Mental Health and HIV/AIDS

Positive mental health have more supporting role of infectious disease. A human positive thought survive very disease and alive well-being and good quality of life. Keyes (2005) reports data from the MIDUS study in the USA which indicates that some 50 per cent of the general population is moderately mentally healthy, 17 per cent are flourishing, 10 per cent are languishing and a further 23 per cent meet the criteria for diagnosable mental disorders such as depression. A Scottish Survey reports some 14 per cent of the population as having 'good mental well-being' (as measured on the Warwick Edinburgh Mental Well-being scale), 73 per cent with average and 14 per cent with poor mental well-being (Braunholtz *et al.*, 2007). Keyes (2005) argues that, compared with those who are flourishing, moderately mentally healthy and languishing adults have significant psychosocial impairment and poorer physical health, lower productivity and limitations to daily living (Keyes, 2004, 2005).

Ishizuka's theory, like that of Rogers, is primarily a clinical one, based on years of experience with patients. Like the humanist Carl Rogers, the positive mental health Lifetrack model was inspired, developed, and tested in daily clinical practice with demanding patients. It evolved from the need to help patients with their lives improve their overall psychological adjustment. Patients inspired the model of positive mental health, put it to the test, and challenged it daily for the last 35 years. Segerstom *et al.* (1998) found that an association between optimism and higher numbers of CD4 (helper) T cell in stressed law school students was mediated partially by the positive mood associated with optimism.

Positive belief also may be connected to physical disease by promoting better health behaviours. People who have a positive sense of self-worth, belief in their own control and optimism about the future may be more likely to practice conscientious health habit and to use services appropriately. Taylor *et al.* (1992) found that men who were unrealistically optimistic about their ability to stave off the progression of the AIDS virus nonetheless practiced better health habit than did their more pessimistic counterparts.

Rom *et al.* (2009) studied have been done regarding positive mental attitude and its effects on health, specifically with people of serious illnesses such as HIV/AIDS, cancer and kidney disease. Cancer specifically has received a lot of attention since Lance Armstrong, along with other survivors, has given their stories. People with positive mental attitude have a significantly higher chance of survival and recovery. Subha *et al.* (2010) studied that a particular type of Positive Self Talk was developed from Frenchman Alexandre Simonnet to fight Panic Attacks. A study comparing people with chronic kidney disease with people kidney disease free showed that there was a significant difference between the groups. The kidney disease free group rated much higher in positive mental attitude. There was no difference found in spirituality and females with chronic kidney disease were found to be significantly more superstitious. Larry (2010) studied done with HIV-positive individuals found that a high health self-efficacy, a task-oriented coping style, and a positive mental attitude were strong predictors or a health-promoting lifestyle which has a significant affect on overall health (coping and surviving).

References

About.com (2006, July 25). *What is Mental Health?*. Retrieved June 1, 2007, from About.com

Aspinwall, L.G., and Staudinger, U.M. (Eds.). (2003). *A psychology of human strengths: Fundamental questions and future directions for a positive psychology.* Washington, DC: American Psychological Association.

Banth, S., and Singh, P. (2011). Positive character strengths in middle-rung army officers and managers in civilian sectors. *Journal of Indian Academy of Applied Psychology*, 37 (2), 320-324.

Banth, S., and Talwar, C. (2010). *Anasakti*, the Hindu Ideal, and its Relationship to Well-Being and Orientations to Happiness. *Journal of Religion and Health.* DOI: 10.1007/s10943-010-9402-3 (retrieved on 29-11-2011).

Barlow, D.H., Durand, V.M., and Steward, S.H. (2090). Abnormal psychology: An integrative approach (Second Canadian Edition). Toronto: Nelson. p.16.

Barry, M.M., Patel, V., Jané-Llopis, E., Raeburn, J., and Mittlemark, M. (2007). Strengthening the evidence base for mental health promotion. In: D.C. McQueen and C.M. Jones (Eds.) *Global Perspectives on Health Promotion.* New York, USA: Springer.

Braunholtz, S., Davidson, S., Myant, K., Ipsos- MORI, and O'Connor, R. (2007) Well? What do You Think? (2006). The Third National Scottish Survey of Public Attitudes to Mental Health, Mental Well-being and Mental Health Problems. Edinburgh, UK: Social Research, Scottish Executive.

Chang, edited by Edward, C. (2001). *Optimism and pessimism implications for theory, research, and practice* (1st ed. Ed.). Washington, DC: American Psychological Association. pp. 101-125.

Clifford Beers Clinic. (2006, October 30). *About Clifford Beers Clinic*. Retrieved June 1, 2007, from CliffordBeers.org

Gable, S.L., and Haidt, J. (2005). What (and why) is positive psychology? *Review of General Psychology*, 9 (2) 103-10.

Hill, Napoleon (1960). *Think and grow rich* (Rev. ed.). Greenwich, Conn.: Fawcett Crest.

Hill, Napoleon; Stone, W. Clement Stone; preface by Og Mandino; with a new introduction by W. Clement (1987). *Success through a positive mental attitude*. New York: Pocket.

Huppert, F.A. and Whittington, J.E. (2003). Evidence for the independence of positive and negative well-being: implications for quality of life assessment. *British Journal of Psychology*, 8, 107-22.

Huppert, F.A. (2005). Positive mental health in individuals and populations. In: F. Huppert, N. Bayliss and B. Keverne (Eds.) *The Science of Well-being*. Oxford, UK: Oxford University Press.

Jahoda, M. (1958). *Current Concepts of Positive Mental Health*. New York, USA: Basic Books.

Johns Hopkins University. (2010). *Origins of Mental Health*. from JHSPH.edu

Keyes, C.L.M. (2002). The mental health continuum: from languishing to flourishing in life. *Journal of Health and Social Research,* 43, 207-22.

Keyes, C.L.M. (2004). The nexus of cardiovascular disease and depression revisited: the complete mental health perspective and the moderating role of age and gender. *Aging and Mental Health,* 8, 266-74.

Keyes, C.L.M. (2005). Mental illness and/or mental health? Investigating axioms of the complete state model of health. *Journal of Consulting and Clinical Psychology,* 73, 539-48.

Kitchener, B.A., and Jorm, A.F. (2002). *Mental Health First Aid Manual.* Centre for Mental Health Research, Canberra. p. 5.

Kovess-Masfety, M., Murray, M. and Gureje, O. (2005) Positive mental health. In: H. Herrman, S. Saxena and R. Moodie (Eds) *Promoting Mental Health: Concepts, Emerging Evidence, Practice.* A report of the World Health Organization, Department of Mental Health and Substance Abuse in collaboration with the Victorian Health Promotion Foundation and University of Melbourne. Geneva, Switzerland: WHO.

Larry, R.S. (2010). "Exploring the relationships between perceived health self-efficacy, coping and health-promoting behaviours among non-substance abusing *vs.* substance abusing patients with HIV disease". *Dissertation Abstracts International: Section B: The Sciences and Engineering,* 71 (1-B): 661.

Lopez, S.J., and Snyder, C.R. (Eds.). (2002). *Positive psychological assessment.* Washington, DC: American Psychological Association.

Mohan, J. (2007). Spiritual psychology and subjective well-being. *Paper presented in International conference on spiritual psychology,* Malaysia.

Mohan, J., Sehgal, M., and Tripathi, A. (2008b). A study of dispositional forgiveness in relation to personality and spiritual well-being among adolescents. *Research Journal: Social Sciences, Panjab University,* 15(1), 127-145.

Mohan, J., Sehgal, M., and Tripathi, A. (2009). The Forgiving personality: Identifying its structure in terms of Happiness and Well-being among Indian youth. *Journal of Well-being,* 3(2), 1-10.

Mohan, J., Sehgal, M., and Tripathi, A. (2010). Gender differences in offense specific and dispositional forgiveness among Indian adolescents. (*In the Edited book on Positive Psychology by* Prof. Jitendra Mohan).

Patel, V. and Prince, M. (1977). Global mental health—a new global health field comes of age. *JAMA,* 303, 1976-77.

Richards, K.C., Campania, C., and Muse-Burke, J.L. (2010). Self-care and Well-being in Mental Health Professionals: The Mediating Effects of Self-awareness and Mindfulness. *Journal of Mental Health Counseling,* 32(3): 247.

Rom, S.A.; Miller, L., and Peluso, J. (2009). Playing the game: Psychological factors in surviving cancer. *International Journal of Emergency Mental Health,* 11(1): 25-36.

Ryff, C., Love, G., and Urry, H. *et al.* (2006). Psychological well-being and ill-being: do they have distinct or mirrored biological correlates? *Psychotherapy and Psychosomatics,* 75, 85-95.

Segerstron, S.C., Taylor, S.E., Kemeny, M.E., and Fahey, J.L. (1998). Optimism is associated with mood, coping and immune change in response to stress. *Journal of Personality and Social Psychology*, 74, 1646-1655.

Seligman, M.E.P., and Csikszentmihalyi, M. (2000). Positive psychology: an introduction. *American Psychologist*, 55(1).

Seligman, M.E.P., Steen, T.A., Park, N., and Peterson, C. (2005). Positive psychology progress: empirical validation of interventions. *American Psychologist,* 60 (5) 410-21.

Social Hygiene in 20th Century Britain Taylor & Francis, pp. 80-83.

Storrie, K; Ahern, K., and Tuckett, A. (2010). A systematic review: Students with mental health problems—a growing problem". *International Jou:nal of Nursing Practice,* 16(1), 1-6. 16(1): 1-16.

Subha, T.G., and Mukherjee, Tilottama (September 2010). Optimism, superstitious beliefs and spirituality in chronic kidney disease. *Indian Journal of Community Psychology,* 6(2): 5-14, 262-274.

Taylor, S.E., Kemeny, M.E., Aspinwall, L.G., Schneider, S.C. Rodriguez, R., and Herbert, M. (1992). Optimism, coping, psychological distress, and high-risk sexual behaviour among men at risk for AIDS. *Journal of Personality and Social Psychology,* 63, 460-473.

World Health Organization (2001). Mental Health: New Understanding, New

Hope. *The World Health Report.* Geneva, Switzerland: World Health Organization.

World Health Organization (2002). *Prevention and Promotion in Mental Health.* Geneva, Switzerland: World Health Organization.

World Health Organization (2004a). *Promoting Mental Health*: Concepts, Emerging Evidence, Practice, Summary Report. A report of the World Health Organization, Department of Mental Health and Substance Abuse in collaboration with the Victorian Health Promotion Foundation and the University of Melbourne. Geneva, Switzerland: World Health Organization.

World Health Organization (2005a). *Mental Health Action Plan for Europe: Facing the Challenges, Building Solutions.* Geneva, Switzerland: World Health Organization.

Zubrick, S. and Kovess-Masfety, M. (2005). Indicators of mental health. In: H. Herrman, S. Saxena and R. Moodie (Eds) *Promoting Mental Health: Concepts, Emerging Evidence, Practice.* A report of the World Health Organization, Department of Mental Health and Substance Abuse in collaboration with the Victorian Health Promotion Foundation and University of Melbourne. Geneva, Switzerland: World Health Organization.

15

Ritual, Religiosity, Spirituality and Health Connection

Teenu Nandal and *Nav Rattan Sharma*

Health of the individual and ultimately of society mirror a complex relationship of mental, physical, spiritual, family, community and environmental factors at large. Health, appears to constitute a new form of idolatry replacing salvation in eternity with fitness in an ever expanding life-span. Achieving health becomes evidence of elegance. There is a strong sense that the body itself has become a sign, a sign which announces the attitudes of an individual. It makes sense that individual define his/her own problems and determine how to effect change to achieving a healthy mind in a healthy body in a healthy society. Health and illness, and the body whose characteristics they are, have remained the site of spiritual, metaphysical forces, agentive powers that fight out a battle between good and evil inside the body. Increasing international attention is now being paid, to keep people well and healthy, to enhance the capacity of individuals and communities, to take control over their lives and to improve their over all health. Literatures suggest that the variables like ritual, religiosity and spirituality play very important role in maintenance of health and well-being of the individual. Efforts are made to create, develop and find out those ways which would work as remedial procedures to face and overcome difficult times. This paper is an attempt to synthesize the recent research about the relationship of health with ritual, religiosity and spirituality in an empirical framework.

The interface of health and spiritual variables is full of hopes and possibilities (Sharma, Charak, and Sharma, 2009). Rituals, religiosity and spirituality are common and far-reaching phenomena; more over they are integral part of numerous cultures and influence people of all ages, socio-economic status, and educational levels and overall health and well-being of the individual. However, although religiosity and spirituality are used interchangeably, these constructs may not be identical (Lindeman, Blomqvist and Takada, 2012). The similarities and differences between these two warrants further research into different areas (Bonelli and Koenig, 2013). It is well established to divide religiosity into three sub-constructs: Intrinsic, Extrinsic, and Quest Religiosity (Batson and Schoenrade, 1991; Maltby and Lewis, 1996; Maltby and Day, 1998), while the construct spirituality is divided into the following sub-constructs: Cognitive Orientation Towards Spirituality, Experiential/ Phenomenological Dimension of Spirituality, Existential Well-being, Paranormal Beliefs, and Religiousness (MacDonald, 2000). Sometimes spirituality is associated with religions or religious belief; sometimes it is seen as quite independent of any religious understanding (Schneiders, 2003). Spirituality is considered as broader concept than religion that may be one expression of spirituality. It is considered more personal, something individuals define for themselves largely free of the rules, regulations, and responsibilities associated with religion. The term spirituality is increasingly used to refer to the personal, subjective side of religious experience. Other forms of spirituality comprise prayer, meditation, interactions with others or nature, and relationship with God or a higher power. A good number of people who practice spirituality go away from the obstacles of caste, religion, race, nationality and gender and observe the whole humanity as a single entity. They may not challenge religion, but they definitely go beyond its barriers. Rituals are considered as '*Karma*' meaning action. In another words rituals are religion in action.

There is substantial literature that connects religion and spirituality to health (Koenig, McCullough, and Larson, 2001). Researchers have suggested various possible psychological, social, and physiological mediators that may account for the religion and/or spirituality-health connection. However, it is possible that the explanation for these effects may also lie in the nature of religion and spirituality themselves. The interest in the relationship of these variables lies behind a continuing debate among researchers about their health benefits. Further follows a keen observation of the current literature regarding the relationship of above said variables.

Rituals and Health

Knowingly or unknowingly everyone follow rituals whether religious or non-religious on daily basis. Their value lies in their inherent ability to facilitate action. In spite of its significance, the role of rituals in mental health and well-being is less explored. Researchers in different areas have recently focused their attention to the relation between rituals and their possibilities for different health issues. The essential role of ritual in religion has been illustrated by numerous researchers (McCauley, 2001). Cultural traditions and practices shape our self and other experiences including those of health and illness (Egede, 2006). Religious ritual is universally used to define the sacred and to separate it from the profane. Of greater importance from a behavioural perspective, the emotional significance of rituals is unexplainable. But recent evolutionary research observations define religion in terms of cognition, focusing on the beliefs rather than the behaviours of religious systems. From a cross-cultural perspective, however, it is ritual that lies at the heart of all religions, and it is participation in ritual that creates believers (Sosis, 2003). Participation in religious ritual results in empirically demonstrated effects on health (Sosis and Ruffle, 2004) and individual health and longevity (Murphy, Ciarrocchi, Piedmont, Cheston and Peyrot, 2000). Religious action and religious way of living offers a very useful insight into the individual to understand his soul and outer world (Kalra, Bhui and Bhugra, 2012).

The research indicates that much of the work is observed on prayer and there are identified several common forms of prayers (petitionary, passive, active, objective, subjective). Different forms of prayers have different objectives. These speak to the multi-dimensionality of prayer and the different outcomes related to specific types of prayers. The use of private prayer as a way of coping is predictive of optimism in the cardiac surgery patients (Ai, Peterson, Bolling and Koenig, 2002). People, who pray for their health, participate in more health promoting behaviours than people who do not pray. The National Health Interview Survey for health habits of people who prayed or do not pray for their health concludes that participants, who prayed, saw a physician more frequently, participated more frequently in vigorous exercise and used more relaxation techniques, support groups, meditation and complementary and alternative medicine therapies (Harrigan, 2009).

Different forms of prayer have different effect on well-being. Adoration, thanks giving and reception prayers had consistently positive relations with well-being, whereas the other forms of prayers (confession, supplication, obligatory) have negative or null relations with the well-being. The prayer types having positive influence appear to be less ego-focused, and more focused on God, whereas the negative types have an opposite nature (Whittington and Scher, 2009).

Review of literature indicates that variables like rituals are influencing people's each aspect of life. Rituals seem to be positively and significantly correlated with life satisfaction, different aspects of holistic health and different factors of subjective well-being.

Literature regarding physiological problems (coronary artery bypass graft, coronary care, acute coronary syndromes, and coronary risk factors), are the centre of attention of the researchers now-a-days. The use of prayer to cope, associates with better post-operative emotional health in patients with coronary artery bypass graft. Older patients are more likely to pray if religion is important to them, whereas younger patients are more likely to pray if they have lower incomes, better pre-operative health, and more education (Ai, Bolling and Peterson, 2000). Patients who indulge into remote, intercessory prayers have lower adverse coronary care unit scores (Harris, Gowda, Kolb, Strychacz, Vacek, Jones, Forker, O'Keefe and McCallister, 2000). Lowest complication rates are observed in patients of acute coronary interventions who are assigned to off-site prayer. People, who regularly pray, have a significantly lower prevalence of multiple coronary risk factors including hypertension (Krucoff, Crater, Green, Maas, Seskevich, Lane, Loeffler, Morris, Bashore and Koenig, 2001).

Religious ritual is positively associates with decreased stress and improved immunological function (Murphy *et al.*, 2000). Bradshaw (2003) establishes that decreases in psychological distress associated with participation in religious ritual may be particularly relevant for the relatively deprived. Under conditions of inequality, religious ritual may, thus, grant direct fitness benefits for participants while simultaneously providing a mechanism for cooperative action. The adaptive function of religion is to ensure cooperation when individuals can achieve net benefits through cooperative action.

Literature supports for effect of religious factors on cardiac health in general populations. Ai, Ladd, Peterson, Cook, Shearer, and Koenig (2010) have observed multifaceted outcomes of religious factors on long-term postoperative tuning concerning prayer and coping with cardiac disease. Preoperative use of prayer for coping, optimism, and hope are predicting lower levels of depression at the follow-up. Subjective religiousness, marital status, and hope are predictive of lower levels of anxiety at the follow-up.

Religion and its underlying beliefs and sub-dimensions including attendance and participation in religious activities have an extremely profound effect on the health of the individual (Krause and Bastida, 2011). Reduced health status, including functional ability combined with limited participation in religious place activities, results in poorer self-rated mental health and more symptoms of depression (Mitchell and Weatherly, 2000). Attending religious activities influences positive health care practices. Church attendance is an important correlate of positive mental health care practices, especially for the uninsured and chronically ill participants (Aaron, Levine and Burstin, 2003). It provides multifaceted physical, emotional, social, and spiritual experiences that promote health through multiple pathways (Idler, Boulifard, Labouvie, Chen, Krause and Contrada, 2008).

Some findings are not consistent with the earlier findings. Kodzi, Gyimah, Emina and Ezeh (2011) state that in elderly population, frequency of religious attendance negatively correlates with health, while the number of close friends, social support, and frequency of community participation positively and independently related to self-reported health.

Even, religious beliefs and activities are common among patients with congestive heart failure and chronic pulmonary disease and are associated with less severe illness and functional disability, fewer prior psychiatric problems, and less psychotropic drug use. Religious activities and attitudes inversely relate to physical illness severity and functional disability, and are less common among patients with prior psychiatric problems, hospitalizations for depression, drinking problems, and those currently taking psychotropic drugs. Religious activities (especially religious attendance) seem connected with greater social support and less depression (Koenig, 2002).

The research, regarding the relationships among race, education, formal as well as informal involvement in the religious activities, and God-mediated control, observe that older white are more likely to have stronger feelings of God-mediated control and older blacks are more likely to sustain their sense of God-mediated control over time (Krause, 2007).

Studies reviewed above regarding the association between ritual and health indicate that many expressions and elements of rituals are helpful in enhancing health and well-being of the individuals.

Religiosity and Health

'Religion' can help human beings to cope in different times in three ways. First, it protects the individual's survival against the depersonalizing influence of environmental procedures. Second, it helps the individual to recognize human imperfections and to mingle realism with optimism. Third, while knowledge gives the individual the physical power to create or to destroy the world, religion gives the ethical force to grow in virtue by nurturing self-control, humility, and freedom from self-centredness. Every religion influences health and illness of the followers and may be a cause of a variety of psychological complains and also help person to face and cope in diverse fields (Behere, Das, Yadav and Behere, 2013). The associations among mental health and differential patterns of religiosity, is observed by enthusiastic and keen research endeavours around the world (Hackney and Sanders, 2003). Variables like religious coping, forgiveness, daily spiritual experiences, religious support and self-rated of religious intensity significantly relate to the mental health status of individuals suffering from different problems (Kane and Jacob, 2010).

Religion may have some different pattern of relations in the health and health behaviours of healthier populations (Nagel and Emch, 2007). Green and Elliot (2010) states that people who identify as religious tend to report better health and happiness, regardless of religious affiliation, religious activities, work and family, social support, or financial status. People with liberal religious beliefs tend to be healthier but less happy than people with fundamentalist beliefs. Abdel-Khalek (2008) monitors that self-ratings of religiosity significantly and positively correlate with the self-ratings of physical health, mental health, and happiness. Boys are significantly higher on religiosity, health, and happiness than girls except anxiety, which is significant and negative (Baroun, 2006). Although some studies demonstrate reduced anxiety rates, others indicate that anxiety levels are heightened in the more religious (Koenig, King and Carson, 2012).

Religious association and significance significantly relate to subjective well-being of the individual (Abdel-Khalek and Lester, 2012; Pokimica, Addai and Takyi, 2011). In younger population, individuals who consider themselves as religious and actually participate at religious events, perceive their own health better and are more satisfied with their life (Pikó and Kovács, 2009). The research reveals that religiosity is shielding for health problems (cigarettes, alcohol, and marijuana use) in violence and emotional distress in younger population (Nonnemaker, McNeely and Blum, 2003). Older adults have higher levels of religious involvement than younger adults (Moreira-Almeida, Pinsky, Zaleski and Laranjeira, 2010).

With the growth in the older population, emerging issues regarding physical and mental health require greater research and clinical attention. An association between self-reported years of incarceration and experienced forgiveness, states that inmates' self-reported religiousness has influenced anxiety, depression, and desire for hastened death. Having a greater number of daily religious experiences and not feeling abandoned by God associate with better emotional health (Allen, Phillips, Roff, Cavanaugh and Day, 2008). Certain existential beliefs or concerns play a very important role in the life of different religious groups. Protestants report better well-being than Catholics and Jews (Cohen and Hall, 2008).

Religion has been found also to moderate the stress-strain relationship and play a significant role in the prediction of well-being (Wildes, Miller, Majors and Ramirez, 2009). Religious well-being may also be considered as an important resource to explore the pathological (affective mentally disordered patients) population (Unterrainer, Schoeggl, Fink, Neuper and Kapfhammer, 2012). A significant three-way interaction between work experience, age, and religiosity in the prediction of well-being is also observed in older and younger Muslim women (Noor, 2008).

Extending previous research concerning the association between religion and psychological health in different religious groups, Lewis, Shevlin, Francis and Quigley (2010) recognize that Protestants group seems significantly higher on psychological health as compared to Catholic group. Females' and Catholics' attendance of religious service seem higher than males and Protestants. Using "atheist" as the reference category, Catholics have higher lifetime odds of single episodes of depression whilst Protestants have higher lifetime odds of anxiety disorder and lower lifetime odds of alcohol use disorders (Park, Hong, Park and Cho, 2012).

Religion and health care are totally connected (Gupta and Chandra, 2004). There is a large amount of literature on religiosity but only a small number of research that have stressed on the influence of religiosity on formal caregivers. Caregivers have a strong sense of religiousness, which plays an important role in their lives, including the type of care they provide to others, their mental health and their quality of life (Jagannathan and Juvva, 2009). Better social functioning, better mental health and fewer anxiety symptoms associates more with organizational religiosity. Prayer (non-organizational religiosity), however, associates with negative results, such as higher stress, poorer general health perceptions and more anxiety symptoms (Lucchetti, Lucchetti, Oliveira, Crispim, Pires, Gorzoni, Panicio, and Koenig, 2013).

Religious involvement seems to have negative associations with post-traumatic stress symptoms (Watlington and Murphy, 2006). Religious resources (support of religious guidance, positive religious coping practices) predict well-being more strongly, while spiritual struggles (troubled relations with God, negative interactions with members, chronic religious doubts) more closely connect with psychological distress (Ellison, Roalson, Guillory, Flannelly and Marcum, 2010).

Religious orientation is a useful construct pertaining to health status and health relevant behaviours and further demonstrates the multidimensional nature of religion. Intrinsic and Non-religious types report the most favourable health perceptions and lowest body mass indexes (Masters and Knestel, 2011). Exploring religiosity, sense of meaning in life, and health behaviour in older adults', Homan and Boyatzis (2010) observe that stronger religiosity and sense of meaning associate with healthier behaviours; however, extrinsic religious orientation associate with decreased rates of healthy behaviour.

Religious moral beliefs help in overcoming post-war psychosocial problems and socialization of the personality, leading to the improvement in mental health. Religious moral beliefs work as mental health protective factors for these individuals. A higher index of religious moral beliefs enabled better control of distress, provide better mental health stability (Hasanovic and Pajevic, 2010).

Research supports the notion that religious coping is linked to better health conditions. Positive religious coping (benevolent religious appraisals, religious forgiveness) reflects a secure relationship with God and associates with improved mental health. In contrast, negative religious coping (reappraisals of God's powers, feeling abandoned or punished by God) reflects a weak relationship with God and associates with worse mental well-being (Pargament, 2010). Negative religious coping (struggling with faith) associates with significantly poorer functioning on depression, distress, mental health, pain, and fatigue (Sherman, Simonton, Latif, Spohn and Tricot, 2005). Positive religious coping is linked to better overall quality of life of the individual (Fabricatore, Handal, Rubio and Gilner, 2004). Coping strategies and social support may mediate the relationship between religiosity and psychological distress in individuals (Steglitz, Ng, Mosha, and Kershaw, 2012).

The presence of health messages in the religious sermons influences deeply the life of the followers. Leader's perception about health promotion is important for members or followers of the same environment for health benefits (Williams, Glanz, Kegler and Davis, 2012).

Research has shown that religion is associated with a wide range of health related behaviours among adults of all ages. Religious salience is significantly related to different health aspects even after controlling for a variety of social, demographic, and health-related aspects. Religious attendance and preventive services are influential in middle-age females with frequent use of more mammograms, Pap smears and self-breast exams (Benjamins, 2007) and correlate of less-risky health behaviours among pregnant and post-partum women (Page, Ellison and Lee, 2009).

The association of religiousness on one hand, and physical health on the other, seem weaker than the psychological one in pathological population, although there exists between them a significant relationship. Patients who categorize themselves as non-religious had severer self-rated and observer-rated health problems and greater medical co-morbidity (Koenig, George and Titus, 2004). People, who pray less, often report a greater number of depressive symptoms, and faith as an important source of strength in life, positively associates with chronic conditions such as asthma or arthritis (Braam, Hein, Deeg, Twisk, Beekman and Tilburg, 2004). Religious involvement among major and minor depression is seemed widespread (Koenig, 2007). Among depressed patients, there is no relationship between religion and depression type, but depression severity is associated with a lower religious attendance, prayer, scripture reading, and lower intrinsic religiosity. Recent research supports that a higher level of general religiosity significantly associates with a lower level of depression (Lucchetti, Lucchetti, Peres, Moreira-Almeida and Koenig, 2012) and confirmed to be a substantial suicidal buffer (Bullock, Nadeau and Renaud, 2012).

Work on schizophrenia is still embryonic; recent studies, however, suggest that religious individuals with psychotic illnesses frequently deploy prayer and Bible reading to help them cope with their voices, and higher levels of religiosity may increase medication compliance (Mohr, Perroud, Gillieron, Brandt, Rieben, Borras and Huguelet, 2011). Religion increase social integration and instilled hope, purpose, and meaning in the lives of outpatients with psychotic illness (schizophrenia) (Mohr, Borras, Nolan, Gillieron, Brandt, Eytan, Leclerc, Perroud, Whetten, Pieper, Koenig, and Huguelet, 2012).

Religiousness stabilized the lives of the disabled, providing meaning for the experience of disability, assistance with coping and strengthening other benefits to the individuals with physical disabilities. Increased assistance of religious place in promoting theological understanding of disability and religious support in caring are important in keeping them feel mentally healthy (Treloar, 2002). Higher level of religious involvement associates with higher levels of social support (Watlington and Murphy, 2006) and better quality of life (Harrison, Edwards, Koenig, Bosworch, Decastro and Wood, 2005).

The above historical evidences prove that religiosity can also comfort people in their time of trouble and misfortune, increase sense of control, enhance feelings of security, and boost self-confidence. Thus, the role of religion in human life is unspoken and unavoidable.

Spirituality and Health

All people are spiritual and by virtue of being human, regardless of age, bio-psycho-social-spiritual beings. Widespread evidence shows that the interest in spirituality is not confined to individuals who attend religious place or who are identified as being religious (Shea, 2000). Spirituality is an integral part of the health and well-being of every individual and relevant in their lives, irrespective of the problem they face or the situation they experience. It becomes the inseparable part of individual psyche. Some people are spiritual, connected to a higher power from which they derive meaning, although not belonging to and participating in institutionalized religion. Cultural factors must be taken into account on levels of beliefs and practices while considering larger picture of variables (Lysne and Wachholtz, 2011). Comprehensive research evidence shows that spiritual beliefs and practices help prevent many physical and mental problems and plays an important role in overall well-being of the individual (Goel, Sharma, Kalia, Kour, Kumar, Kanwalpreet, and Swami, 2006; Nandal, 2011).

Prior research suggests that spirituality and well-being are positively associated (Kashdan and Nezlek, 2012). Growing research has demonstrated a link between spiritual well-being and better health (Holt-Lunstad, Steffen, Sandberg and Jensen, 2011). Spirituality may be a salient quality of life determinant for many individuals (Sawatzky, Ratner and Chiu, 2005). Konopack and McAuley (2012) suggest that spirituality may influence health and well-being *via* an efficacy-mediated path, with strongest effects on mental health status and support previous findings of an efficacy-mediated relationship between physical activity and quality of life, with the exception that self-efficacy moderately associates with physical health status but not mental health status. It suggests that those who are more spiritual and physically active report greater quality of life. The research also concludes that existential well-being was positively related to quality of life for individuals living with HIV (Tuck, McCain and Elswick, 2001). This Non-religious belief (existential worldview) significantly relates to life satisfaction, general health, and social quality of life in persons with spinal cord injury. In case of pathological population the dimensions of religious and spiritual well-being remains high for individuals displaying schizotypy and borderline personality traits (Bennett, Shepherd, and Janca, 2013).

Increase in spirituality associates with increase odds of feeling that life has improved due to a direct effect, and due to indirect effects through healthy beliefs and health status/health concerns (Szaflarski, Ritchey, Leonard, Mrus, Peterman, Ellison, McCullough and Tsevat, 2006). The health of individuals with significant medical conditions appears to be primarily related to positive spiritual beliefs and especially congregational support (Cohen, Yoon, and Johnstone, 2009). Long survival of HIV positive also significantly relate to both, frequency of prayer (positively) and judgmental attitude (negatively) (Ironson, Solomon, Balbin, O'Cleirigh, George, Kumar, Larson, and Woods, 2002). Recent research states that spiritual well-being significantly work on fatigue symptom distress, memory disturbance, loss of appetite, drowsiness, dry mouth, and sadness (Kandasamy, Chaturvedi, and Desai, 2011).

Spirituality is an important resource for coping for many patients dealing with chronic diseases. They help patients' in physical, emotional, social, existential and spiritual needs to contribute to their improvement and recovery. Caring for need (spiritual, existential and psychosocial) is not only relevant to those who are at the last stage of their life but also to those who suffer from long term chronic illnesses (Bussing and Koenig, 2010). Higher levels of spirituality associate with higher levels of religious coping strategies (Watlington and Murphy, 2006). Boscaglia, Clarke, Jobling and Quinn (2005) explore that anxiety is more common for those who do not use positive spiritual coping mechanisms to deal with the serious problems. Research provides evidence that frequent use of spiritual resources, importance of faith, and reliance has significant associations with physical and mental health. In case of research related to elderly, sometimes more emphasis is on attitudes rather than practices as the stronger spiritual variables related to mental health (Meisenhelder and Chandler, 2002).

The perceived sense of closeness to God appears to be particularly valuable to people in difficult situations. Spiritual people report more life satisfaction (Nandal, 2011) and happiness than of no spiritual people. They are more active and hold different health beliefs (Nagel and Emch, 2007). Spirituality provides a sense of direction and meaning in life to the individual (Gockel, 2009). Even religious upbringing, parenting, marriage and agreeableness also associate with spirituality (McCullough, Enders, Brion, and Jain, 2005).

Spirituality comes out as an important predictor of reductions in drug use in drug addicts. Increasing spirituality during drug treatment could improve long term drug treatment outcomes (Conner, Anglin, Annon, and Longshore, 2009).

Spirituality seems to impact worker in the workplace and show an increase in performance/productivity. It has a positive impact on job satisfaction (Bodia and Ali, 2012). Interestingly, one set of researchers found that high levels of spiritual intelligence do not result in high levels of job satisfaction (Rastgar, Davoudi, Oraji and Abbasian, 2012).

Studies have shown that higher spirituality levels are associated with less depression (Lucchetti, Lucchetti, Badan-Neto, Peres, Peres, Moreira-Almeida, Gomes, and Koenig, 2011) and even greater survival (Chida, Steptoe, and Powell, 2009). Hope and Forgiveness may be the strongest negative correlates of anxious/depressive symptoms (Unterrainer *et al.*, 2012). Depressive episodes often lead to a search for spirituality and it may be helpful in overcoming depression or becoming less vulnerable to relapsing. Strong spiritual values positively associate with increased rates of current depressive disorder and decreased rates of current alcohol use disorder (Robinson, Cranford, Webb, and Brower, 2007).

Research supports that incorporating spirituality in therapeutic practice proved very effective (Tripathi and Asthana, 2013). A repeated exposure with spirituality related knowledge and spiritual practices such as Yoga, Meditation and sacred music may help a person to regulate them in terms of day-to-day behaviour patterns (Kumar, 2011). Research states that spirituality also serves an essential positive responsibility while dealing with psychotic (schizophrenia) problems (Danbolt, Moller, Lien and Hestad, 2011). Therapists use spirituality as a tool to meet the goal of the improvement of the patients. People become more spiritual with increase in illness and their spiritual bend is proved helpful for them (Smith and Suto, 2012)

Spiritual ceremonies might serve as a booster for spiritual and mental quality of life (Hewson and Rowold, 2012). The therapeutic implications of including culturally adapted spiritual ceremonies may facilitate an individual's capacity to contain and integrate traumatic memories, promote restorative self-awareness, and engage community support (Agger, Igreja, Kiehle, and Polatin, 2012).

The above historical evidences claim that spirituality is much more than this construct define and deeply influence individual's life and need more keen exploration.

Conclusion

In conclusion, there is by now a wealth of literature examining the relationship of health and rituals, religion, spirituality. Although on balance, it appears that these variables improve health and well-being of the individuals. The spiritual techniques of managing health may be the most frequently used mainstream coping strategy, apart from other traditional methods of coping. The current conclusions broaden the understanding of various psychosocial features faced by people and provide progressive suggestions to improve the quality of life suffering from different problems. Future work in this area needs to look at factors accounting for these associations and most importantly needs to be sensitive to cultural and theological issues in their assessment.

References

Aaron, K.F., Levine, D. and Burstin, H.R. (2003). African American church participation and health care practices. *Journal of General Internal Medicine,* 18(11), 908-913.

Abdel-Khalek, A.M. (2008). Religiosity, health, and well-being among Kuwaiti personnel. *Psychological Reports*, 102(1), 181-184.

Abdel-Khalek, A.M. and Lester, D. (2012). Constructions of religiosity, subjective well-being, anxiety, and depression in two cultures: Kuwait and USA. *International Journal of Social Psychiatry,* 58(2), 138-145.

Agger, I., Igreja, V., Kiehle, R. and Polatin, P. (2012). Testimony ceremonies in Asia: integrating spirituality in testimonial therapy for torture survivors in India, Sri Lanka, Cambodia, and the Philippines. *Transcultural Psychiatry,* 49(3-4), 568-589.

Ai, A.L., Bolling, S.F. and Peterson, C. (2000). The Use of Prayer by Coronary Artery Bypass Patients. *International Journal for the Psychology of Religion,* 10(4), 205-220.

Ai, A.L., Ladd, K.L., Peterson, C., Cook, C.A., Shearer, M. and Koenig, H.G. (2010). Long-term Adjustment After Surviving Open Heart Surgery: The Effect of Using Prayer for Coping Replicated in a Prospective Design. Gerontologist. 50(6), 798-809.

Ai, A.L., Peterson, C. Bolling, S.F. and Koenig, H. (2002). Private prayer and optimism in middle-aged and older patients awaiting cardiac surgery. *Gerontologist,* 42(1), 70-81.

Allen, R.S.; Phillips, L.L.; Roff, L.L.; Cavanaugh, R. and Day, L. (2008). Religiousness/Spirituality and Mental Health Among Older Male Inmates. *The Gerontologist,* 48, 692-697.

Baroun, K.A. (2006). Relations among religiosity, health, happiness, and anxiety for Kuwaiti adolescents. *Psychological Reports*, 99(3), 717-722.

Batson, C.D., and Schoenrade, P.A. (1991). Measuring religion as quest: I validity concerns. *Journal for the Scientific Study of Religion,* 30(4), 416-429.

Behere, P.B., Das, A., Yadav, R. and Behere, A.P. (2013). Religion and mental health. *Indian Journal of Psychiatry,* 55(2), 187-194.

Benjamins, M.R. (2007). Predictors of Preventive Health Care Use Among Middle-aged and Older Adults in Mexico: The Role of Religion. *Journal of Cross-Cultural Gerontology*, 22(2), 221-234.

Bennett, K., Shepherd, J. and Janca, A. (2013). Personality disorders and spirituality. *Current Opinion in Psychiatry,* 26(1), 79-83.

Bodia, M.A. and Ali, H. (2012). Workplace spirituality: A spiritual audit of banking executives in Pakistan. African *Journal of Business Management,* 6(11), 3888-3897.

Bonelli, R.M. and Koenig, H.G (2013). Mental disorders, religion and spirituality 1990 to 2010: a systematic evidence-based review. *Journal of Religion and Health,* 52(2), 657-673.

Boscaglia, N., Clarke, D.M., Jobling, T.W.; and Quinn, M.A. (2005). The contribution of spirituality and spiritual coping to anxiety and depression in women with a recent diagnosis of gynaecological cancer. *International Journal of Gynaecological Cancer,* 15(5), 755-761.

Braam, A.W.; Hein E.; Deeg, D.J.H.; Twisk, J.W.R., Beekman, A.T.F. and Tilburg W.V. (2004). Religious involvement and 6-year course of depressive symptoms in older Dutch Citizens: Results from the longitudinal aging study Amsterdam. *Journal of Aging and Health,* 16(4), 467-489.

Bradshaw, M. (2003). Religion as Compensation for Deprivation: The Interactive Influence of Religion and SES on Psychological Distress. Paper presented at Society for the Scientific Study of Religion, Annual Meeting, October 2003. Norfolk, VA.

Bullock, M., Nadeau, L. and Renaud, J. (2012). Spirituality and Religion in Youth Suicide Attempters' Trajectories of Mental Health Service Utilization: The Year before a Suicide Attempt. *Journal of the Canadian Academy of Child and Adolescent Psychiatry,* 21(3), 186-193.

Bussing, A. and Koenig, H.G (2010). Spiritual needs of patients with chronic diseases. *Religions,* 1, 18-27.

Chida, Y., Steptoe, A. and Powell, L.H. (2009). Religiosity/spirituality and mortality. A systematic quantitative review. *Psychotherapy and Psychosomatics,* 78(2), 81-90.

Cohen, A.B. and Hall, D.E. (2008). Existential Beliefs, Social Satisfaction, and Well-Being Among Catholic, Jewish, and Protestant Older Adults. *International Journal for the Psychology of Religion,* 19(1), 39-54.

Cohen, D., Yoon, D.P. and Johnstone, B. (2009). Differentiating the Impact of Spiritual Experiences, Religious Practices, and Congregational Support on the Mental Health of Individuals with Heterogeneous Medical Disorders. *International Journal for the Psychology of Religion*, 19(2), 121-138.

Conner, B.T., Anglin, M.D., Annon, J., and Longshore, D. (2009). The effect of religiosity and spirituality on drug treatment outcomes. *The Journal of Behavioural Health Services and Research,* 36(2), 189-198.

Danbolt, L.J. Moller, P., Lien, L. and Hestad, K.A. (2011). The Personal Significance of Religiousness and Spirituality in Patients with Schizophrenia. *International Journal for the Psychology of Religion,* 21(2), 145-158.

Egede, L.E. (2006). Race, Ethnicity, Culture, and Disparities in Health care. *Journal of General Internal Medicine,* 21(6), 667-669.

Ellison, C.G, Roalson, L.A., Guillory, J.M., Flannelly, K.J. & Marcum, J.P. (2010). Religious Resources, Spiritual Struggles, and Mental Health in a Nationwide Sample of PCUSA Clergy. *Pastoral Psychology,* 59(3), 287-304.

Fabricatore, A.N., Handal, P.J., Rubio, D.M. and Gilner, F.H. (2004). Stress, Religion, and Mental Health: Religious Coping in Mediating and Moderating Roles. *International Journal for the Psychology of Religion,* 14(2), 91-108.

Gockel, A. (2009). Spirituality and the Process of Healing: A Narrative Study. *International Journal for the Psychology of Religion*, 19(4), 217-230.

Goel, N.K., Sharma, M.K., Kalia, M., Kour, G., Kumar, R., Kanwalpreet, Swami, H.M. (2006). Value of Spiritual Dimension in Health Care System of Chandigarh, Union Territory. *Indian Journal of Community Medicine*, 31(4), 305-306.

Green, M. and Elliott, M. (2010). Religion, Health, and Psychological Well-Being. *Journal of Religion and Health,* 49(2), 149-163.

Gupta, R. and Chandra, H. (2004). Prayers, Mantra and Heart Disease. *South Asian Journal of Preventive Cardiology*, 8(3). http://www.sajpc.org/vol8/vol8_3/prayersmantra.htm

Hackney, C.H. and Sanders, G.S (2003). Religiosity and Mental Health: A Meta-Analysis of Recent Studies. *Journal for the Scientific Study of Religion,* 42(1), 43-55.

Harrigan, J.T. (2009). Health Promoting Habits of People Who Pray for Their Health. *Journal of Religion and Health*, Online First™, 27 October 2009.

Harris, W.S., Gowda, M., Kolb, J.W., Strychacz, C.P., Vacek, J.L., Jones, P.G., Forker, A., O'Keefe, J.H. and McCallister, B.D. (2000). A randomized controlled trial of the effects of remote intercessory prayer on outcomes inpatients admitted to the coronary care unit. *Archives of Internal Medicine,* 159, 2273-2278.

Harrison, M.O., Edwards, C.L., Koenig, H.G., Bosworch, H.B., Decastro, L. and Wood, M. (2005). Religiosity/spirituality and pain in patients with sickle cell disease. *Journal of Nervous and Mental Disease,* 193(4), 250-256.

Hasanoviæ, M., and Pajeviæ, I. (2010). Religious moral beliefs as mental health protective factor of war veterans suffering from PTSD, depressiveness, anxiety, tobacco and alcohol abuse in co-morbidity. *Psychiatria Danubina,* 22(2), 203-210.

Hewson, P.D. and Rowold, J. (2012). Do spiritual ceremonies affect participants' quality of life? A pilot study. *Complementary Therapies in Clinical Practice,* 18(3), 177-181.

Holt-Lunstad, J., Steffen, P.R., Sandberg, J. and Jensen, B. (2011). Understanding the connection between spiritual well-being and physical health: an examination of ambulatory blood pressure, inflammation, blood lipids and fasting glucose. *Journal of Behavioural Medicine*, 34(6), 477-488.

Homan, K.J., and Boyatzis, C.J. (2010). Religiosity, sense of meaning, and health behaviour in older adults. *International Journal for the Psychology of Religion,* 20, 173-186.

Idler, E.L., Boulifard, D.A., Labouvie, E., Chen, Y.Y., Krause, T.J. and Contrada, R.J. (2008). Looking Inside the Black Box of "Attendance at Services": New Measures for Exploring an Old Dimension in Religion and Health Research. *International Journal for the Psychology of Religion,* 19(1), 1-20.

Ironson, G., Solomon, G.F., Balbin, E.G., Cleirigh, C.O., George, A. Kumar, M., Larson, D. and Woods, T.E. (2002). The ironson-woods spirituality/ religiousness index is associated with long survival, health behaviours, less distress, and low cortisol in people with HIV/AIDS. *Annals of Behavioural Medicine,* 24(1), 34-48.

Jagannathan, A. and Juvva, S. (2009). Life after cancer in India: coping with side effects and cancer pain. *Journal of Psychosocial Oncology,* 27(3), 344-360.

Kalra, G., Bhui, K.S. and Bhugra, D. (2012). Sikhism, spirituality and psychiatry. *Asian Journal of Psychiatry*, 5(4), 339-343.

Kandasamy, A., Chaturvedi, S.K. and Desai, G. (2011). Spirituality, distress, depression, anxiety, and quality of life in patients with advanced cancer. *Indian Journal of Cancer*, 48(1), 55-59.

Kane, M.N. and Jacobs, R.J. (2010). Predictors of the Importance of Spiritual and Religious Beliefs Among University Students. *Journal of Religion and Spirituality in Social Work. Social Thought*, 29(1), 49-70.

Kashdan, T.B. and Nezlek, J.B. (2012). Whether, when, and how is spirituality related to well-being? Moving beyond single occasion questionnaires to understanding daily process. *Personality and Social Psychology Bulletin,* 38(11), 1523-1535.

Kodzi, I.A.; Gyimah, S.O.; Emina, J. and Ezeh, A.C. (2011). Religious Involvement, Social Engagement, and Subjective health Status of Older Residents of Informal Neighbourhoods of Nairobi. *Journal of Urban Health,* 88(2), 370-380.

Koenig, H. (2002). Religion, Congestive Heart Failure, and Chronic Pulmonary Disease. *Journal of Religion and Health,* 41(3), 263-278.

Koenig, H.G. (2007). Religion and depression in older medical inpatients. *American Journal of Geriatric Psychiatry*, 15(4), 282-291.

Koenig, H.G., George, L.K. and Titus, P. (2004). Religion, spirituality, and health in medically ill hospitalized older patients. *Journal of the American Geriatrics Society,* 52(4), 554-562.

Koenig, H.G., McCullough, M.E., Larson, D.B. (2001). A history of religion, science and medicine (chapter 2). *Handbook of Religion and Health.* New York, NY: Oxford University Press, pp. 24-49.

Koenig H., King D., and Carson, V. (2012). *Handbook of religion and health* (2nd ed). New York: Oxford University Press.

Konopack, J.F. and McAuley, E. (2012). Efficacy-mediated effects of spirituality and physical activity on quality of life: a path analysis. *Health and Quality of Life Outcomes,* 10:57. Doi: 10.1186/1477-7525-10-57.

Krause, N.M. (2007). Social Involvement in Religious Institutions and God-Mediated Control Beliefs: A Longitudinal Investigation. *Journal for the Scientific Study of Religion,* 46(4), 519-537.

Krause, N. and Bastida, E. (2011). Prayer to the Saints or the Virgin and Health among Older Mexican Americans. *Hispanic Journal of Behavioural Sciences,* 33(1), 71-87.

Krucoff, M.W., Crater, S.W., Green, C.L., Maas, A.C., Seskevich, J.E., Lane, J.D., Loeffler, K.A., Morris, K., Bashore, T.M., and Koenig, H.G (2001). Integrative noetic therapies as adjuncts to percutaneous intervention during unstable coronary syndromes: Monitoring and Actualization of Noetic Training (MANTRA) feasibility pilot. *American Heart Journal,* 142, 760-767.

Kumar, R. (2011). Role of spirituality in human well-being. *Indian Journal of Health and Well-being,* 2(1), 204-206.

Lewis, C.A., Shevlin, M., Francis, L.J. and Quigley, C.F. (2010). The Association Between Church Attendance and Psychological Health in Northern Ireland: A National Representative Survey Among Adults Allowing for Sex Differences and Denominational Difference. *Journal of Religion and Health,* 50, 986-995.

Lindeman, M., Blomqvist, S. and Takada, M. (2012). Distinguishing spirituality from other constructs: not a matter of well-being but of belief in supernatural spirits. *The Journal of Nervous and Mental Disease,* 200(2), 167-173.

Lucchetti, G., Lucchetti, A.L.G., Badan-Neto, A.M., Peres, P.T., Peres, M.F.P., Moreira-Almeida, A., Gomes, C. and Koenig, H.G. (2011). Religiousness affects mental health, pain and quality of life in older people in an outpatient rehabilitation setting. *Journal of Rehabilitation Medicine,* 43(4), 316-322.

Lucchetti, G., Lucchetti, A.L.G., Peres, M.F.P., Moreira-Almeida, A. and Koenig, H. (2012). Religiousness, Health, and Depression in Older Adults from a Brazilian Military Setting. *ISRN Psychiatry,* 2012. doi:10.5402/2012/940747.

Lucchetti, G., Lucchetti, A.L., Oliveira, G.R., Crispim, D., Pires, S.L., Gorzoni, M.L., Panicio, C.R. and Koenig, H.G (2013). Nursing home care: exploring the role of religiousness in the mental health, quality of life and stress of formal caregivers. *Journal of Psychiatric and Mental Health Nursing.* Published online 23 May, 2013. doi: 10.1111/jpm.12092.

Lysne, C.J. and Wachholtz, A.B. (2011). Pain, spirituality and meaning making: What can we learn from the literature? *Religions*, 2, 1-16.

MacDonald, D.A. (2000). Spirituality: Description, measurement and relation to the Five Factor Model of personality. *Journal of Personality*, 68(1), 153-197.

Maltby, J., and Day, L. (1998). Amending a measure of the Quest Religious Orientation: Applicability of the scale's use among religious and nonreligious persons. *Personality and Individual Differences*, 25(3), 517-522.

Maltby, J., and Lewis, C.A. (1996). Measuring intrinsic and extrinsic orientation toward religion: Amendments for its use among religious and non-religious samples. *Personality and Individual Differences*, 21(6), 937-946.

Masters, K.S., and Knestel, A. (2011). Religious orientation among a random sample of community-dwelling adults: Relations with health status and health-relevant behaviours. *The International Journal for the Psychology of Religion*, 21, 63-76.

McCauley, R.N. (2001). Ritual, Memory and Emotion: Comparing Two Cognitive Hypotheses. In *Religion in Mind*, J. Andresen, ed. pp. 115-140. Cambridge University Press: Cambridge.

McCullough, M.E., Enders, C.K., Brion, S.L., and Jain, A.R. (2005). The varieties of religious development in adulthood: A longitudinal investigation of religion and rational choice. *Journal of Personality and Social Psychology*, 89, 78-89.

Meisenhelder, J.B. and Chandler, E.N. (2002). Spirituality and Health Outcomes in the Elderly. *Journal of Religion and Health*, 41(3), 243-252.

Mitchell, J. and Weatherly, D. (2000). Beyond church attendance: Religiosity and mental health among rural older adults. *Journal of Cross-Cultural Gerontology*, 15(1), 37-54.

Mohr, S., Perroud, N., Gillieron, C., Brandt, P.Y., Rieben, I., Borras, L., Huguelet, P. (2011). Spirituality and religiousness as predictive factors of outcome in schizophrenia and schizo-affective disorders. *Psychiatry Res.*, 186, 177-182.

Mohr, S., Borras, L., Nolan, J., Gillieron, C., Brandt, P.Y., Eytan, A., Leclerc, C., Perroud, N., Whetten, K., Pieper, C., Koenig, H.G. and Huguelet, P. (2012). Spirituality and religion in outpatients with schizophrenia: a multi-site comparative study of Switzerland, Canada, and the United States. *International Journal of Psychiatry in Medicine*, 44(1), 29-52.

Moreira-Almeida, A., Pinsky, I., Zaleski, M. and Laranjeira, R. (2010). Religious involvement and sociodemographic factors: a Brazilian national survey. *Revista de Psiquiatria Clinica*, 37(1), 12-15.

Murphy, P.E., Ciarrocchi, J.W., Piedmont, R.L., Cheston, S., and Peyrot, M. (2000). The Relation of Religious Belief and Practices, Depression, and Hopelessness in Persons with Clinical Depression. *Journal of Consulting and Clinical Psychology*, 68, 1102-1106.

Nagel, E. and Emch, S.S. (2007). The Relationship between Spirituality, Health Beliefs, and Health Behaviours in College Students. *Journal of Religion and Health*, 46(1), 141-154.

Nandal, T. (2011). Rituals, Religiosity, Spirituality as Correlates of Health. Unpublished doctoral dissertation, Maharishi Dayanand University, Rohtak.

Nonnemaker, J.M., McNeely, C.A., and Blum, R.W. (2003). Public and Private Domains of Religiosity and Adolescent Health Risk Behaviours: Evidence from the National Longitudinal Study of Adolescent Health. *Social Science and Medicine* 2003, 57(11), 2049-2054.

Noor, N.M. (2008). Work and Women's Well-being: Religion and Age as Moderators. *Journal of Religion and Health,* 47(4), 476-490.

Page, R.L.; Ellison, C.G. and Lee, J. (2009). Does Religiosity Affect Health Risk Behaviours in Pregnant and Postpartum Women? *Maternal and Child Health Journal,* 13(5), 621-632.

Pargament, K.I. (2010). Religion and coping: The current state of knowledge. In *Oxford Handbook of Stress and Coping*; Folkman, S., Ed.; Oxford University Press: Oxford, UK, 2010; 269-288.

Park, J.I., Hong, J.P., Park, S. and Cho, M.J. (2012). The relationship between religion and mental disorders in a Korean population. *Psychiatry Investigation,* 9(1), 29-35.

Rastgar, D.A.A., Davoudi, S.M.M., Oraji, S., and Abbasian, M. (2012). A Study of the Relationship Between Employees Spiritual Intelligence and Job Satisfaction: A Survey in Iran's Banking Industry. *Spectrum,* 1(2), 57-74.

Pikó, B. and Kovács, E. (2009). Is religiosity a protective factor? Social epidemiologic study of adolescent psychological health. *Orvosi Hetilap,* 150(41), 1903-1908.

Robinson, E.A., Cranford, J.A., Webb, J.R., and Brower, K.J. (2007). Six-month changes in spirituality, religiousness, and heavy drinking in a treatment-seeking sample. *Journal of Studies on Alcohol and Drugs,* 68(2), 282-290.

Pokimica, J., Addai, I. and Takyi, B.K. (2011). Religion and Subjective Well-Being in Ghana. *Social Indicators Research,* 106(1), 61-79.

Sawatzky, R., Ratner, P.A. and Chiu, L. (2005). "A meta-analysis of the relationship between spirituality and quality of life." *Social Indicators Research,* 72 (2), 153-188.

Schneiders, S. (2003). Religion vs. Spirituality: A Contemporary Conundrum. Spiritus: *A Journal of Christian Spirituality* 3(2), 163-185.

Sharma, P., Charak, R. and Sharma, V. (2009). Contemporary perspectives on spirituality and mental health. *Indian Journal of Psychological Medicine,* 31(1), 16-23.

Shea, J. (2000). *Spirituality and Health Care*. Chicago: Park Ridge Center for the Study of Health, Faith and Ethics.

Sherman, A.C.; Simonton, S.; Latif, U.; Spohn, R. and Tricot, G. (2005). Religious Struggle and Religious Comfort in Response to Illness: Health Outcomes among Stem Cell Transplant Patients. *Journal of Behavioural Medicine,* 28(4), 359-367.

Smith, S. and Suto, M.J. (2012). Religious and/or spiritual practices: extending spiritual freedom to people with schizophrenia. *Canadian Journal of Occupational Therapy,* 79(2), 77-85.

Sosis, R. (2003). Why Aren't We All Hutterites? Costly Signaling Theory and Religious Behaviour. *Human Nature* 14, 91-127.

Sosis, R. and Ruffle, B. (2004). Ideology, Religion, and the Evolution of Cooperation: Field Experiments on Israeli Kibbutzim. *Research in Economic Anthropology* 23, 87-115.

Steglitz, J. Ng, R., Mosha, J.S. and Kershaw, T. (2012). Divinity and distress: the impact of religion and spirituality on the mental health of HIV-positive adults in Tanzania. *Aids and Behaviour,* 16(8), 2392-2398.

Szaflarski, M., Ritchey, P.N., Leonard, A.C., Mrus, J.M., Peterman, A.H., Ellison, C.G., McCullough, M.E. and Tsevat, J. (2006). Modelling the effects of spirituality/religion patients' perceptions of living with HIV/AIDS. *Journal of General Internal Medicine,* 21(5), S28-S38.

Toussaint, L.L.; Williams, D.R ; Musick, M.A. and Everson, S.A. (2001). Forgiveness and Health: Age Differences in a U.S. Probability Sample. *Journal of Adult Development*, 8(4), 249-257.

Treloar, L.L. (2002). Disability, spiritual beliefs and the church: the experiences of adults with disabilities and family members. *Journal of Advanced Nursing,* 40 (5), 594-603.

Tripathi, M. and Asthana, H.S. (2013). Spirituality and religiosity as coping strategies in terminal illness. *Indian Journal of Health and Well-being,* 4(5), 1180-1184.

Tuck, I., McCain, N.L., and Elswick, R.K. (2001). Spirituality and psychosocial factors in persons living with HIV. *Journal of Advanced Nursing,* 33, 776-783.

Unterrainer, H.F., Schoeggl, H., Fink, A., Neuper, C. and Kapfhammer, H.P. (2012). Soul darkness? Dimensions of religious/ spiritual well-being among mood-disordered inpatients compared to healthy controls. *Psychopathology,* 45(5), 310-316.

Watlington, C.G., and Murphy, C.M. (2006). The roles of religion and spirituality among African American survivors of domestic violence. *Journal of Clinical Psychology,* 62(7), 837-857.

Whittington, B.L. and Scher, S.J. (2009). Prayer and Subjective Well-Being: An Examination of Six Different Types of Prayer. *International Journal for the Psychology of Religion,* 20(1), 59-68.

Wildes, K.A., Miller, A.R., de Majors, S.S. and Ramirez, A.G. (2009). The religiosity/spirituality of Latina breast cancer survivors and influence on health-related quality of life. *Psychooncology*, 18(8), 831-840.

Williams, R.M., Glanz, K., Kegler, M.C. and Davis, E. (2012). A Study of Rural Church Health Promotion Environments: Leaders' and Members' Perspectives. *Journal of Religion and Health,* 51(1), 148-160.

16

Spirituality and Mental Health

Exploring the Relationship

Shilpa Kumari and *Shobhana Joshi*

The term 'spirituality' and 'religiosity' is known to almost all the people and has been part of human experience and human civilization from the beginning. Psychology of religion is not a new field, it is among both the oldest and newest research areas in psychology. It was part of the field of psychology from the beginning. William James (1902, 1961), Edwin Starbuck (1899), G. Stanley Hall (1904, 1917), and George Coe (1900) were some of the scholars who have taken earlier initiation for inquiry within the field of psychology of religion. The famous psychologist William James wrote the varieties of 'Religious Experience' in 1902, shortly after the publication of '*The Psychology of Religion*' (Starbuck, 1899).

"Before the 1990s, the relationship between religion and health was largely an underestimated area of research. Researchers often buried religious variables in the methods and results section of their studies without overtly highlighting them as legitimate areas of health research (e.g. by including them in article or abstracts)" (Miller and Thoresen, 2003).

Researchers have rarely stated specific hypotheses about spiritual/religious measures, and often mentioned relatively strong predictive relationships that have simply appeared in a table, without further mention or discussion (Larson *et al.*, 1992).

Although a lot of important research has been conducted on how spirituality/religion affects mental health (George, Ellison, and Larson, 2002; Hood *et al.*, 1996), but measurements of spiritual/religious constructs which are used in health research are usually poor in quality (Larson *et al.*, 1998).

Psychology of religion flourished until the 1930s but then remain suppressed for about three decades. But now again, a renewed interest in psychology of religion has emerged (Paloutzian, 2002). In the 1990s, this novel area of research began to mature. The quality as well as methodological quality of studies on religion and health improved markedly (Miller and Thoresen, 2003). A number of books and abundant of empirical studies suggest that it is once again an important area in the discipline of psychology (Baston, Schoenrade, and Ventis, 1993; Hood and others, 1996; Paloutzian, 1996; Wulff, 1997). Research initiatives were launched within National Institute of Health (NIH), including extramural programme of National Institute on Aging, the National Institute on Alcohol Abuse and Alcoholism, and the National Centre for Complementary and Alternative Medicine.

Overtime these scholarly and scientific inquiries have accumulated a substantial body of research and information about religiousness and spirituality. Given this increasing knowledge base, it can be assumed that there exist a clear consensus among psychologists about the nature and definition of religiousness and spirituality. But, this is not the fact and definitions of religiousness and spirituality remain relatively inconsistent across researchers (Zinnabauer and Pargament, 2005).

Defining Religion and Spirituality

Religiosity and spirituality are the key concepts in the psychology of religion. "The upsurge in the interest in these constructs has existed over past 15 years by both applied and basic researches" (Emmons and Paloutzian, 2003). However, despite such common usage, these terms have no universally accepted definitions and even today a specific definition of the term religiosity and spirituality remains to be the subject of debate.

Some authors use the terms religion and spirituality interchangeably, while others attribute quite separate and distinct meanings to each term. 'Religion' is often used to describe a system in which beliefs, rituals, sacred text, and accepted public and private behaviours, such a prayer and church attendance, are established and upheld, whereas 'spirituality' is often used to refer to the direct, personal, and individual experience of the sacred (Potts, 1998). The terms religion and spirituality often overlap but studies exploring the differences between spirituality and religion have found that although they are not fully independent, they do not mean the same thing, and have concluded that it may be important to consider them as separate constructs (Woods and Ironson, 1999; Zinnbauer, Pargament, Cole, Rye, Butter, Belavich, Hipp, Scott, and Kadar, 1997). According to Kennedy, Davis, and Taylor (1998), spirituality has been shown to correlate with some religious approaches but, it does not necessarily entail an acceptance of and commitment to an institutionally defined set of beliefs, values and practices.

Spirituality has been defined as, 'An inherent quality of all human beings that drives the search for meaning and purpose in life, involves relationships with oneself, others, and a transcendent dimension' (Hermann, 2000).

The origin of the word religion comes from the transliteration of Latin word "religio" meaning to bind, to bind fast, or to fasten up. It is defined as reverence for God, or gods, or the fear of God. Religion could be best defined as a human attempt to achieve the highest possible good by adjusting life to the strongest and the best power in the universe. This power is usually called as God (Puthengady, 2005). The term 'religion' refers to beliefs, practices and rituals related to a specific established religious tradition. Each religion has some norms which have been expressed in the cultural values of the society as a whole. Religion has been considered as an organized, social phenomena, that is, practiced with within a community with specific traditions (Hadzic, 2011; Idler *et al.*, 2009; Koenig, 2009), whereas spirituality refers to a more subjective experience of religion and a personal relationship to the divine (Jungerman, 2013).

Similarly, William James (1961) had focused on the individual side of religiosity and he has regarded religion as the "feeling, acts, and experiences of individual men in their solitude…in relation to whatever they may consider the divine". According to Kalevi Tamminen (1991), religiousness involved a conscious dependency on a deity or God. Tamminen has also argued that this dependency or commitment is reflected in an individual's experiences, beliefs and personality, motivating the individual to engage in a variety of behaviour, such as devotional behaviours and moral behaviours. Dollahite (1998) has defined religion as "a covenant faith community with teachings and narratives that enhance the search for the sacred and encourage morality".

But some psychologists of religion have tried to differentiate spirituality from religiosity. Spirituality is increasingly used to refer to the personal, subjective side of religious experience (Koenig *et al.*, 2001). Because of this subjectivity spirituality, is conceptually more difficult to define than religion. Benner (1989) defines spirituality as, the human response to God's gracious call to a relationship with himself. Similarly, Vaughan (1991) describes spirituality as "a subjective experience of the sacred" and Doyle (1992) defines it as the search for existential meaning". Spirituality is seen as an "integral part of one's identity", a personal experience of divine and as "unity with the greater world or mystery" (Gall *et al.*, 2011:158). In contrast religion is seen as an external tool through which spiritual state can be access (Jungerman, 2013).

Thus, the terms "religiousness" and "spirituality" have been defined by different psychologists in different ways (Zinnbauer *et al.*, 1997; Zinnbauer *et al.*, 1999; Zinnbauer and Pargament, 2002). Traditionally religion was regarded as a "broad band" construct, which was not differentiated from the spirituality (Hill *et al.*, 2000; Pargament, 1999; Zinnbauer *et al.*, 1997, 1999). And all the religious and spiritual phenomena were included under the broad category of the construct religion, or the terms religion and spirituality have been used interchangeably (Spilka and McIntosh, 1996).

Zinnbauer and Pargament (2005) have devoted a full chapter on religiousness and spirituality in the Handbook of Psychology of Religion and spirituality in which they have discussed about different approaches to understand 'religion' and 'spirituality'. According to them the traditional approach understands the religious phenomena from both substantive and functional perspectives. Substantive approaches define religion by its substance, i.e. the sacred. According to Zinnbauer and Pargament (2005), the definition of religion given by Argyle and Beit-Hallahmi (1975) characterizes this approach as "a system of beliefs in a divine or superhuman power, and practices of worship or other rituals directed towards such a power" (p.1). Thus, traditional approach investigates those emotions, thoughts, behaviours, and relationships, that are explicitly related to a transcendent or imminent power (Bruce, 1996), or that have acquired sacred qualities themselves (Emmons, 1999; Pargament and Maloney, 2002; Zinnbauer and Pargament, 2005).

"Functional approaches examine the purposes religiousness serve in an individual's life. Beliefs, emotions, practices, and experiences are investigated as functional mechanisms that are used to deal with fundamental existential issues, such as meaning, death, suffering, isolation, and injustice (Bruce, 1996; Pargament, 1997)"; (Zinnbauer and Pargament, 2005). According to Zinnbauer and Pargament (2005), the definition of religion given by Baston, Schoenrade, and Ventis (1993) reflects the functional approach: "whatever we as individuals do to come to grips personally with the questions that confront us because we are aware that we and others like us are alive and that we will die" (p. 8).

But now there is a lot of shift in the definition of religion and the most important shift had occurred with the emergence of the construct spirituality. Spirituality has emerged as a distinct construct and has been a major focus of attention in research during the past several decades (Hill *et al.*, 2002; Hood, 2003; Wulff, 1997; Zinnbauer *et al.*, 1999).

"Functional descriptions that were once applied to religion are now becoming the province of spirituality. Spirituality has come to represent individual's effort at reaching a variety of sacred or existential goals in life, such as finding meaning, wholeness, inner potential, and interconnections with others. For example, spirituality is now being depicted as a search for universal truth (Goldberg, 1990) and as a form of belief that relates the individual to the world and gives meaning and definition to existence (Soeken and Carson, 1987). In contrast, religiousness is substantively associated with formal belief, group practice and institutions. As such, it is often portrayed as peripheral to these existential functions (Pargament, 1999)" (Zinnbauer and Pargament, 2005, p. 25).

"Traditional psychological research has also emphasized the personal aspects of religiousness (Miller and Thoresen, 2003) for which the definition of religion by William James is the best example which illustrates the individual focus. Although sociologists of religion include social or communal aspects of religious life in their conceptualizations of the term religion (Zinnbauer and Pargament, 2005)."

Departing from traditional analyses of individual beliefs, emotions, and experiences, many writers in this field are now contrasting the "institutional", "organized", and "social" aspects of religion with the "personal", "transcendent", and "relatedness" qualities of spirituality (Miller and Thoresen, 2003)" (Zinnbauer and Pargament, 2005, p. 25). According to Peteet (1994), Religiousness is defined as "[reflecting] commitments to beliefs and practices characteristic of particular traditions," and spirituality is characterized as "[viewing] the human condition in a larger and/or transcendent context and [being] therefore, concerned with the meaning and purpose of life and with unseen realities, such as one's relationship to a supreme being" (p. 237).

Similarly, a content analysis conducted by Emblen (1992) revealed that religiousness was defined as "a system of organized beliefs and worship which a person practices," and spirituality was defined as "a personal life principle which animates a transcendent quality of relationship with God" (p. 45).

Hill *et al.* (2000) have also used the individual-institutional dimension to distinguish between spirituality and religiousness. They propose that the sacred lie at the core of both constructs, and religion includes "the means and methods of [a] search (for the sacred) that receive validation and support from within an identifiable group of people".

"Similarly, Zinnbauer *et al.* (1997) have also found in their content analysis that personal beliefs in the sacred were common to definitions of both constructs religion and spirituality. But, definitions of religiousness often included references to organizational practice or activities, attendance at services, performance of rituals, church membership or allegiance, commitment or organizational beliefs, or adherence to institutionally based belief connectedness or relationship with sacred beings or forces" (Zinnabauer and Pargament, 2005, p. 26). Thus, conceptualization of the term spirituality, involves some underlying attributes, i.e. transcendence, the existentialism, and sacredness. Definition given by Vaughan *et al.* (1996) who defined spirituality as "a subjective experience that exist both within and outside of traditional religious system" (p. 497) and by Sussman *et al.* (1997), who defined spirituality as "subjectively experiencing a life force" (p. 112). Similarly, definition by Benner (1989), Emblen (1992) exemplifies the various conceptualizations in relation to experiential, relational and existential phenomena and healing practices associated with spirituality (Thoresen, 1999).

Despite the diversity in the conceptual definitions of spirituality, several common defining characteristics can be extracted. The conceptual definitions generally involve a relationship to something that lies beyond physiological, psychological or social human perception or experience. This relational object of spirituality may be described as "divinity", "a higher power", a "divine being", "ultimate reality", "God" or "god-being" (Burkhardt, 1989; Dyson, Cobb, and Forman, 1997; Emblen, 1992; Larson *et al.*, 1998; Reed, 1993; Thoresen, 1999). The experience associated with this relational aspect of spirituality can be described as transcendent or transpersonal in nature (Emblen, 1992; Reed, 1993; Vaughan *et al.*, 1996). Most definitions of spirituality support the notion that spirituality is associated with an existential search for meaning and purpose regarding complex questions about life (Larson *et al.*, 1998; Thoresen, 1999). This search can be directed by religious institutions or by personal life experiences. However, Hill *et al.* (2000) caution that although the existential search appears to provide a fairly clear defining characteristic of spirituality, existentialism in and of itself is not equal to spirituality. Based on an extensive review of literature on spirituality, several researchers suggest that the criterion distinguishing spirituality from other potentially meaningful existential pursuits, ideologies or life-giving practices is its orientation toward the sacred (George *et al.*, 2000; Hill *et al.*, 2000; Larson *et al.*, 1998). Pargament (1999) explains that "the sacred encompasses concepts of God, the divine, and the transcendent, but it is not limited to notions of higher powers. It also includes objects, attributes, or qualities that become sanctified by virtue of their association with or representation of the holy" (p. 12). Sacred refers to those aspects of life that are either transcendent in nature or associated with a transcendent dimension. In addition, the sacred encompasses the transcendent and existential characteristics of spirituality discussed earlier. In consideration of the relational characteristic of spirituality, spirituality can then be defined as involving a relationship with the sacred.

Thus, it can be said that spirituality has been increasingly differentiated from religiosity (Bartoli, 2007). Now, religiosity refers to an organized system of beliefs about the sacred, along with rituals, rules, and other requirements of a belief system endorsed by a group (Fuller, 2001; Pargament, 1997). Whereas, spirituality is increasingly seen as an inner process of connectedness with the sacred, a psychological process internal to the individual (Gallup and Jones, 2000; Sperry and Shafranske, 2005). Although, there is a significant overlap between these two terms, historically spirituality has been experienced through religion but a person engaged in a religious group may or may not have spiritual experiences and a person who has had spiritual experiences may or may not be part of a religious group (Friedman and Pappas, 2007).

Models of Spiritual Development

Although there are many models of spiritual development and broadly it can be categorized into two types: western models and eastern models. Eastern models are also of many types, but here only two models are discussed below:

(i) One of very important models for spiritual development is '*Yogasutras*' given by Patanjali. It is comprised eight limbs or steps which laid the basis for *Ashtang Yoga* which aims at "quiet the mind", transcend one's usual identity and "know God" (Yati, 2009). This *yoga* system proposes many tools for spiritual development; meditation and mindfulness; postures and breathing practices; moderation in lifestyles; and positive virtues such as honesty and not injuring others. Spiritual development is seen as related to attainment of these qualities.

(ii) Other model for spiritual development comes from Buddhist tradition, i.e. the Buddha's "eightfold". As the name suggests, it is comprised eight paths and these paths are aspiring towards right perspective, right intention, right speech, right action, right livelihood, right effort, right awareness and concentration. The first two paths are said to produce wisdom, the next four paths are to change conduct, and the last two paths to improve meditation. These eight paths are not necessarily sequential but are to be developed simultaneously, each supporting the others (Sangharakshita, 2007; Snelling, 1991).

Spirituality and Physical Health

There is a growing body of research that indicates that religion and spirituality are associated with better mental health, particularly among people with chronic and acute illnesses (e.g., Dein and Steigall, 1997; Worthington, Kurusu, McCullough, and Sandage, 1996). Koenig in his review found that approximately 80 per cent of research on R/S and health involves studies on mental health.

In the first edition of the 'Handbook of Religion and Mental Health' Koenig, McCullough, and Larson (2001), identified 110 studies published prior to the year 2000 and 344 studies published between 2000 and 2010 for a total of 454 studies. All these studies explored how R/S helped people to cope with a wide range of illnesses or in a variety of stressful situations. These include people dealing with general medical illness (Koenig, 1998; Pargament, Koenig, Tarakeshwar, and Hahn, 2004), chronic pain (Büssing, Michalsen, Balzat *et al.*, 2009), kidney disease (Tix and Frazier, 1998), diabetes (Zald'ývar and Smolowitz, 1994; Fitchett, Murphy, Kim, Gibbons, Cameron, and Davis, 2004), pulmonary disease (Sodergren, Hyland, Crawford, and Partridge, 2004.), cancer (Yoshimoto, Ghorbani, Baer *et al.*, 2006.; Shaw, Han, Kim *et al.*, 2007), blood disorders (Cooper-Effa, Blount, Kaslow, Rothenberg and Eckman, 2001), heart/cardiovascular diseases (Hughes, Tomlinson, Blumenthal, Davidson, Sketch, and Watkins, 2004; Ai, Park, Bu Huang, Rodgers, and Tice, 2007), dental (Heydecke, Tedesco, Kowalski, and Inglehart, 2004) or vision (Magyar-Russell, Fosarelli, Taylor, and Finkelstein, 2008) problems, neurological disorders (Giaquinto, Spiridigliozzi, and Caracciolo, 2007), HIV/AIDS (Cotton, Puchalski, Sherman *et al.*, 2006), systemic lupus erythematosus (Rinaldi, Ghisi, Iaccarino *et al.*, 2006), irritable bowel syndrome (Kuttner, Chambers, Hardial, Israel, Jacobson, and Evans, 2006), musculoskeletal disease (Abra´ıdo-Lanza, V´asquez, and Echeverr´ıa, 2004), caregiver burden (Rabins, Fitting, Eastham, and Zabora, 1990; Folkman, Chesney, Cooke, Boccellari, and Collette, 1994 Hebert, Dang, and Schulz, 2007), psychiatric illness (Tepper, Rogers, Coleman, and Malony 2001, Bosworth, Park, McQuoid, Hays, and Steffens, 2003), bereavement (Murphy, Johnson, and Lohan, 2003; Brown, Nesse, House, and Utz, 2004), end-of-life issues (Idler, Kasl, and Hays, 2001; Emanuel, Fairclough, Wolfe, and Emanuel, 2004), overall stress (Koenig, Cohen, Blazer *et al.*, 1992; Larson, Hansen, and Moneta, 2006; Pienaar, Rothmann, and Van Devijver, 2007), natural disasters (Smith, 1996; Hollifield, Hewage, Gunawardena, Kodituwakku, Bopagoda, and Weerarathnege, 2008), war (Pargament, Ishler, Dubow *et al.*, 1994. Scholte, Olff, Ventevogel *et al.,* 2004) or acts of terrorism (Schuster, Stein, Jaycox *et al.*, 2001), and miscellaneous adverse life situations (Ellison and Taylor, 1996; Pargament, Koenig and Perez, 1999; Nooney and Woodrum, 2002.). In the overwhelming majority of studies, people reported that R/S was helpful.

Similarly, Pargament and many psychologists (Bickel *et al.*, 1998; Pargament, 1997; Koenig, Pargament, and Nielsen, 1998; Pargament, Kendell, Hathaway, Gravengoed, Newman, and Jones, 1988) have found that positive religious ways of coping, such as seeking spiritual support and connection, and the use of collaborative religious coping (in which the individual is seen as being an active partner with God in problem solving) under highly stressful life events including physical ill health, are related to better quality of life and lower levels of depression, anxiety, and anger. In contrast, negative religious ways of coping, such as reappraisal of God's power and nature as punishing, being angry with God, religious doubts, and the use of self-directing coping (in which the individual takes on total responsibility for problem solving), have negative psychological effects, including higher levels of depression and trait anxiety, and lower levels of self-esteem and mood.

One possible explanation for the positive effects of religion on coping behaviour could be that religion may provide people a sense of suffering, a sense of meaning about the occurrence of life events, because many studies have found that religion and spirituality provide meaning and purpose in life (Hall, 1998; Tebbi *et al.*,1987; Woods and Ironson, 1999) both among the general population as well as among medically ill people (e.g., cancer and HIV patients). Ai, Dunkle, Paterson, and Boiling (1998);

Baumeister (1991); Bickel *et al.*, (1998) have also found that meaningfulness of life and religion have been found to be negatively related to depression and anxiety. Several researchers have also demonstrated that higher levels of spiritual well-being are associated with lower levels of psychological distress variables, such as, depression, hopelessness, desire for hastened death, and suicidal ideation among severely ill patients receiving palliative care (Hills, Paice, Cameron, and Shott, 2005). Silverstri, Knittig, Zoller and Nietert (2003) have conducted a study on 100 patients with newly diagnosed advanced lung cancer and found that patients ranked faith in God just beneath their oncologists' recommendations, as the most important factor in their decisions about treatment. Another cross-sectional study on advanced cancer patients found that spiritual well-being was correlated with quality-of-life measures (Fisch, Titzer, and Kristeller, 2003). Similarly, in a survey of outpatients with cancer reported that 40 per cent wanting help in 'finding meaning in life', 42 per cent in 'finding hope,' and 51 per cent in 'overcoming fears.' (Moadel, Morgan, Fatone, Grennan, Carter, Laruffa, *et al.,* 1999). Chaturvedi, Shenoy, Prasad Senthilnathan, and Premlatha (1996) found that peace of mind, spiritual satisfaction, and social satisfaction were considered to be very important in nearly two-thirds of the cancer patients.

A vast majority of studies reported statistically significant positive association and a handful of studies have reported negative associations and some studies reported no associations between religious involvement and mental health.

Spirituality and Mental Health

Koenig *et al.* (2001) have located at least 40 studies that have examined relationships between R/S and hope, among those, 29 (73%) reported only significant positive relationships with degree of hope and no studies found an inverse relationship. Of the six highest quality studies, half found a positive relationship (Sethi and Seligman, 1994; Murphy, Ciarrocchi, Piedmont, Cheston, Peyrot, and Fitchett, 2000; Ai, Park, Bu Huang, Rodgers, and Tice, 2007).

A total of 32 studies examining relationships between R/S and optimism were found and of those, 26 (81%) reported significant positive relationships (Koenig *et al.*, 2001). Of the 11 best studies, eight (73%) reported significant positive relationships (Idler and Kasl, 1997; Krause, 2002; Ai, Peterson, Bolling, and Koenig, 2002; Krause, 2006). Similarly, with hope, no studies reported inverse relationships. At least 45 studies have examined relationships of R/S with meaning and purpose, and 42 (93%) reported significant positive relationships. These studies were often in populations where there was a challenge to having meaning and purpose, such as in people with chronic disabling illness. Of the 10 studies with quality ratings of 7 or higher, all 10 reported significant positive associations (Francis, 2002; Skrabski, Kopp, Ozsa, R′ethelyi, and Rahe, 2005; Krause, 2009; Krause, 2010).

Koenig (2012) had found overall, 444 studies which have examined relationships between R/S and depression, dating back to the early 1960s. Among those studies, 272 (61%) reported significant inverse relationships between R/S and depression (including nine studies at a trend level), and 28 (6%) studies found positive relationships between R/S and depression (including two studies at a trend level). Of the 178 studies with the highest methodological rigour, 119 (67%) reported inverse relationships of R/S and depression (Kennedy, Kelman, Thomas, and Chen, 1996; Koenig, Cohen, Blazer *et al.*,1992; Koenig, George, and Peterson, 1998; Musick, Koenig, Hays, and Cohen, 1998; Propst, Ostrom, Watkins, Dean, and Mashburn, 1992; Strawbridge, Shema, Cohen, and Kaplan, 2001; Koenig, 2007; Van Voorhees, Paunesku, Kuwabara *et al.*, 2008; Ellison and Flannelly, 2009; Krause, 2009; Payman, K. George, and Ryburn, 2008) and 13 (7%) found positive relationships of R/S with depression (Spiegel, Bloom, and Gottheil, Pargament, Koenig, Tarakeshwar, and Hahn, 2004; Braam, Delespaul, Beekman *et al.*, 2004; Wijngaards-De Meij, Stroebe, Schut *et al.*, 2005; Solomon, Gelkopf, and Bleich, 2005; Eliassen, Taylor, and Lloyd, 2005; Bormann, Gifford, Shively *et al.*, 2006; Benjamins, 2007; Branco, 2007; Braam, Deeg, Poppelaars, Beekman, and Van Tilburg, 2007; Andersson, 2008; Miller, Forcehimes, Leary, and LaNoue, 2008; Maselko and Buka, 2008). Of 70 prospective cohort studies, 39 (56%) reported that greater R/S predicted lower levels of depression or faster remission of depression, whereas seven (10%) predicted worse future depression and seven (10%) reported mixed results (both significant positive and negative associations depending on R/S characteristic). Of 30 clinical trials, 19 (63%) found that R/S interventions produced better outcomes than either standard treatment or control groups. Two studies (7%) found standard treatments were superior to R/S interventions (Bormann, Gifford, Shively *et al.,* 2006; Miller, Forcehimes, O'Leary, and LaNoue, 2008) and one study reported mixed results.

Moreover, individual studies in stressed populations, particularly persons with serious medical illness, find a more substantial impact for religion on the prevalence and course of depression.

For example, 1000 depressed medical inpatients over age 50 with either congestive heart failure or chronic pulmonary disease were identified with depressive disorder using the Structured Clinical Interview for Depression (Koenig, 2007). The religious characteristics of these patients were compared to those of 428 non-depressed patients. Depressed patients were significantly more likely to indicate no religious affiliation, more likely to indicate—spiritual but not religious, less likely to pray or read scripture, and scored lower on intrinsic religiosity. These relationships remained robust after controlling for demographic, social and physical health factors. Among the depressed patients, severity of depressive symptoms was also inversely related to religious indicators.

Investigators followed 865 of these depressed patients for 12 to 24 weeks, examining factors influencing speed of remission from depression (Koenig, 2007). The most religious patients (those who attended religious services at least weekly, prayed at least daily, read the Bible or other religious scriptures at least three times weekly, and scored high on intrinsic religiosity) remitted from depression over 50 per cent faster than other patients (Hazard Ratio = 1.53, 95 per cent confidence intervals 1.20-1.94), controlling for multiple demographic, psychosocial, psychiatric, and physical health predictors of remission. Several other studies have likewise shown a positive impact for religion on course of depression (Koenig, Cohen, Blazer *et al.*, 1992; Koenig, George, Peterson, 1998; Braam, Beekman, Deeg, 1997).

A number of clinical trials have also examined the effects of R/S interventions on anxiety levels. Overall, at least 299 studies have examined this relationship, and of those, 147 (49%) studies reported inverse association of R/S (three at a trend level) with anxiety, whereas 33 (11%) studies reported positive relationship between R/S and anxiety, i.e. greater anxiety in those who were more R/S. Of the latter, however, only one was a prospective study, one was a randomized clinical trial, and 31 (94%) were cross-sectional studies (where it was not clear whether R/S caused anxiety or whether anxiety increased R/S as a coping response to the anxiety). Of the 67 studies with quality ratings of seven or higher, 38 (55%) reported inverse relationships (Williams, Larson, Buckler, Heckmann, and Pyle, 1991; Koenig, Fpord, George, Blazer, and Meador,1993; Azhar, Varma, and Dharap, 1994; Razali, Hasanah, Aminah, and Subramaniam, 1998; Cardozo, Bilukha, Gotway Crawford *et al.*, 2004; Chen, 2005; Zehnder, Prchal, Vollrath, and Landolt, 2006; Wachholtz and Pargament, 2008; Hill, Burdette, Ellison, and Musick, 2006; Foley, Baillie, Huxter, Price, and Sinclair,) and seven (10%) found positive relationships (greater anxiety among the more R/S) (Zeidner and Hammer, 1992; Martz 2004; Solomon, Gelkopf, and Bleich 2005; Miller, Forcehimes, O'Leary, and LaNoue, 2008; Hollifield, Hewage, Gunawardena, Kodituwakku, Bopagoda, and Weerarathnege, 2008; Meisenhelder and Marcum Meisenhelder and Marcum, 2009). Among these 299 studies were 239 cross-sectional studies, 19 prospective cohort studies, 9 single-group experimental studies, and 32 randomized clinical trials. Of the 19 longitudinal studies, 9 (47%) reported that R/S predicted a lower level of anxiety over time; one study (5%) found an increase in anxiety (among women undergoing abortion for fetal anomaly) (Korenromp, Page-Christiaens, Van den Bout, Mulder, and Visser, 2009), seven reported no association, and two reported mixed or complex results. Of the nine experimental studies, seven (78%) found a reduction in anxiety following an R/S intervention (before *versus* after comparison). Of the 32 randomized clinical trials, 22 (69%) reported that an R/S intervention reduced anxiety more than a standard intervention or control condition, whereas one study (3%) found an increase in anxiety following an R/S intervention in persons with severe alcohol dependence (Miller, 2008).

Studies provide evidence for strong links between spirituality, religion and mental health, but it is difficult to determine how these connections occur without in-depth qualitative research. A number of proposed mediators are described below:

(i) Ellison (1991) suggested four main ways in which religiosity may enhance various aspects of well-being: (1) through social participation and support; (2) through establishing a close personal relationship to God or a divine other; (3) by providing systems of meaning to explain existence; and (4) through the promotion of healthy lifestyle choices.

(ii) According to Koenig (2012) Religion/Spirituality influences mental health through following mechanisms: (1) religion acts as a coping mechanisms as it provides powerful cognitions that gives a sense of meaning to difficult life circumstances and a sense of purpose, subjective sense of control over events. (2) Every religion has some rules and regulations about living life and to treat others within a social group and religion also promotes healthy life style. (3) Religion promotes human virtues such as honesty, forgiveness, gratefulness, patience, and dependability, emphasize love for others, compassion, and altruistic acts etc. Which help to maintain and enhance social relationships.

Implications

The research reviewed reflects that spiritual practice can provide meaning, a sense of control, mindfulness, reduced anxiety, and a positive outlook on life. So, spirituality can be incorporated into mental care by allowing patients to discuss the role of spirituality on their psychological well-being (Dalmida, 2006). Some of the implications are discussed below.

Mindfulness

The root of mindfulness practices lies in Buddhism. The goal of mindfulness is to cultivate attention to the present moment in a non-judgmental way. It is theorized that mindfulness-based stress reduction (MBSR) programmes, as well as other meditative practices contribute to well-being by reducing mental preoccupation with daily stressors (Carmody *et al.*, 2008). Spiritual practices such as contemplative prayer, mindfulness meditation, and rituals produce a calming effect and are positively associated with mental health (Baetz and Towes, 2009). According to Foster (2004) there has been strong evidence regarding practice of mindfulness, meditation and *yoga* relaxation meditation in mental health and the benefits that these spiritual practices have on psychological well-being.

Mindfulness can also assist clients by helping them accept their situations and find solutions instead of being affected by them (Strosahl and Robinson, 2008). Research has shown that mindfulness-based therapies are effective treatments for a variety of mood disorders. Studies show that mindfulness-based interventions reduced depressive symptoms in adults with mental disorders (Klainin-Yobas *et al.*, 2011). Hofmann *et al.* (2010) conducted an effect size analysis of mindfulness-based interventions and found that such therapies were moderately effective in improving mood and anxiety. Mindfulness-based therapies have also shown promise in preventing substance use and addiction relapse (Appel and Kim-Appel, 2009).

Prayer

A number of studies reveal that prayer can significantly reduce depression and anxiety (Boelens *et al.*, 2009; Anastasi and Newberg, 2008; O'Laoire, 1997). Boelens *et al.*, conducted a study to investigate the effect of person-to-person prayer on perceived depression and anxiety. After randomization to a prayer (intervention) or control group, participants completed Hamilton Rating Scales for Depression and Anxiety. The intervention group received six hour-long prayer sessions weekly while those in the control group received none. Rating scales were repeated after the six weeks and a month later. At completion, participants receiving the intervention showed significant improvement of depression, anxiety and optimism compared to controls ($p < 0.01$ in all cases) and maintained these improvements ($p < 0.01$) for at least 1 month after the final prayer session. Anastasi and Newberg (2008) studied the impact of religious ritual prayer (reciting the Rosary) on thirty Catholic college students. The intervention group participated in a one-time recitation of the Rosary in a campus chapel, while the control group watched a video with religious content. Pre-test and post-test questionnaires were administered for both state and trait anxiety. Results showed a significant improvement in state anxiety (27%; $p = 0.004$) within the Rosary intervention group between pre- and post-test means. A significant reduction was also found in the post-test state anxiety scores for the Rosary intervention group compared to the control group ($p = 0.035$). The ritualized, repetitive nature of the Rosary, not provided by the religious-content video, may give participants a greater sense of calm.

Positive Outlook

Another popular way that psychologists have combine psychology and spirituality during therapy has been by encouraging positive thinking (Matteson, 2008). This technique has shown positive results while working with multiple mental health disorders (Lukoff, 2007). Faith, in general, may promote virtues such as compassion, hope and forgiveness, resulting in better physical and mental health (Hadzic, 2011; Hill and Pargament, 2003). Both belief in a loving God (or higher power) along with a positive worldview, are associated with improved health status, consistent with psychoneuroimmunological models of health (Campbell and Yoon, 2010).

Conclusion

The field of religion, spirituality and health is growing rapidly. The majority of studies have shown that religion and/or spirituality can have a positive impact on mental health or well-being, as well as on physical health. A large number of research shows that people who are more spiritual/religious have better mental health and adapt more quickly to health problems compared to those who are less spiritual/religious. This effect may occur through a number of proposed mechanisms. For example, spiritual beliefs may fill their life with a sense of meaning and purpose; mindfulness, prayer and meditation can provide a calming effect; and spiritual virtues such as compassion, hope and forgiveness can promote a more positive worldview. Also, spiritual beliefs and practices can be used in medical care setting which helps patients to cope with illness and other stressful life changes. Thus, it is very important for mental health professionals to be aware of their patient's religious, spiritual and cultural beliefs such that they can be assisted according to the relevance of needs.

This review focuses on a number of different trends to define religiosity and spirituality which gives some positive signs to understand and differentiate between the terms religion and spirituality.

References

Abra´1do-Lanza, A.F., V´asquez, E., and Echeverr´1a, S.E. (2004). "En las Manos de Dios [in God's Hands]: religious and other forms of coping among Latinos with arthritis," *Journal of Consulting and Clinical Psychology*, 72, 1, 91-102.

Ai, A.L., Dunkle, R.E., Paterson, C., and Boiling, S.F. (1998). "The role of private prayer in psycho logical recovery among midlife and aged patients following cardiac surgery". *The Gerontologist,* 38, 591-601.

Ai, A.L., Park, C.L., Bu Huang, Rodgers, W., and Tice, T.N. (2007). "Psychosocial mediation of religious coping styles: a study of short-term psychological distress following cardiac surgery," *Personality and Social Psychology Bulletin*, 33(6), 867-882.

Ai, A.L., Peterson, C., Bolling, S.F., and Koenig, H. (2002). "Private prayer and optimism in middle-aged and older patients awaiting cardiac surgery," *Gerontologist*, 42(1), 70-81.

Anastasi, M.W., and Newberg, A.B. (2008). "A Preliminary Study of the Acute Effects of Religious Ritual on Anxiety." *The Journal of Alternative and Complementary Medicine,* 14(2), 163-165.

Andersson, G. (2008). "Chronic pain and praying to a higher power: useful or useless?" *Journal of Religion and Health*, 47(2), 176-187.

Argyle, M. and Beit-Hallahmi, B. (1975). *The Social Psychology of Religion.* London: Routledge.

Azhar, M.Z., Varma, S.L., and Dharap, A.S. (1994). "Religious psychotherapy in anxiety disorder patients," *Acta Psychiatrica Scandinavica*, Vol. 90, No. 1, pp. 1-3.

B¨ussing, A., Michalsen, A., and Balzat, H.J. *et al.* (2009). "Are spirituality and religiosity resources for patients with chronic pain conditions?" *Pain Medicine*, 10(2), 327-339.

Baetz, M., Bowen R., Jones G. (2006). "How spiritual values and worship attendance relate to psychiatric disorders in the Canadian population." *Canadian Journal of Psychiatry,* 51, 654-661.

Baston, C.D., Schoenrade, P., and Ventis, W.L. (1993). *Religion and the Individual: A Social-Psychological Perspective*, New York: Oxford University Press.

Baumeister, R.F. (1991). *Meanings of Life*. New York: Guilford Press.

Benjamins, M.R. (2007). "Predictors of preventive health care use among middle-aged and older adults in Mexico: the role of religion," *Journal of Cross-Cultural Gerontology*, 22(2), 221-234.

Benner, D.G. (1989). "Toward a psychology of spirituality: implications for personality and psychotherapy." *Journal of Psychology and Christianity,* 5, 19-30.

Bickel, C.O., Ciarrocchio, J.W., Sheers, N.J., Estadt, B.K., Powell, D.A., and Pargament, K.I. (1998). "Perceived stress, religious coping styles, and depressive affect". *Journal of Psychology and Christianity,* 17, 33-42.

Bickel, C.O., Ciarrocchio, J.W., Sheers, N.J., Estadt, B.K., Powell, D.A., and Pargament, K.I. (1998). "Perceived stress, religious coping styles, and depressive affect". *Journal of Psychology and Christianity,* 17, 33-42.

Boelens, P.A., Reeves, R.R., Replogle, W.H., and Koenig, H.G. (2009). "A randomized trial of the effect of prayer on depression and anxiety. "*International Journal of Psychiatry in Medicine,* 39(4), 377-392.

Bormann, J.E., Gifford, A.L., Shively, M. *et al.*, (2006). "Effects of spiritual mantram repetition on HIV outcomes: A randomized controlled trial," *Journal of Behavioural Medicine*, 29(4), 359-376.

Bosworth, H.B., Park, K.S., McQuoid, D.R., Hays, J. C, and Steffens, D.C. (2003). "The impact of religious practice and religious coping on geriatric depression," *International Journal of Geriatric Psychiatry*, 18, 10, 905-914.

Braam, A.W., Beekman, A.T. F., and Deeg, D.G.H. *et al.* (1997). "Religiosity as a protective of prognostic factor of depression in later life; results from a community study in The Netherlands". *Acta Psychiatr Scand,* 96, 199-205.

Braam, A.W., Deeg, D.J. H., Poppelaars, J.L., Beekman, A.T. F. and Van Tilburg, W. (2007). "Prayer and depressive symptoms in a period of secularization: patterns among older adults in the Netherlands," *American Journal of Geriatric Psychiatry*, 15(4), 273-281.

Braam, A.W., Delespaul, P., Beekman, A.T. *et al.* (2004). "National context of healthcare, economy and religion, and the association between disability and depressive symptoms in older Europeans: results from the EURODEP concerted action," *European Journal of Ageing*, 1 (1), 26-36.

Branco, K.J. (2007). "Religious activities, strength from faith, and social functioning among African American and white nursing home residents," *Journal of Religion, Spirituality and Aging*, 19(4), 3-20.

Brown, S.L., Nesse, R.M., House, J.S., and Utz, R.L. (2004). "Religion and emotional compensation: results from a prospective study of widowhood," *Personality and Social Psychology Bulletin*, 30, 9, 1165-1174.

Bruce, S. (1996). *Religion in the Modern World: From Cathedrals to Cults.* Oxford, UK: Oxford University Press.

Burkhardt, M.A. (1989). Spirituality: An analysis of the concept. *Holistic Nursing Practice,* 3(3), 69-77.

Campbell, J.D., Yoon, D.P., Johnstone, B. (2010). "Determining Relationships Between Physical Health and Spiritual Experience, Religious Practices, and Congregational Support in a Heterogeneous Medical Sample." *Journal of Religion in Health,* 49(3), 3-17.

Cardozo, L.B., Bilukha, O.O., Gotway Crawford C.A., *et al.* (2004). "Mental health, social functioning, and disability in postwar Afghanistan," *Journal of the American Medical Association*, 292(5), 575-584.

Chaturvedi, S.K., Shenoy, A., Prasad, K.M., Senthilnathan, S.M., Premlatha, B.S. (1996). "Concerns, Coping and Quality of life in head and neck Cancer Patients". *Support Care Cancer,* 4, 186-90.

Chen, Y.Y. (2005). "Written emotional expression and religion: effects on PTSD symptoms," *International Journal of Psychiatry in Medicine*, 35 (3), 273-286.

Coe, G.A. (1900). *The Spiritual Life: Studies in the Science of Religion.* New York: Eaton and Mains.

Cotton, S., Puchalski, C.M., and Sherman S.N. *et al.*, (2006). "Spirituality and religion in patients with HIV/AIDS," *Journal of General Internal Medicine*, 21 (5), 5-13.

Dein, S., and Stygall, J. (1997). "Does being religious help or hinder coping with chronic illness: A critical literature review". *Palliative Medicine,* 11, 291-298.

Dollahite, D.C. (1998). Fathering, faith and spirituality. *Journal of Men's Studies, 7*, 3-15.

Doyle, D. (1992). "Have we looked beyond the physical and psychosocial?" *Journal of Pain and Symptom Management,* 7, 302-311.

Dyson, J., Cobb, M. and Forman, D. (1997). The meaning of spirituality: A literature review. *Educator*, 20, 4, 303-306.

Eliassen, A.H., Taylor, J., and D.A. Lloyd, D.A. (2005). "Subjective religiosity and depression in the transition to adulthood," *Journal for the Scientific Study of Religion*, 44(2), 187-199.

Ellison, C.G and Flannelly, K.J. (2009). "Religious involvement and risk of major depression in a prospective nationwide study of African American adults," *Journal of Nervous and Mental Disease*, 197(8), 568-573.

Ellison, C.G and Taylor, R.J. (1996). "Turning to prayer: social and situational antecedents of religious coping among African Americans," *Review of Religious Research*, 38(2), 111-131.

Ellison, C.G. (1991). "Religious Involvement and Subjective Well-Being". *Journal of Health and Social Behaviour*, 32(3), 80-99.

Emanuel, E.J., Fairclough, D.L., Wolfe, P., and Emanuel, L.L. (2004). "Talking with terminally ill patients and their caregivers about death, dying, and bereavement: is it stressful? Is it helpful?" *Archives of Internal Medicine*, 164(18), 1999-2004.

Emblen, J.D. (1992). Religion and spirituality defined according to current use in nursing literature. *Journal of Professional Nursing*, 8(1), 41-47.

Emmons, R.A. and Paloutzian, R.F. (2003). The psychology of religion. *Annual Review of Psychology*, 54, 377-402.

Fisch, M.J., Titzer, M.L., Kristeller, J.L. (2003). "Assessment of quality of life in outpatients with advanced cancer: the accuracy of clinician estimations and the relevance of spiritual well-being—a Hoosier Oncology Group study." *Journal of Clinical Oncology*, 21, 2754-2759.

Fitchett, G., Murphy, P.E., Kim, J., Gibbons, J.L., Cameron, J.R. and Davis, J.A. (2004). "Religious struggle: prevalence, correlates and mental health risks in diabetic, congestive heart failure, and oncology patients," *International Journal of Psychiatry in Medicine*, 34(2), 179-196.

Foley, E. Baillie, A., Huxter, M., Price, M., and Sinclair, E. (2010). "Mindfulness-based cognitive therapy for individuals whose lives have been affected by cancer: a randomized controlled trial," *Journal of Consulting and Clinical Psychology*, 78(1), 72-79.

Folkman, S., Chesney, M.A., Cooke, M., Boccellari, A., and Collette, L. (1994). "Caregiver burden in HIV-positive and HIV negative partners of men with AIDS," *Journal of Consulting and Clinical Psychology*, 62, 4, 746-756.

Foster, T.M. (2004). *Yoga: Physical, mental, emotional and spiritual impact*. California State University, Sacramento.

Francis, L.J. (2000). "The relationship between bible reading and purpose in life among 13-15-year-olds," *Mental Health, Religion and Culture*, 3, 33-36.

Gall, T.L., Malette, J., Guirguis-Younger, M. (2011). Spirituality and Religiousness: A Diversity of Definitions. *Journal of Spirituality in Mental Health*, 13(3), 158-181.

George, L.K., Ellison, C.G., and Larson, D.B. (2002). Explaining the relationship between religious involvement and health. *Psychological Inquiry*, 13(3), 190-200.

George, L.K., Larson, D.B., Koenig, H.G., and McCullough, M.E. (2000). "Spirituality and health: What we know, what we need to know". *Journal of Social and Clinical Psychology*, 19(1), 102-116.

Giaquinto, S., Spiridigliozzi, C., and Caracciolo, B. (2007). "Can faith protect from emotional distress after stroke?" *Stroke*, 38(3), 993-997.

Goldberg, R.S. (1990). "The transpersonal element in spirituality and psychiatry". *Psychiatric Residents Newsletter*, 10, 9.

Hadzic, M. (2011). "Spirituality and Mental Health: Current Research and Future Directions". *Journal of Spirituality in Mental Health,* 13(4), 223-235.

Hall, B.A. (1998). "Patterns of spirituality in persons with advanced HIV disease." *Research in Nursing and Health,* 21, 143-153.

Hall, G.S. (1904). *Adolescence: Its Psychology and its Relations to Physiology, Anthropology, Sociology, Sex, Crime, Religion, and Education* (2 Vols.). New York: Appleton.

Hall, G.S. (1917). *Jesus the Christ, in Light of Psychology*. New York: Doubleday.

Hebert, R.S., Dang, Q., and Schulz, R. (2007). "Religious beliefs and practices are associated with better mental health in family caregivers of patients with dementia: findings from the reach study," *American Journal of Geriatric Psychiatry*, 15(4), 292-300.

Hermann, C. (2000). "A guide to the spiritual needs of elderly cancer patients." *Geriatric Nursing,* 21, 324-325.

Hill, P.C., Pargament, K.I., Hood, R.W., McCullough, M.E., Swyers, J.P., Larson, D.B. *et al.* (2000). "Conceptualizing religion and spirituality: Points of commonality, points of departure." *Journal for the Theory of Social Behaviour,* 30(1), 51-77.

Hill, T.D., Burdette, A.M., Ellison, C.G., and Musick, M.A. (2006). "Religious attendance and the health behaviours of Texas adults," *Preventive Medicine*, 42 (4), 309-312.

Hills, J., Paice, J.A., Cameron, J.R., Shott, S. (2005). "Spirituality and distress in palliative care consultation." *Journal of Palliative Medicine,* 8, 782.

Hood, R.W. (2003). The relationship between religion and spirituality. *Defining religion: investigating the boundaries between the sacred and secular religion and the social order,* 10, 241-265.

Hood, R.W., Spilka, B., Hunsberger, B., and Gorsuch, R.L. (1996). *The Psychology of Religion: An Empirical Approach*. New York: Guilford Press.

Hofmann, S.G, Sawyer, A.T., Witt, A.A., and Oh, D. (2010). "The effect of mindfulness-based therapy on anxiety and depression: A meta-analytic review." *Journal of Consulting and Clinical Psychology*, 78(2), 169.

Hollifield, M., Hewage, C., Gunawardena, C.N., Kodituwakku, P., Bopagoda, K., and Weerarathnege, K. (2008). "Symptoms and coping in Sri Lanka 20-21 months after the 2004 tsunami," *British Journal of Psychiatry*, 192 (1), 39-44.

Hollifield, M., Hewage, C., Gunawardena, C.N., Kodituwakku, P., Bopagoda, K., and Weerarathnege, K. (2008). "Symptoms and coping in Sri Lanka 20-21 months after the 2004 tsunami," *British Journal of Psychiatry*, 192(1), 39-44.

Holt, C.L. and McClure, S.M. (2006). "Perceptions of the Religion-Health Connection Among African American Church Members." *Qualitative Health Research,* 16, 268-281.

Hughes, J.W., Tomlinson, A., Blumenthal, J.A., Davidson, J., Sketch, M.H., and Watkins, L.L. (2004). "Social support and religiosity as coping strategies for anxiety in hospitalized cardiac patients," *Annals of Behavioural Medicine*, 28, 3, 179-185.

Idler, E.L and Kasl, S.V. (1997). "Religion among disabled and non-disabled persons I: cross-sectional patterns in health practices, social activities, and well-being," *Journals of Gerontology B*, 52(6), 294-305, 1997.

Idler, E.L., Kasl, S.V., and Hays, J.C. (2001). "Patterns of religious practice and belief in the last year of life," *Journals of Gerontology B*, 56, (6), 326-334.

James, W. (1961). *The varieties of religious experience*. New York: Collier Books.

James, A., and Wells, A. (2003). Religion and mental health: towards a cognitive-behavioural framework. *British Journal of Health Psychology*, 8, 359-376.

Jungerman, J.M. (2013). "Qualitative perspective on spirituality and mental health." Thesis for MPH in Behavioural Science and Health Education.

Kennedy, J.E., Davis, R.C., and Taylor, B.G. (1998). "Changes in spirituality and well-being among victims of sexual assault." *Journal for the Scientific Study of Religion*, 37, 322-328.

Kennedy, G.J., Kelman, H.R., Thomas, C., and Chen, J. (1996). "The relation of religious preference and practice to depressive symptoms among 1,855 older adults," *Journals of Gerontology*, 51, 301-308.

Klainin-Yobas, P., Cho, M.A.A., and Creedy, D. (2012). "Efficacy of mindfulness-based interventions on depressive symptoms among people with mental disorders: A meta-analysis." *International Journal of Nursing Studies*, 49(1), 109-121.

Koenig, H.G. (1998). "Religious beliefs and practices of hospitalized medically ill older adults," *International Journal of Geriatric Psychiatry*, 13, 213-224.

Koenig, H.G. (2007). "Religion and remission of depression in medical in patients with heart failure/pulmonary disease," *Journal of Nervous and Mental Disease*, 195 (5), 389-395.

Koenig, H.G. (2007). "Religion and depression in older medical inpatients." *American Journal of Geriatric Psychiatry*, 15, 282-291.

Koenig, H.G. (2009). "Research on Religion, Spirituality, and Mental Health: A Review." *The Canadian Journal of Psychiatry*, 54(5), 283-291.

Koenig, H.G. (2012). *Religion, spirituality and health: The research and clinical implications.* International Scholarly Research Network Psychiatry.

Koenig, H.G., Cohen, H.J. and Blazer, D.G. *et al.*, (1992). "Religious coping and depression among elderly, hospitalized medically ill men," *American Journal of Psychiatry*, 149(12), 1693-1700.

Koenig, H.G., Cohen, H.J., and Blazer D.G. *et al.*, (1992). "Religious coping and depression among elderly, hospitalized medically ill men," *American Journal of Psychiatry*, 149(12), 1693-1700.

Koenig, H.G., Cohen, H.J., Blazer, D.G., *et al.* (1992). "Religious coping and depression among elderly, hospitalized medically ill men." *American Journal of Psychiatry*, 149, 1693-1700.

Koenig, H.G., Fpord, S.M., George, L.K., Blazer, D.G., and Meador, K.G. (1993). "Religion and anxiety disorder: an examination and comparison of associations in young, middle-aged, and elderly adults," *Journal of Anxiety Disorders*, 7 (4), 321-342.

Koenig, H.G., George, L.K., and Peterson, B.L. (1998). "Religiosity and remission of depression in medically ill oder patients," *American Journal of Psychiatry*, 155 (4), 536-542.

Koenig, H.G., McCullough, M.E., and Larson, D.B. (2001). *Handbook of Religion and Health.* NY: Oxford University Press, pp. 118-143, 216-217, 527-530.

Koenig, H.G., Pargament, K.L., and Nielsen, J. (1998). "Religious coping and health status in medically ill hospitalized older adults." *The Journal of Nervous and Mental Disease,* 186, 513-521.

Korenromp, M.J., Page-Christiaens, G.C. M.L., van den Bout, J., Mulder, E.J.H. and Visser, G.H.A. (2009). "Adjustment to termination of pregnancy for fetal anomaly: a longitudinal study in women at 4, 8, and 16 months," *American Journal of Obstetrics and Gynaecology*, 201(2), 160-e1-160-e7,

Krause, N. (2002). "Church-based social support and health in old age: exploring variations by race," *Journals of Gerontology B.*, 57 (6), 332-347.

Krause, N. (2006). "Religious doubt and psychological well-being: a longitudinal investigation," *Review of Religious Research*, 47, 287-302.

Krause, N. (2009). "Meaning in life and mortality," *Journal of Gerontology B*, supplement, 64, 517-S527.

Krause, N. (2009). "Religious involvement, gratitude, and change in depressive symptoms over time," *International Journal for the Psychology of Religion*, 19(3), 155-172.

Krause, N. (2010). "God-mediated control and change in self-rated health," *International Journal for the Psychology of Religion*, 20, 267-287.

Kuttner, L., Chambers, C.T., Hardial, J., Israel, D.M., Jacobson, M. and Evans, K. (2006). "A randomized trial of yoga for adolescents with irritable bowel syndrome," *Pain Research and Management*, 11, 4, 217-223.

Larson, D.B., Sawyers, J.P., and McCullough, M.E. (1998). *Scientific research on spirituality and health: A report based on the Scientific Progress in Spirituality Conferences.* New York: John M. Templeton Foundation.

Larson, R.W., Hansen, D.M., and Moneta, G. (2006). "Differing profiles of developmental experiences across types of organized youth activities," *Developmental Psychology*, 42 (5), 849-863.

Lukoff, D. (2007). "Spirituality in the Recovery from Persistent Mental Disorders." *Southern Medical Association.* Vol. 100, No. 6.

Magyar-Russell, G., Fosarelli, P., Taylor, H., and Finkelstein, D. (2008). "Ophthalmology patients' religious and spiritual beliefs: an opportunity to build trust in the patient-physician relationship," *Archives of Ophthalmology*, 126, 9, 1262-1265.

Martz, E. (2004). "Death anxiety as a predictor of posttraumatic stress levels among individuals with spinal cord injuries," *Death Studies*, 28(1), 1-17.

Maselko, J. and Buka, S. (2008). "Religious activity and lifetime prevalence of psychiatric disorder," *Social Psychiatry and Psychiatric Epidemiology*, 43 (1), 18-24.

Matteson, D.R. (2008). *Exploring the Spiritual: Paths for Counselors and Psychotherapists*. New York: Routledge.

Meisenhelder, J.B., Marcum, J.P. (2009). "Terrorism, posttraumatic stress, coping strategies, and spiritual outcomes". *Journal of Religion and Health*, 48(1), 46-57.

Meisenhelder, M.J. and Marcum, J.P. (2009). "Adjustment to termination of pregnancy for fetal anomaly: a longitudinal study in women at 4, 8, and 16 months," *American Journal of Obstetrics and Gynaecology*, 201 (2), 160-e1-160-e7.

Miller, J.J., Fletcher, K., Kabat-Zinn, J. (1995). "Three-year follow-up and clinical implications of a mindfulness meditation-based stress reduction intervention in the treatment of anxiety disorders." *General Hospital Psychiatry,* 17(3), 192-200.

Miller, W.R., Forcehimes, A., O'Leary, M.J., and LaNoue, M.D. (2008). "Spiritual direction in addiction treatment: two clinical trials," *Journal of Substance Abuse Treatment*, 35(4), 434-442.

Miller, W.R. and Thoresen, C.E. (2003). "Spirituality, religion, and health: An emerging research field. " *American Psychologist,* 58, 24-35.

Moadel, A., Morgan, C., Fatone, A., Grennan, J., Carter, J., Laruffa, G., *et al.* (1999). "Seeking meaning and hope: Self-reported spiritual and existential needs among an ethnically-diverse cancer patient population." *Psychooncology*, 8:378-85.

Murphy, P.E., Ciarrocchi, J.W., Piedmont, R.L., Cheston, S., Peyrot, M. and Fitchett, G (2000). "The relation of religious belief and practices, depression, and hopelessness in persons with clinical depression," *Journal of Consulting and Clinical Psychology*, Vol. 68, No. 6, pp. 1102-1106.

Murphy, S.A., Johnson, L.C., and Lohan, J. (2003). "Finding meaning in a child's violent death: a five-year prospective analysis of parents' personal narratives and empirical data," *Death Studies*, 27, 5, 381-404.

Musick, M.A., Koenig, H.G., Hays, J.C. and Cohen, H.J. (1998). "Religious activity and depression among community dwelling elderly persons with cancer: The moderating effect of race," *Journals of Gerontology*, 53 (4), 218-S227.

Nooney, J. and Woodrum, E. (2002). "Religious coping and church based social support as predictors of mental health outcomes: testing a conceptual model," *Journal for the Scientific Study of Religion*, 41 (2), 359-368.

Pargament, K.I. (1997). *The Psychology of religion and coping: Theory, research, and practice*. New York: Guilford Press.

Pargament, K.I. (1999). "The psychology of religion and spirituality? Yes and no." *International Journal for the Psychology of Religion,* 9(1), 3-14.

Pargament, K.I., Ishler, K., Dubow E. *et al.* (1994). "Methods of religious coping with the Gulf War: Cross-sectional and longitudinal analyses," *Journal for the Scientific Study of Religion.*

Pargament, K.I., Kendell, J., Hathaway, W., Gravengoed, N., Newman, J.M., and Jones, W. (1988). "Religion and the problem-solving process: Three styles of coping." *Journal for the Scientific Study of Religion,* 27, 90-104.

Pargament, K.I., Koenig, H.G. and Perez, L.M. (1999). "A comprehensive measure of religious coping: development and initial validation of the RCOPE," *Journal of Clinical Psychology*, 56(4), 519-543.

Pargament, K.I., Koenig, H.G., Tarakeshwar, N., and Hahn, J. (2004). "Religious coping methods as predictors of psychological, physical and spiritual outcomes among medically ill elderly patients: a two-year longitudinal study," *Journal of Health Psychology*, 9(6), 713-730.

Payman, V., George, K. and Ryburn, B. (2008). "Religiosity of depressed elderly inpatients," *International Journal of Geriatric Psychiatry*, 23(1), 16-21.

Peteet, J.R. (1994). Approaching spiritual problems in psychotherapy: A conceptual framework. *Journal of Psychotherapy Practice and Research,* 3, 237-245.

Pienaar, J., Rothmann, S., and Van Devijver, F.J. R. (2007). "Occupational stress, personality traits, coping strategies, and suicide ideation in the South African police service," *Criminal Justice and Behaviour*, 34(2), 246-258.

Potts, R.G. (1998). "Spirituality, religion, and the experience of illness." In P. Camic and S. Knight (Eds.) *Clinical handbook of health psychology* (pp. 495-522). Seattle: Hogrefe and Huber.

Propst, L.R., Ostrom, R., Watkins, P., Dean, T., and Mashburn, D. (1992). "Comparative efficacy of religious and non-religious cognitive-behavioural therapy for the treatment of clinical depression in religious individuals," *Journal of Consulting and Clinical Psychology*, 60 (1), 94-103.

Puthangady, A. (2005). "The psychology of religious fundamentalism." *Journal of Dharma,* 30(2).

Rabins, P.V., Fitting, M.D., Eastham, J., and Zabora, J. (1990). "Emotional adaptation over time in care-givers for chronically ill elderly people," *Age and Ageing*, 19, 3, 185-190.

Razali, R.M., Hasanah, C.I., Aminah, K., and Subramaniam, M. (1998). "Religious-sociocultural psychotherapy in patients with anxiety and depression," *Australian and New Zealand Journal of Psychiatry*, 32(6), 867-872.

Reed, J. (1991). "Self-transcendence and mental health in oldest-old adults." *Nursing Research,* 39, 355-359.

Reed, P.G. (1993). "An emerging paradigm for the investigation of spirituality in nursing." *Religion*, 33(4), 347-361.

Rinaldi, S., Ghisi, M., and Iaccarino, L. *et al.* (2006). "Influence of coping skills on health-related quality of life in patients with systemic lupus erythematosus," *Arthritis Care and Research*, 55, 3, 427-433.

Rovers, M. and Kocum, L. (2010). "Development of a Holistic Model of Spirituality." *Journal of Spirituality in Mental Health,* 12(1).

Sangharakshita. (2007). *The Buddha's noble eightfold path.* London, UK: Windhorse.

Sawatzky, R., Ratner, P.A, and Chiu, L. (2005). "A Meta-Analysis of the Relationship Between Spirituality and Quality of Life." *Social Indicators Research,* 72, 153-188.

Scholte, W.F., Olff, M., Ventevogel, P. *et al.* (2004). "Mental health symptoms following war and repression in Eastern Afghanistan," *Journal of the American Medical Association*, 292(5), 585-593.

Schuster, M.A., Stein, B.D., Jaycox, L.H. *et al.* (2001). "A national survey of stress reactions after the September 11, 2001, terrorist attacks," *New England Journal of Medicine*, 345(20), 1507-1512.

Sethi, S. and Seligman, M.E.P. (1994). "The hope of fundamentalists," *Psychological Science*, 5, 58-59.

Shaw, B., Han, J.Y., and Kim, E. *et al.* (2007). "Effects of prayer and religious expression within computer support groups on women with breast cancer," *Psycho-Oncology*, 16(7), 676-687.

Silverstri, G.A., Knittig, S., Zoller, J.S., Nietert, P.J. (2003). "Importance of faith on medical decisions regarding cancer care." *Journal of Clinical Oncology,* 2, 1379-1382.

Skrabski, A., Kopp, M., Ozsa, S.R., Ethelyi, J.R. and Rahe, R.H. (2005). "Life meaning: an important correlate of health in the Hungarian population," *International Journal of Behavioural Medicine*, 12, 78-85.

Smith, B.W. (1996). "Coping as a predictor of outcomes following the 1993 midwest flood," *Journal of Social Behaviour and Personality*, 11(2), 225-239.

Smith, T.B., McCullough, M.E., and Poll, J. (2003). "Religiousness and depression: evidence for a main effect and the moderating influence of stressful life events." *Psychological Bulletin,* 129, 614-636.

Snelling, J. (1991). *The Buddhist handbook: A complete guide to Buddhist schools of teaching, practice, and history*. Rochester, NY: Inner Traditions.

Sodergren, S.C., Hyland, M.E., Crawford, A., and Partridge, M.R. (2004). "Positivity in illness: self-delusion or existential," *British Journal of Health Psychology*, 9(2), 163-174.

Soeken, K.L. and Carson, V.J. (1987). "Responding to the spiritual needs of the chronically ill." *Nursing Clinics of North America,* 22, 603-611.

Solomon, Z. Gelkopf, M., and Bleich, A.(2005). "Is terror genderblind? Gender differences in reaction to terror events," *Social Psychiatry and Psychiatric Epidemiology*, 40(12), 947-954.

Speca, M., Carlson, L.E., Goodey, E., *et al.* (2000). "A randomized, wait-list controlled clinical trial: The effect of a mindfulness meditation-based stress reduction programme on mood and symptoms of stress in cancer outpatients." *Psychosomatic Medicine,* 62, 613-622.

Spiegel, D., Bloom, J.R., and Gottheil, E. (1983). "Family environment as a predictor of adjustment to metastatic breast carcinoma," *Journal of Psychosocial Oncology*, Vol. 1, No. 1, 33-44.

Spilka, B. and McIntosh, D.N. (1996). Religion and spirituality: the known and the unknown. Paper presented at the annual conference of the American Psychological Association, Toronto, Canada.

Starbuck, E.D. (1899). *The Psychology of Religion.* New York: Scribner.

Strawbridge, W.J., Shema, S.J., Cohen, R.D., and Kaplan, G.A. (2001). "Religious attendance increases survival by improving and maintaining Good health behaviours, mental health, and social relationships," *Annals of Behavioural Medicine*, vol. 23(1), 68-74.

Strosahl, K. and Robinson, P. (2008). *The mindfulness and acceptance workbook for depression.* Oakland: New Harbinger.

Tepper, L., Rogers, S.A., Coleman, E.M., and Malony, H.N. (2001). "The prevalence of religious coping among persons with persistent mental illness," *Psychiatric Services*, 52, 5, 660-665.

Thoresen, C.E. (1999). "Spirituality and health: Is there a relationship?" *Journal of Health Psychology,* 4, 291-300.

Tix, A.P. and Frazier, P.A. (1998). "The use of religious coping during stressful life events: main effects, moderation, and mediation," *Journal of Consulting and Clinical Psychology*, 66(2), 411-422.

Tlebbi, C., Mallon, J., Richard, M., and Bigler, L. (1987). "Religiosity and locus of control in adoles cent cancer patients." *Psychological Reports,* 683-696.

Toneatto, T., Nguyen, L. (2007). "Does mindfulness meditation improve anxiety and mood symptoms? A review of the controlled research." *Canadian Journal of Psychiatry,* 52, 260-266.

Van Voorhees, B.W., Paunesku, D., and Kuwabara, S.A. *et al.*, (2008). "Protective and vulnerability factors predicting new-onset depressive episode in a representative of U.S. adolescents," *Journal of Adolescent Health*, 42(6), 605-616.

Vaughan, F. (1991). "Spiritual issues in psychotherapy." *Journal of Transpersonal Psychology,* 23, 105-119.

Vaughan, F., Wittine, B., and Walsh, R. (1996). Transpersonal psychology and the religious person. In E.D. Shafranske (Ed.), *Religion and the clinical practice of psychology* (pp. 483-510). Washington, DC: American Psychological Association.

Wachholtz, A.B. and Pargament, K.I. (2008). "Migraines and meditation: does spirituality matter?" *Journal of Behavioural Medicine*, Vol. 31, No. 4, pp. 351-366.

Wijngaards-De Meij, L., Stroebe, M., Schut, H. *et al.* (2005). "Couples at risk following the death of their child: Predictors of grief *versus* depression." *Journal of Consulting and Clinical Psychology*, 73(4), 617-623.

Williams, D.R., Larson, D.B., Buckler, R.E., Heckmann, R.C., and Pyle, C.M. (1991). "Religion and psychological distress in a community sample," *Social Science and Medicine*, 32(11), 1257-1262.

Woods, T.E., and Ironson, G.H. (1999). "Religion and spirituality in the face of illness. How cancer, cardiac, and HIV patients describe their spirituality/ religiosity." *Journal of Health Psychology,* 4, 393-412.

Worthington, E.L., Kurusu, T.A., McCullough, M.E., and Sandage, S.J. (1996). "Empirical research on religion and psychotherapeutic processes and outcomes: A 10-year review and research prospectus." *Psychological Bulletin,* 119, 348-487.

Wulff, D. (1997). *Psychology of Religion: Classical and Contemporary.* New York: Wiley.

Yati, N.C. (2009). *Principles and Practices of Patanjali's Yoga Sutras.* New Delhi, India: D.K. Printworld.

Yoshimoto, S.M., Ghorbani, S., and Baer, J.M. *et al.* (2006). "Religious coping and problem-solving by couples faced with prostate cancer," *European Journal of Cancer Care*, 15(5), 481-488.

Zald′ývar, A. and Smolowitz, J. (1994). "Perceptions of the importance placed on religion and folk medicine by non-Mexican-American Hispanic adults with diabetes." *The Diabetes.*

Zehnder, D., Prchal, A., Vollrath, M., and Landolt, M.A. (2006). "Prospective study of the effectiveness of coping in pediatric patients," *Child Psychiatry and Human Development*, 36(3), 351-368.

Zeidner, M. and Hammer, A.L. (2004). "Coping with missile attack: resources, strategies, and outcomes," *Journal of Personality*, Vol. 60, No. 4, pp. 709-746, 1992.

Zinnabauer, B.J. and Pargament, K.I. (2002). "Capturing the meanings of religiousness and spirituality: one way down from a definitional tower of Babel." *Research in the Social Scientific Study of Religion,* 13, 23-54.

Zinnabauer, B.J. and Pargament, K.I. (2005). "Religiousness and spirituality." In *Handbook of the Psychology of Religion and Spirituality*, edited by Raymond F. Paloutzian and Crystal L. Park. The Guilford Press: New York, London.

Zinnabauer, B.J., Pargament, K.I., and Scott, A.B. (1999). "The emerging meanings of religiousness and spirituality: problems and prospects." *Journal of Personality,* 67, 889-919.

Zinnbauer, B.J., Pargament, K.I., Cole, B., Rye, M.S., Butter, E.M., Belavich, T.G., Hipp, K.M., Scott, A.B., and Kadar, J.L. (1997). "Religion and spirituality: Unfuzzying the fuzzy." *Journal for the Scientific Study of Religion,* 36, 549-564.

17

Preventing Mental Disorders and Promoting Mental Health

Challenges Ahead

Anubhuti Dubey

Mental health is one of the biggest challenges faced by every country currently. Mental health problems affect at least one in four people at some point in time in their lives. Prevention of mental disorders and promotion of mental health are distinct but overlapping aims. Rapidly changing social and environmental conditions in countries around the world make it quite difficult for health professionals and health planners to pay attention to needs of those who are "well". These professionals are often preoccupied with the immediate problems of those who have a disease. Actually, mental health is everybody's business. Particularly important are the decision-makers in governments at local and national levels whose actions affect mental health. Some of the key messages in prevention of mental disorders and promotion of mental health are as follows—

1. The World Health Organization's (WHO) definition of health (1947) is "*a state of complete physical, mental and social well-being and not merely the absence of disease or infirmity*" clearly affirms that mental health is visibly a vital element of this definition. Hence, there is no health without mental health.
2. Mental health is crucial to individuals, families and societies and it is the basis for well-being and effective functioning for an individual and for a community. Empowerment and advocacy are important mechanisms to address these issues.
3. As the physical health and illness are determined by multiple

and interacting social, psychological and biological factors so is the mental health and mental illnesses.

4. Research evidences suggest linkages in mental health and behaviour. A range of mental, social and behavioural health problems may intermingle so as to exaggerate their influence on behaviour and well-being. Social problems of substance abuse, violence, and abuses of women and children on the one hand, and chronic health problems such as heart disease, depression and anxiety on the other, are more rampant and demanding to cope with in conditions of high unemployment, low income, limited education, stressful work conditions, gender discrimination, unhealthy lifestyle and human rights violations etc.
5. Effective public health interventions programmes can improve mental health of families and communities. Furthermore, a climate that value and safeguards basic civil, political, economic, social and cultural rights is elementary to the promotion of mental health.
6. The widespread stigma attached to mental health problems jeopardizes the development and implementation of mental health policy. Stigma is the main cause of discrimination and exclusion.

A comprehensive approach to the treatment of individuals experiencing severe mental illness includes biological issues, social, cultural and contextual issues.

Attending to some of the biological issues involves psychiatric care with appropriate medication by a physician and treatment team who understand the illness and its treatment, careful monitoring of intended effects and side effects, identification of new and physical and mental/ emotional problems as they emerge, attention to both acute and residual symptoms as they emerge, elimination of toxic chemicals and unnecessary drugs, and a balanced nutritional diet.

Focusing on social issues in intervention and treatment incorporates assistance in the development of survival skills including psychosocial and occupational rehabilitation. In addition, help in the development of communication and problem solving skills for the client and significant others and in the construction of a supportive social network.

Noticing on Cultural and Contextual issues suggest that in multicultural societies the underutilization of services relate to the stigma of mental health in the some culture and the cultural mistrust of mental health counsellors and the mental health system. In many cultures, there is a strong stigma that is attached to mental health and treatment of psychological conditions. The stigma not only attaches itself to the individual who is ill, it also attaches itself to the family (Aloud and Rathur, 2009; Hsu and Alden, 2008). The belief that mental problems are attributed to a lack of faith, spirit possession, bad *karma*, and the evil eye is strongly engrained in many non-Western cultures. This may encourage families and individuals to avoid seeking help for their psychological problems for fear that they will shame their family or that they are revealed as being weak. Some cultures also believe that admitting to having a mental health problem is a form of loss of face and shameful (Aloud and Rathur, 2009; Cauce *et al.*, 2002; Vogel, Wade, and Hackler, 2007).

Mental Health Promotion in India

At the time of independence roughly no mental health services were there in India (Thornicroft and Szmukler, 2001; Thornicroft, Tansella and Law, 2008). In 1947, India had only 10000 psychiatric beds for a population of over 300 million, compared to the UK, which, with one-tenth of the population of India, had over 150000 psychiatric beds (Srinivasa Murthy, 2011). The first 2 decades of independent India were dedicated to almost doubling-up the number of mental hospital beds and humanizing the services at hospitals (Sharma, 1990). Fascinatingly, one of the most significant innovations took place in a mental hospital setting was the sincere participation of families in the care of mentally ill persons. In Amritsar, Dr. Vidya Sagar started this initiative of involving families (at that point of time) when families were considered 'toxic' to the mentally ill and were not involved in the care of the mentally ill (Srinivasa Murthy, 2007). The next major development was in 1975, when a new initiative to integrate mental health with general health services, also referred to as the community psychiatry initiative, was adopted to develop mental health services (Isaac *et al.*, 1986). Further, The National Mental Health Programme (NMHP) was formulated in 1982 to develop a national-level initiative for mental healthcare based on the community psychiatry approach (Srinivasa Murthy, 2000). Besides these a large number of other community programmes to focus on a wide variety of mental health needs of the community through initiatives on suicide prevention, care of the elderly, substance use and disaster mental healthcare, and by setting up of day care centres, half-way homes, long stay homes and rehabilitation facilities took place (Patel and Thara, 2003; Gururaj and Isaac, 2004; Srinivasa Murthy, 2006).

Challenges Ahead

Health services are not provided equitably to people with mental disorders. A number of studies have reported on untreated patients in the community (Janardhan and Raghunandan, 2009; Philip *et al.*, 2003). Some of the major challenges for mental healthcare in India includes large 'unmet need' for mental healthcare in the community; poor understanding of psychological distress as requiring medical intervention in the general population; limited acceptance of modern medical care for mental disorders among the general population; limitations in the availability of mental health services (professionals and facilities) in the public health services; poor utilization of available services by the ill population and their families; problems in recovery and reintegration of persons with mental illnesses and lack of institutionalized mechanisms for organization of mental healthcare (Srinivasa Murthy, 2011).

Some of the initiatives to meet the challenges in mental disorder prevention, promotion and care so for in India are—National Mental Health Programme, advocacy and awareness programmes, the recognition of the human rights of the mentally ill by the National Human Rights Commission (NHRC), rehabilitation facilities have increased, the budget has doubled in many mental health institutions, humanizing mental hospitals, development of general hospital psychiatry units, community-level services, family support programmes, use of traditional systems of care, legislation, public mental health education, private sector psychiatry and epidemiological and intervention researches.

The road for prevention of mental disorder and promotion of mental health is long and difficult as far as the population of India is concerned. Hence, there is a grave need to develop and evaluate psychosocial interventions that can be integrated into management a range of mental health problems. Health-care systems should be strengthened to improve delivery of mental health care, by focusing on existing programmes and activities, such as those which address the prevention and treatment of HIV, gender-based violence; integrated management of childhood mental illnesses and child nutrition; and innovative management programmes. Mental health promotion needs to target the whole population, including people with mental health problems and their carers. The development and implementation of effective plans to promote mental health will enhance mental well-being for all.

References

Aloud, N. and Rathur, A. (2009). "Mental health and psychological services among Arab Muslim populations." *Journal of Muslim Mental Health*, 4, 79-103.

Cauce, A.M., Domenech-Rodriguez, M., Paradise, M., Cochran, B.N., Shea, J.M., Srebnik, D. *et al.* (2002). "Cultural and contextual influences in mental health help-seeking behaviour: A focus on ethnic minority youth." *Journal of Consulting and Clinical Psychology,* 70, 44-55.

Gururaj, G., and Isaac, M.K. (2004). "Psychiatric epidemiology in India: Moving beyond numbers." In: Agarwal S.P., (ed). *Mental Health: An Indian Perspective.* New Delhi: Directorate General of Health Services; 2004: 37-61.

Hsu, L. and Alden, L. (2008). "Cultural influences on willingness to seek treatment for social anxiety in Chinese and European-heritage students." *Cultural Diversity and Ethnic Minority Psychology,* 3, 215-223.

Isaac, M.K., Chandrasekar, C.R., Srinivasa Murthy, R., and Karur, B.V. (1986). "Decentralised training for PHC medical officers of a district. The Bellary approach." In Verghese, A. (eds.). *Continuing Medical Education,* Vol. VI. Calcutta: Indian Psychiatric Society.

Janardhan, A. and Raghunandan, S. (2009). *Caregivers in Community Mental Health—A Research Study*. Bangalore: Basic Needs (India).

Patel, V., and Thara, R. (eds) (2003). *Meeting Mental Health Needs in Developing Countries: NGO Innovations in India*. New Delhi: Sage (India).

Philip, M., Gangadhar, B.N., Jagadisha, Velayudhan, L., and Subbakrishna, D.K. (2003). "Influence of duration of untreated psychosis on the short-term outcome of drug-free schizophrenia patients." *Indian Journal of Psychiatry,* 45, 158-60.

Sharma, S. (1990). *Mental Hospitals in India.* New Delhi: Directorate General of Health Services, Government of India.

Srinivasa Murthy, R. (2011). "Mental health initiatives in India (1947-2010)." *The National Medical Journal of India,* Vol. 24 (2), 98-107.

Srinivasa Murthy, R. (2000). "Community mental health in India." In *Mental health in India—Essays in Honour of Prof. N.N. Wig.* Bangalore: Peoples Action for Mental Health. 150-76.

Srinivasa Murthy, R. (2007). "Family and mental health care in India." *Alumni J Christian Medical College,* 41:19-30.

Srinivasa Murthy, R. (eds.) (2006). *Mental Health by the People.* Bangalore, Peoples Action for Mental Health.

Thornicroft, G.J., and Szmukler, G. (2001). *Textbook of Community Psychiatry*. Oxford: Oxford University Press.

Thornicroft, G., Tansella, M., and Law, A. (2008). Steps, challenges and lessons in developing community mental health care. *World Psychiatry*, 7, 87-92.

Vogel, D., Wade, N., and Hackler, A. (2007). "Perceived public stigma and the willingness to seek counselling: The mediating roles of self-stigma and attitudes toward counselling." *Journal of Counselling Psychology*, 54, 40-50.

Index